Handbook on
Obsessive–Compulsive and Related Disorders

Handbook on
Obsessive–Compulsive
and Related Disorders

Edited by

Katharine A. Phillips, M.D.

Professor of Psychiatry and Human Behavior,
Alpert Medical School of Brown University;
Senior Research Scientist and Director,
Body Dysmorphic Disorder Program, Rhode Island Hospital,
Providence, Rhode Island

Dan J. Stein, M.D., Ph.D.

Professor and Chair, Department of Psychiatry,
University of Cape Town,
Cape Town, South Africa

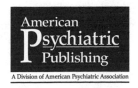

American **P**sychiatric Publishing

A Division of American Psychiatric Association

Washington, DC
London, England

Copyright © 2015 American Psychiatric Association
ALL RIGHTS RESERVED

Manufactured in the United States of America on acid-free paper
19 18 17 16 15   5 4 3 2 1
First Edition

Typeset in Rotis Sans Serif Std and Warnock Pro.

American Psychiatric Publishing
A Division of American Psychiatric Association
1000 Wilson Boulevard
Arlington, VA 22209-3901
www.appi.org

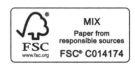

Library of Congress Cataloging-in-Publication Data
Handbook on obsessive-compulsive and related disorders / edited by Katharine A. Phillips, Dan J. Stein.
    p. ; cm.
  Includes bibliographical references and index.
  ISBN 978-1-58562-489-8 (pbk. : alk. paper)
  I. Phillips, Katharine A., editor. II. Stein, Dan J., editor.
  [DNLM: 1. Obsessive-Compulsive Disorder. WM 176]
  RC533
  616.85'227—dc23

                                       2015003076

British Library Cataloguing in Publication Data
A CIP record is available from the British Library.

Contents

Contributors

Jonathan S. Abramowitz, Ph.D.
Professor and Associate Chair, Department of Psychology, University of North Carolina, Chapel Hill, North Carolina

Naomi A. Fineberg, M.B.B.S., M.A., M.R.C.Psych.
Consultant Psychiatrist, Highly Specialized Obsessive Compulsive Disorder and Body Dysmorphic Disorder Service, Hertfordshire Partnership University NHS Foundation Trust, Welwyn Garden City; Visiting Professor, Postgraduate Medicine, University of Hertfordshire, College Lane, Hatfield, Hertfordshire, United Kingdom

Jon E. Grant, J.D., M.D., M.P.H.
Professor, Department of Psychiatry and Behavioral Neuroscience, Pritzker School of Medicine, University of Chicago, Chicago, Illinois

Eric Hollander, M.D.
Director, Autism and Obsessive Compulsive Spectrum Program and the Anxiety and Depression Research Program, and Clinical Professor of Psychiatry and Behavioral Sciences, Albert Einstein College of Medicine and Montefiore Medical Center; and Director, Spectrum Neuroscience and Treatment Institute, New York, New York

David C. Houghton, M.S.
Department of Psychology, Texas A&M University, College Station, Texas

Sukhwinder Kaur, M.B.B.S., M.R.C.Psych.
Research Psychiatrist, Highly Specialized Obsessive Compulsive Disorder and Body Dysmorphic Disorder Service, Hertfordshire Partnership University NHS Foundation Trust, Welwyn Garden City, Hertfordshire, United Kingdom

Sangeetha Kolli, M.B.B.S., M.R.C.Psych.
Consultant Psychiatrist, Highly Specialized Obsessive Compulsive Disorder and Body Dysmorphic Disorder Service, Hertfordshire Partnership University NHS Foundation Trust, Welwyn Garden City, Hertfordshire, United Kingdom

David Mataix-Cols, Ph.D.
Professor of Child and Adolescent Psychiatric Science, Department of Clinical Neuroscience, Karolinska Institutet, Stockholm, Sweden

Tara Mathews, Ph.D.
Assistant Professor of Psychology in Psychiatry, Weill Cornell Medical College, New York, New York

Davis Mpavaenda, Dip.C.B.T., B.A.B.C.P. Accred., Masters Health Law
Consultant Cognitive Behavioural Therapist, Highly Specialized Obsessive Compulsive Disorder and Body Dysmorphic Disorder Service, Hertfordshire Partnership University NHS Foundation Trust, Welwyn Garden City, Hertfordshire, United Kingdom

Ashley E. Nordsletten, Ph.D.
Postdoctoral Research Fellow, Department of Clinical Neuroscience, Karolinska Institutet, Stockholm, Sweden

Brian L. Odlaug, M.P.H.
Visiting Researcher, Department of Public Health, Faculty of Health and Medical Sciences, University of Copenhagen, Copenhagen, Denmark

Mayumi Okuda, M.D.
Instructor in Psychiatry, Department of Psychiatry, College of Physicians and Surgeons of Columbia University, New York, New York

Katharine A. Phillips, M.D.
Professor of Psychiatry and Human Behavior, Alpert Medical School of Brown University; Senior Research Scientist and Director, Body Dysmorphic Disorder Program, Rhode Island Hospital, Providence, Rhode Island

Samar Reghunandanan, M.B.B.S., M.D., M.R.C.Psych.
Research Psychiatrist, Highly Specialized Obsessive Compulsive Disorder and Body Dysmorphic Disorder Service, Hertfordshire Partnership University NHS Foundation Trust, Welwyn Garden City, Hertfordshire, United Kingdom

Lillian Reuman, M.A.
Graduate Student, Department of Psychology, University of North Carolina, Chapel Hill, North Carolina

H. Blair Simpson, M.D., Ph.D.
Professor of Psychiatry at Columbia University Medical Center, Columbia University; Director of the Anxiety Disorders Clinic and the Center for OC and Related Disorders, New York State Psychiatric Institute, New York, New York

Ivar Snorrason, M.A.
Department of Psychology, University of Wisconsin–Milwaukee, Milwaukee, Wisconsin

Dan J. Stein, M.D., Ph.D.
Professor and Chair, Department of Psychiatry, University of Cape Town, Capetown, South Africa

Michelle Tricamo, M.D.
Assistant Professor of Psychiatry, Weill Cornell Medical College, New York, New York

John T. Walkup, M.D.
Professor of Psychiatry, Weill Cornell Medical College, New York, New York

Douglas W. Woods, Ph.D.
Professor and Department Head, Department of Psychology, Texas A&M University, College Station, Texas

Disclosures of Competing Interests

The following contributors to this book have indicated a financial interest in or other affiliation with a commercial supporter, a manufacturer of a commercial product, a provider of a commercial service, a nongovernmental organization, and /or a government agency, as listed below:

Naomi A. Fineberg, M.B.B.S., M.A., M.R.C.Psych.—*Research support:* AstraZeneca, Cephalon, ENCP, GlaxoSmithKline, Lundbeck, Medical Research Council (UK), National Institute for Health Research (UK), Servier, Wellcome Foundation; *Consultant:* GlaxoSmithKline, Lundbeck, Novartis, Servier, Transcept; *Honararia for lectures at scientific meetings:* AstraZeneca, Bristol-Myers Squibb, Jazz Pharmaceuticals, Lundbeck, Servier; *Financial support to attend scientific meetings:* Bristol-Myers Squibb, British Association for Psychopharmacology, Cephalon, ECNP, International College of OC Spectrum Disorders, International Society for Addiction, Janssen, Lundbeck, Novartis, Royal College of Psychiatrists, Servier, World Health Organization.

Jon E. Grant, J.D., M.D., M.P.H.—*Research grants:* National Center for Responsible Gaming, Forest, National Institute of Mental Health, Roche; *Royalties:* American Psychiatric Publishing, McGraw-Hill, Oxford University Press, W.W. Norton; *Other compensation:* yearly compensation from Springer Publishing for acting as Editor-in-Chief, *Journal of Gambling Studies.*

Eric Hollander, M.D.—*Research grant:* Brainsway, Roche; *Consultant:* Roche, Shire.

David Mataix-Cols, Ph.D.—Served as advisor to the DSM-5 Obsessive-Compulsive Spectrum Sub-Work Group of the Anxiety, Obsessive-Compulsive Spectrum, Posttraumatic and Dissociative Disorders Work Group.

Brian L. Odlaug, M.P.H.—*Research grant:* Trichotillomania Learning Center; *Consultant:* Lundbeck; *Royalties:* Oxford University Press.

Katharine A. Phillips, M.D.—*Research support and/or salary support:* Forest (medication only, for a study sponsored and funded by NIMH), National Institute of Mental Health (salary and research funding), Transcept (research funding); *Consultant:* Janssen Research and Development; *Honoraria, royalties, or travel reimbursement:* Guilford Press, Merck Manual, Oxford University Press, speaking or grant reviewing honoraria and/or travel reimbursement from academic and federal institutions and from professional organizations, UpToDate; *Royalties* (potential): American Psychiatric Publishing, The Free Press.

H. Blair Simpson, M.D., Ph.D.—*Research funds for clinical trials:* Janssen (2006–2012), Transcept (2011–2013), Neuropharm (2009); *Scientific advisory board:* Pfizer (for Lyrica, 2009–2010), Jazz Pharmaceuticals (for Luvox CR, 2007–2008); *Consultant:* Quintiles (on therapeutic needs for OCD, September 2012); *Royalties:* Cambridge University Press, UpToDate.

Dan J. Stein, M.D., Ph.D.—*Consultant:* Biocodex (paid to institution); Novartis; Servier (paid to institution); *Advisory board:* Eli Lilly, Lundbeck, Novartis; *Speakers' bureau:* Eli Lilly, GlaxoSmithKline, Lundbeck, Servier; *Other financial or material support:* Pfizer.

John T. Walkup, M.D.—*Grant funding:* Hartwell Foundation, Tourette Syndrome Association; *Free drug/placebo from the following pharmaceutical companies* (for National Institute of Mental Health–funded studies): Abbott (in 2005); Eli Lilly (in 2003), Pfizer (in 2007). *One-time consultation:* Shire (in 2011); *Paid speaker:* Tourette Syndrome–Centers for Disease Control and Prevention outreach educational programs, American Academy of Child and Adolescent Psychiatry, American Psychiatric Association; *Royalties* (for books on Tourette syndrome): Guilford Press, Oxford University Press; *Unpaid advisor:* Anxiety Disorders Association of America, *Consumer Reports,* Trichotillomania Learning Center.

Douglas W. Woods, Ph.D.—*Royalties:* American Psychiatric Publishing, Guilford Press, Oxford University Press.

The following contributors to this book have indicated no competing interests to disclose during the year preceding manuscript submission:

Jonathan S. Abramowitz, Ph.D.	Mayumi Okuda, M.D.
David C. Houghton, M.S.	Lillian Reuman, M.A.
Ashley E. Nordsletten, Ph.D.	Ivar Snorrason, M.A.

Foreword

Handbook *on Obsessive-Compulsive and Related Disorders* examines obsessive-compulsive and related disorders (OCRDs) as a new chapter in the *Diagnostic and Statistical Manual of Mental Disorders,* 5th Edition (DSM-5; American Psychiatric Association 2013). This book is quite timely, because for the first time in our field, obsessive-compulsive disorder (OCD) is no longer in the chapter on anxiety disorders and is instead grouped with other related conditions, which are now known as *obsessive-compulsive and related disorders.* I am quite pleased to see this development and believe that this will have a profound impact not only on clinical utility—how clinicians conceptualize, diagnose, and treat patients with these conditions—but also on how researchers conduct relevant research. The DSM-5 approach to OCRDs perhaps also resonates, at least to some extent, with constructs that have been proposed by the National Institute of Mental Health in its Research Domain Criteria framework.

The book provides a "behind the scenes" examination of the concept of OCRDs; all of the chapters but one are authored or coauthored by individuals who were involved in the development of DSM-5 as Obsessive-Compulsive Spectrum Sub-Work Group members, advisors, or authors of published reviews that examined possible changes for DSM-5. This book covers disorders in the new DSM-5 OCRD chapter: OCD, body dysmorphic disorder (previously a somatoform disorder), hoarding disorder (a new disorder), trichotillomania (hair-pulling disorder) (previously an impulse-control disorder not elsewhere classified), and excoriation (skin-picking) disorder (a new disorder). It also includes discussions of other conditions, such as tic disorders, illness anxiety disorder, and obsessive-compulsive personality disorder; these disorders are not included in the DSM-5 OCRD chapter, but they were considered for inclusion in that chapter during the DSM-5 development process.

The concept of OCRDs is certainly not new. My first book on this topic, *Obsessive-Compulsive Related Disorders* (Hollander 1993), was published more than 20 years ago and drew attention to many of these conditions and to this spectrum concept. More recent work has highlighted a broader impulsivity-compulsivity concept (see, e.g., Fineberg et al. 2010). The OCRDs have both similarities with and important differences from OCD in terms of their phenomenology, comorbidity, family history, brain circuitry, and treatment response. This category was seen as evolving from our understanding of compulsivity as a symptom dimension arising from tightly regulated brain circuits (cortical-striatal-thalamic-cortical circuits) that give rise to a spectrum of partially overlapping diagnostic entities.

The Research Planning Agenda for DSM-5, which preceded the formal development of DSM-5, systematically examined the relationship between various putative OCRDs and OCD in terms of a number of cross-cutting issues. The proceedings of that process were published as *Obsessive-Compulsive Spectrum Disorders: Refining the Research Agenda for DSM-V* (Hollander et al. 2011). This research planning agenda laid very useful groundwork for the formal development of DSM-5. This development included a comprehensive process of literature reviews; weighing of available evidence by the Obsessive-Compulsive Spectrum Sub-Work Group members and advisors as well as the larger DSM-5 work group of which it was a component; field trials; and input and review by many other individuals, groups, and organizations. Evidence that was culled from this extensive process ultimately resulted in the inclusion of the new chapter on OCRDs in DSM-5.

The DSM-5 OCRD chapter is a great step forward, and this book's editors (who were chair and sub-work group chair of the DSM-5 work group that was responsible for the OCRDs) are to be congratulated for their able stewardship of the DSM-5 process, which generated diagnostic criteria and text for these disorders that are clearer, more internally consistent, more precise, and better supported by the existing data than were the DSM-IV (American Psychiatric Association 1994) categories and chapter structure. Future DSM efforts might reconsider whether a broader conceptualization of compulsivity is possible that could include impulsive-compulsive disorders, obsessive-compulsive personality disorder, tic disorders, and autism spectrum disorder. Nevertheless, this book presents a unique collection of chapters and key literature reviews from DSM-5 OCRD sub-work group members and advisors that support decisions regarding boundary issues for OCRDs.

The Research Domain Criteria process has highlighted the need to understand how fundamental brain circuits drive psychopathological symptom domains, and I can think of no area where emerging basic science and animal models can better be directly translated into novel experimental therapeutics than the OCRDs, as suggested by exciting findings in optogenetics, deep brain stimulation, transcranial magnetic stimulation, and immune-inflammatory mechanisms. Nevertheless, when we consider the broadest conceptualization of "compulsivity," there remains a very large unmet need for both services and research investment. The OCRDs contribute enormous financial costs to our society, and research networks are needed that can begin to examine real-world questions such as predicting who is at risk for negative outcomes and high costs for care. I hope you enjoy reading these chapters and that you find the book useful for your clinical practice and research endeavors.

Eric Hollander, M.D.

References

American Psychiatric Association: Diagnostic and Statistical Manual of Mental Disorders, 4th Edition. Washington, DC, American Psychiatric Association, 1994

American Psychiatric Association: Diagnostic and Statistical Manual of Mental Disorders, 5th Edition. Arlington, VA, American Psychiatric Association, 2013

Fineberg NA, Potenza MN, Chamberlain SR, et al: Probing compulsive and impulsive behaviors, from animal models to endophenotypes: a narrative review. Neuropsychopharmacology 35(3):591–604, 2010 19940844

Hollander E: Obsessive-Compulsive Related Disorders. Washington, DC, American Psychiatric Press, 1993

Hollander E, Zohar J, Sirovatka PJ, et al: Obsessive-Compulsive Spectrum Disorders: Refining the Research Agenda for DSM-V. Washington, DC, American Psychiatric Publishing, 2011

CHAPTER 1

Introduction and Major Changes for the Obsessive–Compulsive and Related Disorders in DSM-5

Katharine A. Phillips, M.D.
Dan J. Stein, M.D., Ph.D.

The obsessive-compulsive and related disorders (OCRDs) are common and often severe disorders. Many patients with OCRDs suffer tremendously, and their symptoms usually cause substantial impairment in psychosocial functioning. Some patients commit suicide. Yet these distressing and impairing disorders often go undetected in clinical settings. Patients often suffer in silence and without receiving adequate care. Many are ashamed of their symptoms and reluctant to reveal them to a clinician. In addition, clinicians may be relatively less familiar with the OCRDs, especially those disorders that were not included in DSM prior to DSM-5 (hoarding disorder and excoriation [skin-picking] disorder) (American Psychiatric Association 2013). It is important to screen patients for OCRDs, diagnose these disorders when present, and provide evidence-based treatment, as such intervention can have a substantial impact on patients' lives—robustly improving their symptoms, psychosocial functioning, and quality of life.

This book provides a clinically focused overview of the OCRDs, with an emphasis on their clinical features, assessment, diagnosis, and treatment. We hope that this information will directly influence and improve patient care. In addition, more broadly, this book provides comprehensive and cutting-edge coverage of the field of OCRDs. For example, chapters include information on important features such as prevalence and developmental and gender-related considerations as well as cutting-edge information on these disorders' etiologies and pathophysiologies. Research on OCRDs is elucidating factors that may contribute to the development and maintenance of these conditions; this, in turn, may pave the way to more effective treatments and perhaps, ultimately, even their prevention. This volume is timely, given that significant research has been done on these disorders in recent years. In addition, this research was systematically reviewed as part of the DSM-IV (American Psychiatric Association 1994) revision process, and for the first time these disorders now appear in a separate chapter in DSM.

This book covers all of the disorders in the DSM-5 chapter on OCRDs: obsessive-compulsive disorder (OCD), classified as an anxiety disorder in DSM-IV; body dysmorphic disorder (BDD), classified as a somatoform disorder in DSM-IV; hoarding disorder, new to DSM-5; trichotillomania (hair-pulling disorder), classified as an impulse-control disorder not elsewhere classified in DSM-IV; excoriation (skin-picking) disorder, new to DSM-5; substance/medication-induced obsessive-compulsive and related disorder; obsessive-compulsive and related disorder due to another medical condition; other specified obsessive-compulsive and related disorder; and unspecified obsessive-compulsive and related disorder. The last four conditions are analogous to those included in other chapters of DSM-5. "Other specified OCRD" and "unspecified OCRD" are similar to DSM-IV's "not otherwise specified" category.

This book also includes chapters on several disorders that were strong candidates for inclusion in the new OCRD chapter but were ultimately placed in other chapters in DSM-5. Because these disorders have been viewed by many experts as related to OCD, and thus as OCRDs, and because they may perhaps be included in the OCRD chapter in future editions of current psychiatric classifications, we have included chapters on them in this book. These include tic disorders (classified as neurodevelopmental disorders in DSM-5), illness anxiety disorder (a new version of hypochondriasis that is classified in the somatic symptom and related disorders chapter of DSM-5), and obsessive-compulsive personality disorder (classified in the personality disorders chapter).

We are especially pleased that virtually all of the chapters in this book are authored or coauthored by individuals who were substantially involved in the work of the DSM-5 Obsessive-Compulsive Spectrum Disorders Sub-Work Group, part of the DSM-5 Work Group on Anxiety, Obsessive-Compulsive Spectrum, Posttraumatic, and Dissociative Disorders, which was responsible for changes to these disorders for DSM-5. These authors contributed tirelessly to the DSM-5 development effort as sub-work group members, advisors, or authors of literature reviews that were commissioned by the work group to inform recommendations for DSM-5. Thus, these authors have a deep understanding of the DSM-5 development process, the changes that were made for DSM-5, and the rationale for and clinical relevance of these changes.

Some of the most exciting changes that were made in DSM-5 are the inclusion of the new disorders already noted as well as inclusion of the new chapter on OCRDs. In this introduction, we discuss the concept of OCRDs, why a new OCRD chapter was added to DSM-5, how it was decided which disorders to include in this chapter, why the concept of OCRDs is important for patient care, and some pros and cons of the new chapter. In this introduction we also cover why and how new individual disorders were added and some of the most important changes to individual OCRDs. We then discuss useful screening and severity measures that clinicians can use to assist in identifying, monitoring, and treating these disorders, and we end by briefly noting what each chapter in this handbook covers.

Why and How the New Diagnostic Category of Obsessive–Compulsive and Related Disorders Was Included in DSM–5

Although the OCRD chapter is new to DSM-5, the concept of a group of disorders that appear related to OCD is not new. This concept has been discussed in the literature and investigated for several decades, often under the rubric of "obsessive-compulsive spectrum disorders." Although in psychiatry the term *spectrum* has been used to mean many things, the concept of the obsessive-compulsive spectrum has been used to refer to a group of disorders that are characterized by repetitive thoughts and/or behaviors and that are presumed to be related to OCD while also being distinct disorders (Phillips 2002; Stein and Hollander 1993). *Spectrum* also builds on the idea that similar underlying psychobiological mechanisms may account for these similar symptoms—that a continuum of genotypes, endophenotypes, or other related constructs leads to the various symptom dimensions seen in clinical practice (Hyman 2002; Insel et al. 2010).

Implicit in this concept has been the idea that such disorders might be grouped together in the same chapter in DSM. DSM-IV contained 16 chapters of disorders, such as schizophrenia and other psychotic disorders, mood disorders, and anxiety disorders. A chapter on OCRDs was not included in DSM-IV because at that time (the early 1990s), not enough empirical work had been done on this topic. However, by the time the DSM-5 development process officially began in 2007, substantial research on the OCRDs had been done and the inclusion of a separate chapter about them was considered. Indeed, which chapters should be included in DSM-5 overall—including, possibly, a new OCRD chapter—and which disorders should be in each of those chapters were major points of deliberation during the DSM-5 development process.

At first glance, this issue might not seem very important or clinically relevant. Indeed, how disorders are grouped together in DSM does not influence who receives a particular diagnosis (i.e., caseness), because groupings do not affect diagnostic criteria. Nonetheless, this issue does have some important implications for practice. For example, disorders that are classified together in the same chapter of DSM are generally thought to be related to one another and thus to perhaps have shared pathophysiology and etiology (although for most disorders, much remains to be learned about etiology and pathophysiology). Furthermore, optimally grouping disorders into chapters may usefully guide clinical assessment and treatment approaches—for example, by reminding clinicians to pay particular attention to differentiating disorders in the same chapter from one another. Alternative groupings, such as listing all disorders in DSM randomly or in alphabetical order, would not have such clinically useful implications. In addition, related disorders may be highly comorbid with one another, so clinicians should inquire about the possible presence of other OCRDs in a patient who has one of them. These disorders may also have an increased prevalence in family members, which should prompt clinicians to look for them in the patient if one (or more) is present in a family member or vice versa. The OCRDs also have some shared evaluation and treatment elements.

When considering what the overall metastructure of DSM-5 should look like (i.e., what chapters of disorders should be included) and which disorders should be included within each chapter, the DSM-5 work groups and the DSM-5 Task Force were guided by several principles: 1) the way disorders are grouped together into chapters in DSM should have clinical utility—that is, the groupings should be helpful to clinicians in formulating diagnoses, assessing patients, enhancing communication with patients and among clinicians, and selecting appropriate interventions; 2) the approach should have face validity; and 3) the approach should be evidence based and reflect the apparent relatedness of disorders to one another (First et al. 2004; Phillips et al. 2010). Eleven validators were used to examine the apparent relatedness of disorders to one another: shared symptom similarity, high comorbidity among disorders, course of illness, familiality, genetic risk factors, environmental risk factors, neural substrates, biomarkers, temperamental antecedents, cognitive and emotional processing abnormalities, and treatment response (Phillips et al. 2010). These validators were based on and an extension of those proposed by Robins and Guze in 1970 and subsequently amended by others (Kendler et al. 2002). Similarities and differences between disorders were examined in each validator domain.

The more similar disorders are in terms of these 11 validators, the more likely they are to be related to one another and thus grouped together in the same chapter in DSM-5. For example, OCD and BDD have some similarities in treatment response, with serotonin reuptake inhibitors (SRIs) appearing selectively efficacious for both disorders (Hollander et al. 1999; Ipser et al. 2009; Koran et al. 2007; Phillips and Hollander 2008). Research on the phenomenology of OCRDs as well as on other validators, using a range of different methodologies—including functional brain imaging, epidemiological approaches, and evidence from animal research on habits—also offers support for the relatedness of the OCRDs to OCD and to some of the other disorders within the chapter as well (Joel et al. 2008; Stein and Lochner 2006). (The application of latent structure statistical methods [e.g., factor analysis and latent class analysis] to inform decisions about the structure of DSM and groupings of disorders was considered but had limitations [Wittchen et al. 2009a, 2009b], especially when applied to the OCRDs, and thus these methods were given less weight.)

Validators such as these, along with face validity and clinical utility, were first considered at the DSM-5 Research Planning Conference on Obsessive-Compulsive Spectrum Disorders in 2006, before the formal development of DSM-5 began (Hollander et al. 2007, 2011; Mataix-Cols et al. 2007; Wittchen et al. 2009b). From the results of this conference, as well as the results from an international survey of OCD experts (Mataix-Cols et al. 2007), it was concluded that the obsessive-compulsive spectrum concept had merit and should be included as a new chapter of disorders in DSM-5 (Hollander et al. 2007). Participants in the planning conference and the survey also made recommendations about which disorders to include in this chapter. The DSM-5 work group subsequently commissioned more in-depth literature reviews, considered data published after the planning conference and survey, examined data from the DSM-5 field trials and from secondary data analyses of existing data sets, sought input from many individuals and groups, considered thousands of comments posted online at dsm5.org, and used other methods to make its final recommendations regarding this grouping of disorders (Hollander et al. 2011; Phillips et al. 2010).

Various theoretical approaches have also been applied to the OCRD concept that complement those just discussed. Certain animal habits that could be considered "motoric" or "lower-order, repetitive behaviors" have some phenomenological and psychobiological overlap with tics, hair pulling in trichotillomania (hair-pulling disorder), and compulsive skin picking in excoriation (skin-picking) disorder (Joel et al. 2008; Stein et al. 2010a). These behaviors may be undertaken to modulate self-arousal (Stein et al. 2010a). The more complex symptoms of cognitively focused OCRDs (OCD, BDD, and hoarding disorder), which could be considered "cognitive" or "higher-order" obsessive-compulsive symptoms (Feusner et al. 2009), may focus on harm, cleanliness, order, hoarding of possessions, appearance (appeal to potential mates), and health—all of which may be related to evolutionarily based needs. The compulsions that occur in these disorders may be seen as a means of reducing anxiety induced by triggering obsessions or of neutralizing future threat (Stein et al. 2010b).

After considering up-to-date evidence based on the 11 validators—as well as face validity, clinical utility, and recommendations from the previously mentioned DSM-5 Research Planning Conference and international survey—the DSM-5 sub-work group and work group concluded that a number of putative OCRDs appeared to be more closely related to OCD than to other near-neighbor disorders and that there was merit to including an OCRD group of disorders in DSM-5. Furthermore, through discussions on the harmonization of DSM-5 and ICD-11, the DSM-5 work group reached some consensus on a joint metastructure, which supported the inclusion of a separate chapter of OCRDs in both systems. The work group recommended including within this category several cognitively focused ("higher-order") disorders—OCD, BDD, and hoarding disorder—characterized by both obsessional thoughts and compulsive behaviors, as well as several motorically focused ("lower-order") disorders—trichotillomania (hair-pulling disorder) and excoriation (skin-picking) disorder—characterized by stereotypic behaviors but not obsessions.

Ultimately, in collaboration with other DSM-5 work groups, the recommendation was to classify tic disorders, illness anxiety disorder, and obsessive-compulsive personality disorder in other chapters. Notably, however, a tic specifier was recommended for OCD, to remind clinicians of the importance of assessing tics in patients with this disorder. Although some evidence based on the 11 validators, as well as clinical utility and face validity considerations, supported the inclusion of tics in the OCRD chapter, their relatedness to OCD was less strongly supported. All of these recommendations (as well as proposed changes to other sections of DSM-IV) were subsequently reviewed and approved by the DSM-5 Task Force and ultimately the American Psychiatric Association Board of Trustees.

Initially, it was thought that DSM-5 would be limited to 10 chapters of disorders. Thus, the DSM-5 Work Group on Anxiety, Obsessive-Compulsive Spectrum, Posttraumatic, and Dissociative Disorders initially proposed that DSM-5 include a chapter entitled "Anxiety and Obsessive-Compulsive and Related Disorders," with two subgroups, one for anxiety disorders and one for OCRDs (Stein et al. 2010b). This proposal reflected, for example, OCD's close relationship to the anxiety disorders (where it was classified in DSM-IV) and BDD's close relationship to social anxiety disorder (both disorders are characterized by high levels of social anxiety and avoidance) (Phillips et al. 2010; Stein et al. 2010). However, later during the DSM-5 development process, it became clear that more than 10 chapters of disorders (as required by a decimal coding system) could be included (as per an alphanumeric coding system) (Stein et al. 2011). This led to the recommendation that the anxiety disorders and the OCRDs be placed in separate chapters. Indeed, despite their similarities, these disorders do have some differences. For example, the brain imaging literature has emphasized that the amygdala and related circuitry play a key role in a number of anxiety disorders but that OCD and perhaps BDD seem to be mediated by cortico-striatal-thalamic-cortical circuitry. These disorders also have important differences in terms of effective treatment approaches (Stein et al. 2010b). There are also important differences between the motoric OCRDs, which are characterized by stereotypic behaviors but do not have a prominent cognitive component, and the anxiety disorders.

It should be emphasized that in DSM-5, unlike DSM-IV, the order in which chapters are listed reflects their apparent relatedness to one another, with more closely related disorders in adjacent chapters (Stein et al. 2011). Thus, the OCRD chapter immediately follows the anxiety disorders chapter, reflecting the close relationship between some of the disorders in these two chapters (Stein et al. 2010b).

Relevance of the New OCRD Chapter to Patient Care

Inclusion of the new OCRD chapter in DSM-5 has several important clinical implications. First, grouping these disorders together in the same chapter draws attention to similarities in their key clinical features of obsessions, preoccupations, and/or driven repetitive behaviors. As previously noted, the repetitive behaviors can involve complex compulsions (in OCD, BDD, and hoarding disorder), which are often triggered by obsessions/preoccupations and are often intended to reduce anxiety, or simple motoric behaviors (in trichotillomania (hair-pulling disorder) and excoriation [skin-picking] disorder), which are often triggered by specific stimuli, including particular emotional states, and may serve to regulate arousal. The simple motoric behaviors of both trichotillomania (hair-pulling disorder) and excoriation (skin-picking) disorder are difficult to control, and both these disorders respond to the cognitive-behavioral technique known as habit reversal. OCD and BDD share prominent obsessions/preoccupations and compulsive behaviors that are performed in response to the obsessions/preoccupations; they also share apparent selective response to SRIs and the frequent need for high doses of SRIs.

Another clinical implication of the new chapter is that many OCRDs may be highly comorbid with one another and have an increased prevalence in family members. Thus, as previously noted, if an OCRD is present, clinicians should inquire about the presence of OCRDs in family members and comorbid OCRDs in the patient. Another clinical implication of grouping these disorders together in one chapter is that similar assessment measures may be used. The Level 1 and Level 2 measures that are included in DSM-5 may be used to screen for the presence of these disorders (American Psychiatric Association 2013). Once an OCRD is diagnosed, adaptations of the Yale-Brown Obsessive Compulsive Scale (Y-BOCS) (Goodman et al. 1989; Keuthen et al. 2001; O'Sullivan et al. 1995; Phillips et al. 1997) or the Florida Obsessive-Compulsive Inventory (FOCI) for OCD (Storch et al. 2007) may be used to assess these disorders' severity and change in severity over time.

It is important to emphasize, however, that these disorders have clinically important differences from OCD and from one another. They are not all simply OCD or subtypes of OCD. For example, compared with OCD, BDD is characterized by poorer insight, higher rates of comorbid major depressive disorder and possibly substance use disorders, and higher rates of suicidality (Phillips et al. 2012). Hoarding disorder, which in the past has been considered a form of OCD, has been shown to have a number of important differences from forms of OCD characterized by other symptom dimensions, such as harm avoidance and symmetry concerns (Mataix-Cols et al. 2010).

A common clinical error is to treat all OCRDs with treatments for OCD. Unfortunately, this approach often leads to unsuccessful treatment outcomes. For example, unlike OCD, hoarding disorder does not respond well to simple exposure and response (ritual) prevention. More complex interventions (e.g., those that include work on decision making) are usually needed, and a major focus on motivational interviewing is often required in order to enhance patients' willingness to engage and stay in treatment. Similarly, cognitive-behavioral approaches for BDD are more complex and intensive than those for OCD, requiring, for example, a greater focus on cognitive interventions, perceptual (mirror) retraining, and integration of behavioral experiments into exposure exercises, which often focus on social avoidance. Because of the poorer insight usually seen in BDD (compared with OCD), motivational interviewing techniques are more often needed to engage and retain BDD patients in treatment. Treatment for trichotillomania (hair-pulling disorder) and excoriation (skin-picking) disorder requires the use of habit reversal. Although SRIs are well established as being selectively efficacious for OCD, and probably also for BDD, their effectiveness for hoarding disorder, trichotillomania (hair-pulling disorder), and excoriation (skin-picking) disorder is less clear. As another example, BDD may respond differently than OCD to some SRI augmentation strategies (Phillips and Hollander 2008).

Thus, it is important to differentiate the OCRDs from one another and to use treatment approaches that are specific to each of them. These caveats also apply to other chapters of disorders in DSM. For example, the eating disorders anorexia nervosa and bulimia nervosa, which DSM classifies in the same chapter, typically respond quite differently to pharmacotherapy. Patients with bulimia may respond robustly to a variety of medications, whereas those with anorexia nervosa usually respond fairly poorly to medication. As another example, effective psychotherapy and medications for different personality disorders may meaningfully differ.

Some Pros and Cons of the New OCRD Diagnostic Category

There is no perfect way to categorize disorders in DSM-5; the field is not one that allows nature to be carved precisely at its joints (Phillips et al. 2010). The current knowledge in the field is also relatively limited. Thus, the current DSM-5 metastructure almost certainly does not reflect the true relatedness of disorders to one another. The 11 validators, both individually and in the aggregate, provide only a partial perspective on how closely related disorders are to one another. In addition, data from different validating domains, such as familiality and treatment response, may sometimes conflict, and it is unclear whether some validators should be weighted more heavily than others. Furthermore, studies that directly compare disorders with multiple other disorders across validators to examine their relative relatedness are often lacking. Until the field better understands psychiatric disorders, including their etiology and pathophysiology, we are left with these imperfect, although useful, indicators of disorder relatedness.

Any particular approach to the metastructure has pros and cons, and there are both advantages and disadvantages to including the new OCRD chapter in DSM-5. For example, some OCRDs may not be closely related to one another (e.g., trichotillomania (hair-pulling disorder) and hoarding disorder), although this is probably also the case for disorders in other chapters in DSM-5. As a more specific example, there are some apparent differences in neuroimaging findings across some OCRDs, although these findings could be considered to have some convergence in that they involve related corticostriatal networks that mediate different functions (motoric vs. cognitive vs. affective). Another potential disadvantage is that classifying OCD and BDD separately from the anxiety disorders may imply that they are not related to the anxiety disorders. However, as noted earlier, the fact that the OCRD chapter directly follows the anxiety disorders chapter highlights the close relationships between some of the disorders in these two chapters (Stein et al. 2011). The exclusion of several putative OCRDs from the OCRD chapter, including tic disorders, illness anxiety disorder (hypochondriasis), and perhaps some others as well, may be another disadvantage of the current grouping. Some might consider the chapter name too "OCD-centric" (although, of note, this name does not include the name of the disorder OCD). Perhaps most important to note is that treatment approaches to these disorders differ in some meaningful ways, and, as mentioned previously, grouping them in the same chapter should not be inferred to mean that they should all be treated as though they are OCD.

On the other hand, this new grouping of disorders fixes some major problems that were present in DSM-IV. When DSM-IV was developed in the early 1990s, little research had been done on most of the OCRDs, and the field had only a very limited understanding of the relationships among them. Since then, it has become increasingly apparent that BDD, for example, seems to have many more similarities to OCD than to somatoform disorders, such as somatization disorder and conversion disorder, with which it was classified in DSM-IV (McKay et al. 1997; Phillips et al. 2010). Importantly, there are overlaps in the recommended treatment approach for OCD and BDD (although important differences as well, especially for cognitive-behavioral interventions). Similarly, ongoing research suggests that trichotillomania (hair-pulling disorder) has more similarities to OCD than to impulse-control disorders such as pyromania and intermittent explosive disorder, with which it was classified in DSM-IV (Stein et al. 2010a).

As previously noted, this new OCRD chapter has some advantages for purposes of diagnosis, differential diagnosis, and assessment, given similarities in these disorders' clinical features of prominent obsessions, preoccupations, and/or driven repetitive behaviors. Keep in mind, however, that although the same general approach can be used for screening and assessment of severity, each disorder must be assessed and identified separately—most importantly because treatment approaches differ. In addition, inclusion of this new chapter may encourage clinicians and researchers to screen for all OCRDs in patients who present with an OCRD and to screen family members for multiple OCRDs as well. On the other hand, clinicians should keep in mind that the disorders most commonly comorbid with most of the OCRDs (e.g., major depressive disorder) are in other DSM chapters, although these high comorbidity rates in part reflect the high base rate of some non-OCRDs.

In our view, the DSM-5 conceptualization of OCRDs, including their inclusion in a separate chapter, is an advance over DSM-IV. However, additional studies on the validators are needed, as are studies that directly compare multiple disorders across multiple validators to assess their relative similarities and differences. Indeed, our hope is that the DSM-5 chapter on OCRDs will encourage such work to proceed and will also give impetus to other kinds of needed research, such as the epidemiology of OCRDs. Although DSM-5 aimed to incorporate emerging knowledge on underlying mechanisms, additional research on such mechanisms is clearly required in order to clarify disorder relatedness. The 11 validators include domains that may be relevant to underlying mechanisms, such as genetics and cognitive-affective processing, but more detailed work in areas such as these is needed (Hyman 2007; Insel et al. 2010). The National Institute of Mental Health Research Diagnostic Criteria initiative is expected to be helpful in this regard. Given the complexity of psychopathology more generally, and of the OCRDs in particular, a range of validators (rather than any single validator) and a range of categorical and dimensional constructs (Stein and Lochner 2006), drawing on both proximal and distal explanations (Nesse and Stein 2012), will likely be required in order to develop and ensure an increasingly scientifically valid and clinically useful approach to our future nomenclature.

New Disorders in the OCRD Chapter

In our view, the OCRD chapter includes some of the most important and interesting new disorders in DSM-5: hoarding disorder and excoriation (skin-picking) disorder. Prior to the inclusion of these disorders in DSM-5, our impression is that clinicians often overlooked them in their clinical practice and did not screen patients for them. Furthermore, diagnostic criteria were not available, so that when clinicians had the impression that hoarding behavior or skin-picking behavior might be present and problematic, it was difficult to identify and diagnose these conditions. In turn, these diagnostic limitations impeded the development and implementation of appropriate treatment. Hoarding disorder was often diagnosed and treated as if it were OCD; the problem was that OCD treatments (SRIs and exposure and response prevention) often do not effectively treat hoarding disorder. Our impression is that excoriation (skin-picking) disorder was missed altogether or perhaps diagnosed as an impulse-control disorder not elsewhere classified, which offered little direction for treatment. We hope that the addition of these disorders to DSM-5 will substantially improve patient care by helping clinicians to better identify and diagnose them and, in turn, to apply treatments discussed in this book. The new diagnostic criteria sets will also encourage clinically relevant research.

DSM-5 had a very high threshold for adding new disorders to the nomenclature. Rigorous guidelines had to be met, evidence that the guidelines were met had to be extensively documented, and the work groups' recommendation for inclusion of a new disorder had to be vetted and approved by additional committees that ensured that the guidelines were met. Great care was taken to avoid labeling normal human cognition or behavior as a mental disorder. Guidelines for adding a new disorder to DSM-5 included whether the condition met guidelines for a mental disorder; was a behavioral or psychological syndrome or pattern that occurs in an individual, the consequences of which are clinically significant distress or disability; was not merely an expectable response to common stressors or losses or a culturally sanctioned response to a particular event; reflected an underlying psychobiological dysfunction; was not solely a result of social deviance or conflicts with society; had diagnostic validity using one or more sets of diagnostic validators; and had clinical utility. Additional considerations were whether there was a need for the category; whether the diagnosis was sufficiently distinct from other diagnoses; whether there were proposed diagnostic criteria with clinical face validity, reliability, and adequate sensitivity and specificity; and whether the proposed diagnostic criteria could be easily implemented in a typical clinical interview and reliably operationalized or assessed for research purposes.

Hoarding disorder and excoriation (skin-picking) disorder met these guidelines. For example, they are common and severe conditions that are not better explained by any other disorder in DSM. Both disorders have a long historical tradition in the clinical literature and have been rigorously studied for decades. From a clinical perspective, there was a clear and pressing need for their inclusion in DSM. Regarding the availability of proposed diagnostic criteria, hoarding disorder criteria similar to those that were eventually included in DSM-5 had been well studied by investigators for several decades. Furthermore, proposed diagnostic criteria for hoarding disorder were included in the DSM-5 field trials, which supported their reliability and clinical utility. In addition, the DSM-5 Obsessive-Compulsive Spectrum Sub-Work Group sponsored field studies that further examined reliability of the proposed criteria and their perceived acceptability and usefulness to clinicians. Proposed diagnostic criteria for trichotillomania (hair-pulling disorder) and excoriation (skin-picking) disorder were also examined in field studies commissioned by the sub-work group, ensuring inclusion of empirically supported criteria in DSM-5.

We should also note that the diagnosis of "other specified OCRD" includes some interesting and often severe variations of OCRDs that for the most part were not highlighted or included in DSM-IV. It is worth becoming familiar with these clinical presentations so they can be addressed in treatment.

Some of the Most Important Changes for Individual OCRDs

DSM-5 required that changes to diagnostic criteria be carefully considered. Work groups were cognizant of the fact that DSM is a manual to be used by clinicians and so should be implementable, that recommendations should be research based, and that continuity with previous editions should be maintained where possible. Although it was initially proposed that there be no a priori constraints on the degree of change between DSM-IV and DSM-5, it was also recognized that the empirical evidence for any change should be in proportion to the magnitude of the change; that is, the larger and more significant the change, the stronger should be the required level of support. Proposed changes to the OCRDs were based on extensive reviews of the literature, which were published in a special issue of the journal *Depression and Anxiety* and in other scientific journals. Proposed changes were also focused on the validators mentioned earlier and included discussions of problems with existing criteria, possible advantages of proposed changes, and possible disadvantages of such changes. Here we discuss the changes made to OCD, BDD, and trichotillomania (hair-pulling disorder), the disorders in the OCRD chapter that were already included in DSM-IV.

Before discussing changes to these individual disorders, we must first comment on the new insight specifier in the OCRD chapter. This important addition to DSM-5 was made to the three OCRDs with a prominent cognitive component: OCD, BDD, and hoarding disorder. This change has substantial implications for patient care. The use of a similar insight specifier across these three disorders provides one example of how certain aspects of the clinical approach are similar across these conditions and also different from those used for other conditions. Thus, a specifier of "with absent insight/delusional beliefs" is used when patients with OCD are completely convinced that the OCD beliefs are true, when patients with BDD are completely convinced that the BDD beliefs are true, and when patients with hoarding disorder are completely convinced that hoarding-related beliefs and behaviors are not problematic despite evidence to the contrary. In each of these cases, current recommendations are for clinicians to begin medication treatment with standard first-line therapies (i.e., SRIs) for the relevant OCRD and to refrain from using standard interventions for psychotic disorders (i.e., antipsychotics as monotherapy).

For OCD, the majority of changes proposed to the criteria set can be characterized as clarification of the DSM-IV criteria (Leckman et al. 2010). Thus, for example, the definition of obsession now uses the term *urge* rather than *impulse* in order to avoid confusion with the impulse-control disorders. Similarly, DSM-5 clarifies that obsessions cause marked anxiety or distress "in most individuals," because research studies have found that such anxiety or distress is not present in all patients with OCD. A further example is the insertion of "e.g." just before the phrase "take more than 1 hour per day" in the phrase that defines "time-consuming," to indicate that this guideline is not absolutely fixed; OCD can be considered time consuming even if it occupies only 55 minutes a day. The criterion differentiating symptoms of OCD from symptoms of other mental disorders was clarified and expanded in order to optimize differential diagnosis. The insight specifier for OCD was expanded to include good or fair insight, poor insight, and absent insight/delusional beliefs, and a tic-related specifier was added. Although OCD patients have symptoms on a number of characteristic dimensions, these are described in the DSM-5 text rather than listed as specifiers.

For BDD, a number of clarifications were also included (Phillips et al. 2010). For example, in criterion A, the phrase "imagined defect" was replaced with "perceived defect or flaws...are not observable or appear slight to others." The DSM-IV phrase was confusing to patients with poor insight, and the DSM-5 version is more neutral in tone. In addition, the criterion differentiating BDD symptoms from symptoms of other mental disorders was clarified in order to optimize differentiation from eating disorders. Perhaps the most important change to the BDD criteria set, however, was the inclusion of a new criterion on repetitive behaviors (e.g., mirror checking, excessive grooming, skin picking, reassurance seeking) or mental acts (e.g., comparing appearance with that of others in response to the appearance concerns). This change reflects accumulating research that virtually all patients presenting with BDD preoccupations have such repetitive behaviors at some point in their disorder and is consistent with a conceptualization of BDD as an OCRD. An insight specifier was added, as was a muscle dysmorphia specifier.

For trichotillomania (hair-pulling disorder), a number of changes for DSM-5 were again clarifications of the diagnostic criteria. For example, in Criterion A, which covers hair pulling and resultant hair loss, the term *noticeable* was omitted, as there are different patterns of hair loss, some more noticeable than others, and because many patients disguise their hair loss. The largest change to the criteria set, however, was replacing the criterion that had described a preceding increase in tension prior to hair pulling and a subsequent sense of relief or gratification after hair pulling with a criterion noting repeated attempts to decrease or stop hair pulling. This change was based on research showing that not all patients with chronic hair-pulling symptoms describe preceding tension or subsequent relief/gratification and that patients who do and do not meet this criterion have few, if any, clinical differences (e.g., levels of comorbidity, levels of impairment). In addition, a DSM-5-commissioned field study found that patients with chronic hair-pulling symptoms invariably had made repeated attempts to decrease or stop hair pulling.

Measures to Screen for and Assess OCRDs

DSM-5 includes new self-report assessment measures, which emphasize the value of a dimensional approach to diagnosis. These cross-cutting symptom measures assess domains of psychopathology and are modeled on general medicine's review of systems. It is important to emphasize, however, that these questions should *not* be used as a "gateway" to making diagnoses. In other words, if patients do not endorse symptoms in these measures, clinicians should nonetheless screen patients for the OCRDs.

The cross-cutting symptom measures have two levels (see appendix to this chapter). *Level 1* questions address 13 symptom domains in adults that cover a broad range of psychopathology (12 symptom domains in children and adolescents). *Level 2* questions assess particular domains in greater detail. The measures are intended to be employed at the initial assessment and then used to track the course of symptoms over time.

The tenth domain of the Level 1 cross-cutting symptom measure in adults probes for OCRD symptoms using two questions. The first question addresses "unpleasant thoughts, urges, or images that repeatedly enter your mind." The second question addresses "feeling driven to perform certain behaviors or mental acts over and over again." Each question is rated on a five-point Likert scale with respect to the past 2 weeks, with anchor points of none (not at all), slight (rare, less than a day or two), mild (several days), moderate (more than half the days), and severe (nearly every day). The tenth domain of the Level 1 cross-cutting symptom measure for children and adolescents comprises four questions addressing different OCD symptom dimensions (thoughts about harm, checking behaviors, contamination concerns, doing things in a certain way).

Ratings of mild or greater severity on the questions in this domain should prompt additional inquiry, for which the Level 2 questions can be used. The Level 2 cross-cutting symptom measure provided by DSM-5 for the OCRDs is adapted from part B of the FOCI Severity Scale (Storch et al. 2007) (see appendix to this chapter). This scale comprises five items, which address time occupied by the symptoms, distress caused by the symptoms, difficulty in controlling symptoms, avoidance caused by the symptoms, and interference associated with the symptoms. Each item is rated on a five-point Likert scale ranging from none to extreme. The DSM-5 work group adapted the

FOCI to assess the symptoms of BDD, hoarding disorder, trichotillomania (hair-pulling disorder), and excoriation (skin-picking) disorder. These brief self-rated scales were intended to be consistent in content and structure across the disorders, to reflect DSM-5 criteria, and to provide a dimensional symptom severity rating. In a large nonclinical sample, they each demonstrated a single factor structure, strong internal consistency, and convergent validity (LeBeau et al. 2013). However, their psychometric properties should be further examined, especially in clinical samples.

Clinician-rated symptom severity scales are available for each of the OCRDs. The Y-BOCS for OCD is widely used to assess OCD symptoms at initial presentation and over time (Goodman et al. 1989). The first part of the scale (the Y-BOCS Symptom Checklist) screens for a range of obsessions and compulsions. The second part of the scale comprises five items for obsessions and five items for compulsions, again addressing time occupied by the symptoms, interference caused by the symptoms, distress caused by the symptoms, attempts to resist the symptoms, and difficulty in controlling symptoms. Each item is again rated on a five-point Likert scale ranging from none to extreme. Similar clinician-rated scales have been developed for assessing symptom severity in BDD, hoarding disorder, trichotillomania (hair-pulling disorder), and excoriation (skin-picking) disorder and are discussed in more detail in later chapters.

What Each Chapter in This Book Covers

Chapters on individual disorders in this handbook cover key clinical aspects of each disorder. Each chapter begins with a description of the disorder's phenomenology, including DSM-5 diagnostic criteria and changes from DSM-IV, and illustrates this symptomatology using clinical cases. Given the underrecognition and underdiagnosis of the OCRDs, our view is that these sections are particularly important, and we hope that they will help clinicians to recognize these conditions.

The chapters then go on to describe associated clinical features, including comorbidity, course and prognosis, functional impairment and suicidality, developmental considerations, gender-related issues, and cultural aspects/considerations. Each of these sections is clinically important insofar as it contributes to optimizing differential diagnosis and patient assessment. Sections on differential diagnosis and assessment further consolidate the information already provided.

Each of the chapters also provides information on epidemiology, etiology, and pathophysiology. Research in these areas is again helpful in optimizing clinicians' approach to assessment and intervention and provides a solid foundation from which to initiate treatment planning. Authors include, when appropriate, a discussion of environmental factors, genetic factors, neurocircuitry, and neurochemistry.

Finally, each chapter includes a section on pharmacotherapy and psychotherapy. There have been significant advances in the treatment of OCRDs in recent decades, with a growing evidence base of randomized controlled trials now available. Contributing authors summarize these data and provide guidance on first-line clinical interventions, the use of augmentation strategies and combined treatment modalities, and the approach to the patient with treatment-resistant illness. Where appropriate, authors also cover interventions such as neurosurgery and transcranial magnetic stimulation. Each chapter then concludes by providing a set of key clinical points and recommended readings.

Acknowledgments

Katharine Phillips was chair of the DSM-5 Work Group on Anxiety, Obsessive-Compulsive Spectrum, Posttraumatic, and Dissociative Disorders. Dan Stein was chair of the Obsessive-Compulsive Spectrum Sub-Work Group. We wish to acknowledge the substantive inputs and tireless efforts of other members of the work group: Scott Rauch, Blair Simpson, and, at the start of the process, Eric Hollander. In addition, we relied significantly on the work of many advisors, namely Damiaan Denys, Brian Fallon, Wayne Goodman, Jon Grant, Nancy Keuthen, David Mataix-Cols, Harrison Pope, Steven Rasmussen, Sanjaya Saxena, Harvey Singer, John Walkup, Douglas Woods, and Joseph Zohar. We wish to thank Joseph Bienvenu for leading a DSM-5 commissioned data analysis; Naomi Fineberg, Jamie Feusner, and James Leckman for leading DSM-5-commissioned reviews; David Mataix-Cols for leading field studies on hoarding disorder; and Christine Lochner and colleagues for leading field studies on trichotillomania (hair-pulling disorder) and excoriation (skin-picking) disorder. We are grateful to many other OCRD experts for contributing to literature reviews that informed recommendations for changes to DSM-IV and for responding to surveys that we sent out to the field. We are also grateful to the thousands of clinicians and patients who left comments on the sub-work group's proposals on the DSM-5 Web site. Finally we wish to gratefully acknowledge support from American Psychiatric Association staff, including Seung-Hee Hong.

References

American Psychiatric Association: Diagnostic and Statistical Manual of Mental Disorders, 4th Edition. Washington, DC, American Psychiatric Association, 1994

American Psychiatric Association: Diagnostic and Statistical Manual of Mental Disorders, 5th Edition. Arlington, VA, American Psychiatric Association, 2013

Feusner JD, Hembacher E, Phillips KA: The mouse who couldn't stop washing: pathologic grooming in animals and humans. CNS Spectr 14(9):503–513, 2009 19890232

First MB, Pincus HA, Levine JB, et al: Clinical utility as a criterion for revising psychiatric diagnoses. Am J Psychiatry 161(6):946–954, 2004 15169680

Goodman WK, Price LH, Rasmussen SA, et al: The Yale-Brown Obsessive Compulsive Scale, II: validity. Arch Gen Psychiatry 46(11):1012–1016, 1989 2510699

Hollander E, Allen A, Kwon J, et al: Clomipramine vs desipramine crossover trial in body dysmorphic disorder: selective efficacy of a serotonin reuptake inhibitor in imagined ugliness. Arch Gen Psychiatry 56(11):1033–1039, 1999 10565503

Hollander E, Kim S, Zohar J: OCSDs in the forthcoming DSM-V. CNS Spectr 12(5):320–323, 2007 17585430

Hollander E, Zohar J, Sirovatka P, et al (eds): Obsessive-Compulsive Spectrum Disorders: Refining the Research Agenda for DSM-V. Washington, DC, American Psychiatric Publishing, 2011

Hyman SE: Neuroscience, genetics, and the future of psychiatric diagnosis. Psychopathology 35(2–3):139–144, 2002 12145499

Hyman SE: Can neuroscience be integrated into the DSM-V? Nat Rev Neurosci 8(9):725–732, 2007 17704814

Insel T, Cuthbert B, Garvey M, et al: Research domain criteria (RDoC): toward a new classification framework for research on mental disorders. Am J Psychiatry 167(7):748–751, 2010 20595427

Ipser JC, Sander C, Stein DJ: Pharmacotherapy and psychotherapy for body dysmorphic disorder. Cochrane Database Syst Rev (1):CD005332, 2009 19160252

Joel D, Stein DJ, Schreiber R: Animal models of obsessive compulsive disorder: from bench to bedside via endophenotypes and biomarkers, in Animal and Translational Models for CNS Drug Discovery, Vol 1. Edited by McArthur R, Borsini F. Amsterdam, The Netherlands, Elsevier, 2008, pp 133–164

Kendler KS, Gardner CO, Prescott CA: Toward a comprehensive developmental model for major depression in women. Am J Psychiatry 159(7):1133–1145, 2002 12091191

Keuthen NJ, O'Sullivan RL, Ricciardi JN, et al: The Massachusetts General Hospital (MGH) Hairpulling Scale, 1: development and factor analyses. Psychother Psychosom 64(3–4):141–145, 1995 8657844

Keuthen NJ, Wilhelm S, Deckersbach T, et al: The Skin Picking Scale: scale construction and psychometric analyses. J Psychosom Res 50(6):337–341, 2001 11438115

Koran LM, Hanna GL, Hollander E, et al: Practice guideline for the treatment of patients with obsessive-compulsive disorder. Am J Psychiatry 164(7 suppl):5–53, 2007 17849776

LeBeau RT, Mischel E, Simpson HB, et al: Preliminary assessment of obsessive-compulsive spectrum disorder scales for DSM-5. J Obsessive Compuls Relat Disord 2:114–118, 2013

Leckman JF, Denys D, Simpson HB, et al: Obsessive-compulsive disorder: a review of the diagnostic criteria and possible subtypes and dimensional specifiers for DSM-V. Depress Anxiety 27(6):507–527, 2010 20217853

Mataix-Cols D, Pertusa A, Leckman JF: Issues for DSM-V: how should obsessive-compulsive and related disorders be classified? Am J Psychiatry 164(9):1313–1314, 2007 17728412

Mataix-Cols D, Frost RO, Pertusa A, et al: Hoarding disorder: a new diagnosis for DSM-V? Depress Anxiety 27(6):556–572, 2010 20336805

McKay D, Neziroglu F, Yaryura-Tobias JA: Comparison of clinical characteristics in obsessive-compulsive disorder and body dysmorphic disorder. J Anxiety Disord 11(4):447–454, 1997 9276787

Nesse RM, Stein DJ: Towards a genuinely medical model for psychiatric nosology. BMC Med 10(1):5, 2012 22244350

O'Sullivan RL, Keuthen NJ, Hayday CF, et al: The Massachusetts General Hospital (MGH) Hairpulling Scale, 2: reliability and validity. Psychother Psychosom 64(3–4):146–148, 1995 8657845

Phillips KA: The obsessive-compulsive spectrums. Psychiatr Clin North Am 25(4):791–809, 2002 12462861

Phillips KA, Hollander E: Treating body dysmorphic disorder with medication: evidence, misconceptions, and a suggested approach. Body Image 5(1):13–27, 2008 18325859

Phillips KA, Hollander E, Rasmussen SA, et al: A severity rating scale for body dysmorphic disorder: development, reliability, and validity of a modified version of the Yale-Brown Obsessive Compulsive Scale. Psychopharmacol Bull 33(1):17–22, 1997 9133747

Phillips KA, Stein DJ, Rauch SL, et al: Should an obsessive-compulsive spectrum grouping of disorders be included in DSM-V? Depress Anxiety 27(6):528–555, 2010 20533367

Phillips KA, Pinto A, Hart AS, et al: A comparison of insight in body dysmorphic disorder and obsessive-compulsive disorder. J Psychiatr Res 46(10):1293–1299, 2012 22819678

Robins E, Guze SB: Establishment of diagnostic validity in psychiatric illness: its application to schizophrenia. Am J Psychiatry 126(7):983–987, 1970 5409569

Stein DJ, Hollander E: The spectrum of obsessive-compulsive related disorders, in Obsessive-Compulsive Related Disorders. Edited by Hollander E. Washington, DC, American Psychiatric Press, 1993, pp 241–272

Stein DJ, Lochner C: Obsessive-compulsive spectrum disorders: a multidimensional approach. Psychiatr Clin North Am 29(2):343–351, 2006 16650712

Stein DJ, Fineberg NA, Bienvenu OJ, et al: Should OCD be classified as an anxiety disorder in DSM-V? Depress Anxiety 27(6):495–506, 2010a 20533366

Stein DJ, Grant JE, Franklin ME, et al: Trichotillomania (hair pulling disorder), skin picking disorder, and stereotypic movement disorder: toward DSM-V. Depress Anxiety 27(6):611–626, 2010b 20533371

Stein DJ, Craske MG, Friedman MJ, et al: Meta-structure issues for the DSM-5: how do anxiety disorders, obsessive-compulsive and related disorders, post-traumatic disorders, and dissociative disorders fit together? Curr Psychiatry Rep 13(4):248–250, 2011 21603904

Storch EA, Kaufman DA, Bagner D, et al: Florida Obsessive-Compulsive Inventory: development, reliability, and validity. J Clin Psychol 63(9):851–859, 2007 17674398; corrected in J Clin Psychol 63(12):1265, 2007

Wittchen HU, Beesdo K, Gloster AT: The position of anxiety disorders in structural models of mental disorders. Psychiatr Clin North Am 32(3):465–481, 2009a 19716987

Wittchen HU, Beesdo-Baum K, Gloster AT, et al: The structure of mental disorders re-examined: is it developmentally stable and robust against additions? Int J Methods Psychiatr Res 18(4):189–203, 2009b 20033884

Appendix

The American Psychiatric Association (APA) is offering a number of "emerging measures" for further research and clinical evaluation. These patient assessment measures were developed to be administered at the initial patient interview and to monitor treatment progress. They should be used in research and evaluation as potentially useful tools to enhance clinical decision making and not as the sole basis for making a clinical diagnosis. Instructions, scoring information, and interpretation guidelines are provided; further background information can be found in DSM-5. The APA requests that clinicians and researchers provide further data on the instruments' usefulness in characterizing patient status and improving patient care at www.dsm5.org/Pages/Feedback-Form.aspx.

DSM-5 Self-Rated Level 1 Cross-Cutting Symptom Measure—Adult[1]

DSM-5 Self-Rated Level 1 Cross-Cutting Symptom Measure—Adult

Name: _____ Age: _____ Sex: ❑ Male ❑ Female Date:_____

If this questionnaire is completed by an informant, **what is your relationship with the individual?** _____

In a typical week, approximately how much time do you spend with the individual? _____ **hours/week**

Instructions: The questions below ask about things that might have bothered you. For each question, circle the number that best describes how much (or how often) you have been bothered by each problem during the **past TWO (2) WEEKS**.

	During the past **TWO (2) WEEKS**, how much (or how often) have you been bothered by the following problems?	None Not at all	Slight Rare, less than a day or two	Mild Several days	Moderate More than half the days	Severe Nearly every day	Highest Domain Score (clinician)
I.	1. Little interest or pleasure in doing things?	0	1	2	3	4	
	2. Feeling down, depressed, or hopeless?	0	1	2	3	4	
II.	3. Feeling more irritated, grouchy, or angry than usual?	0	1	2	3	4	
III.	4. Sleeping less than usual, but still have a lot of energy?	0	1	2	3	4	
	5. Starting lots more projects than usual or doing more risky things than usual?	0	1	2	3	4	
IV.	6. Feeling nervous, anxious, frightened, worried, or on edge?	0	1	2	3	4	
	7. Feeling panic or being frightened?	0	1	2	3	4	
	8. Avoiding situations that make you anxious?	0	1	2	3	4	
V.	9. Unexplained aches and pains (e.g., head, back, joints, abdomen, legs)?	0	1	2	3	4	
	10. Feeling that your illnesses are not being taken seriously enough?	0	1	2	3	4	
VI.	11. Thoughts of actually hurting yourself?	0	1	2	3	4	
VII.	12. Hearing things other people couldn't hear, such as voices even when no one was around?	0	1	2	3	4	
	13. Feeling that someone could hear your thoughts, or that you could hear what another person was thinking?	0	1	2	3	4	
VIII.	14. Problems with sleep that affected your sleep quality over all?	0	1	2	3	4	
IX.	15. Problems with memory (e.g., learning new information) or with location (e.g., finding your way home)?	0	1	2	3	4	
X.	16. Unpleasant thoughts, urges, or images that repeatedly enter your mind?	0	1	2	3	4	
	17. Feeling driven to perform certain behaviors or mental acts over and over again?	0	1	2	3	4	
XI.	18. Feeling detached or distant from yourself, your body, your physical surroundings, or your memories?	0	1	2	3	4	
XII.	19. Not knowing who you really are or what you want out of life?	0	1	2	3	4	
	20. Not feeling close to other people or enjoying your relationships with them?	0	1	2	3	4	
XIII.	21. Drinking at least 4 drinks of any kind of alcohol in a single day?	0	1	2	3	4	
	22. Smoking any cigarettes, a cigar, or pipe, or using snuff or chewing tobacco?	0	1	2	3	4	
	23. Using any of the following medicines ON YOUR OWN, that is, without a doctor's prescription, in greater amounts or longer than prescribed [e.g., painkillers (like Vicodin), stimulants (like Ritalin or Adderall), sedatives or tranquilizers (like sleeping pills or Valium), or drugs like marijuana, cocaine or crack, club drugs (like ecstasy), hallucinogens (like LSD), heroin, inhalants or solvents (like glue), or methamphetamine (like speed)]?	0	1	2	3	4	

---

[1]This measure can be reproduced without permission by researchers and by clinicians for use with their patients. Rights holder: American Psychiatric Association. To request permission for any other use beyond what is stipulated above, contact: www.appi.org/CustomerService/Pages/Permissions.aspx.

Instructions to Clinicians

The DSM-5 Level 1 Cross-Cutting Symptom Measure is a self- or informant-rated measure that assesses mental health domains that are important across psychiatric diagnoses. It is intended to help clinicians identify additional areas of inquiry that may have significant impact on the individual's treatment and prognosis. In addition, the measure may be used to track changes in the individual's symptom presentation over time.

This adult version of the measure consists of 23 questions that assess 13 psychiatric domains, including depression, anger, mania, anxiety, somatic symptoms, suicidal ideation, psychosis, sleep problems, memory, repetitive thoughts and behaviors, dissociation, personality functioning, and substance use. Each item inquires about how much (or how often) the individual has been bothered by the specific symptom during the past 2 weeks. If the individual is of impaired capacity and unable to complete the form (e.g., an individual with dementia), a knowledgeable adult informant may complete the measure. The measure was found to be clinically useful and to have good test-retest reliability in the DSM-5 Field Trials that were conducted in adult clinical samples across the United States and in Canada.

Scoring and Interpretation

Each item on the measure is rated on a 5-point scale (0=none or not at all; 1=slight or rare, less than a day or two; 2=mild or several days; 3=moderate or more than half the days; and 4=severe or nearly every day). The score on each item within a domain should be reviewed. Because additional inquiry is based on the highest score on any item within a domain, the clinician is asked to indicate that score in the "Highest Domain Score" column. A rating of mild (i.e., 2) or greater on any item within a domain (except for substance use, suicidal ideation, and psychosis) may serve as a guide for additional inquiry and follow up to determine if a more detailed assessment for that domain is necessary. For substance use, suicidal ideation, and psychosis, a rating of slight (i.e., 1) or greater on any item within the domain may serve as a guide for additional inquiry and follow-up to determine if a more detailed assessment is needed. The DSM-5 Level 2 Cross-Cutting Symptom Measures may be used to provide more detailed information on the symptoms associated with some of the Level 1 domains (see Table 1 below).

Frequency of Use

To track change in the individual's symptom presentation over time, the measure may be completed at regular intervals as clinically indicated, depending on the stability of the individual's symptoms and treatment status. For individuals with impaired capacity, it is preferable that the same knowledgeable informant completes the measures at follow-up appointments. Consistently high scores on a particular domain may indicate significant and problematic symptoms for the individual that might warrant further assessment, treatment, and follow-up. Clinical judgment should guide decision making.

Table 1: Adult DSM-5 Self-Rated Level 1 Cross-Cutting Symptom Measure: domains, thresholds for further inquiry, and associated Level 2 measures for adults ages 18 and over

Domain	Domain Name	Threshold to guide further inquiry	DSM-5 Level 2 Cross-Cutting Symptom Measure available online
I.	Depression	Mild or greater	LEVEL 2—Depression—Adult (PROMIS Emotional Distress—Depression—Short Form)[1]
II.	Anger	Mild or greater	LEVEL 2—Anger—Adult (PROMIS Emotional Distress—Anger—Short Form)[1]
III.	Mania	Mild or greater	LEVEL 2—Mania—Adult (Altman Self-Rating Mania Scale)
IV.	Anxiety	Mild or greater	LEVEL 2—Anxiety—Adult (PROMIS Emotional Distress—Anxiety—Short Form)[1]
V.	Somatic Symptoms	Mild or greater	LEVEL 2—Somatic Symptom—Adult (Patient Health Questionnaire 15 Somatic Symptom Severity [PHQ-15])
VI.	Suicidal Ideation	Slight or greater	None
VII.	Psychosis	Slight or greater	None
VIII.	Sleep Problems	Mild or greater	LEVEL 2—Sleep Disturbance - Adult (PROMIS—Sleep Disturbance—Short Form)[1]
IX.	Memory	Mild or greater	None
X.	Repetitive Thoughts and Behaviors	Mild or greater	LEVEL 2—Repetitive Thoughts and Behaviors—Adult (adapted from the Florida Obsessive-Compulsive Inventory [FOCI] Severity Scale [Part B])
XI.	Dissociation	Mild or greater	None
XII.	Personality Functioning	Mild or greater	None
XIII.	Substance Use	Slight or greater	LEVEL 2—Substance Abuse—Adult (adapted from the NIDA-modified ASSIST)

[1]The PROMIS Short Forms have not been validated as an informant report scale by the PROMIS group.

LEVEL 2—Repetitive Thoughts and Behaviors—Adult (adapted from the Florida Obsessive-Compulsive Inventory [FOCI] Severity Scale [Part B])[2]

LEVEL 2—Repetitive Thoughts and Behaviors—Adult[*]
*Adapted from the Florida Obsessive-Compulsive Inventory (FOCI) Severity Scale (Part B)

Name: _____   Age: ____   Sex: ☐ Male ☐ Female   Date:_____

If the measure is being completed by an informant, what is your relationship with the individual receiving care? _____

In a typical week, approximately how much time do you spend with the individual receiving care? _____ hours/week

Instructions: On the DSM-5 Level 1 cross-cutting questionnaire that you just completed, you indicated that *during the past 2 weeks* you have been bothered by "unwanted repeated thoughts, images, or urges" and/or "being driven to perform certain behaviors or mental acts over and over" at a mild or greater level of severity. The questions below ask about these feelings in more detail and especially how often you have been bothered by a list of symptoms **during the past 7 days.** Please respond to each item by marking (✓ or x) one box per row.

During the past <u>SEVEN (7) DAYS</u>….						Clinician Use
						Item Score
1. On average, how much *time* is occupied by these thoughts or behaviors each day?	☐ 0—None	☐ 1—Mild (Less than an hour a day)	☐ 2—Moderate (1 to 3 hours a day)	☐ 3—Severe (3 to 8 hours a day)	☐ 4—Extreme (more than 8 hours a day)	
2. How much *distress* do these thoughts or behaviors cause you?	☐ 0—None	☐ 1—Mild (slightly disturbing)	☐ 2—Moderate (disturbing but still manageable)	☐ 3—Severe (very disturbing)	☐ 4—Extreme (overwhelming distress)	
3. How hard is it for you to *control* these thoughts or behaviors?	☐ 0—Complete control	☐ 1—Much control (usually able to control thoughts or behaviors)	☐ 2—Moderate control (sometimes able to control thoughts or behaviors)	☐ 3—Little control (infrequently able to control thoughts or behaviors)	☐ 4—No control (unable to control thoughts or behaviors)	
4. How much do these thoughts or behaviors cause you to *avoid* doing anything, going anyplace, or being with anyone?	☐ 0—No avoidance	☐ 1—Mild (occasional avoidance)	☐ 2—Moderate (regularly avoid doing these things)	☐ 3—Severe (frequent and extensive avoidance)	☐ 4 - Extreme (nearly complete avoidance; house-bound)	
5. How much do these thoughts or behaviors *interfere* with school, work, or your social or family life?	☐ 0—None	☐ 1—Mild (slight interference)	☐ 2— Moderate; (definite interference with functioning, but still manageable)	☐ 3—Severe (substantial interference)	☐ 4—Extreme (near-total interference; incapacitated)	
					Total/Partial Raw Score:	
					Prorated Total Raw Score (if 1 item is left unanswered):	
					Average Total Score:	

---

[2]This material can be reproduced without permission by clinicians for use with their own patients. Any other use, including electronic use, requires written permission from Dr. Goodman. Rights holder: © 1994 Wayne K. Goodman, M.D., and Eric Storch, Ph.D. To request permission for any other use beyond what is stipulated above, contact the rights holder.

Instructions to Clinicians

The DSM-5 Level 2—Repetitive Thoughts and Behavior—Adult measure is an adapted version of the 5-item Florida Obsessive-Compulsive Inventory (FOCI) Severity Scale (Part B) that is used to assess the domain of repetitive thoughts and behaviors in individuals age 18 and older. The measure is completed by an individual prior to a visit with the clinician. If the individual receiving care is of impaired capacity and unable to complete the form (e.g., an individual with dementia), a knowledgeable informant may complete the measure. Each item asks the individual (or informant) to rate the severity of the individual's repetitive thoughts and behaviors **during the past 7 days**.

Scoring and Interpretation

Each item on the measure is rated on a 5-point scale (i.e., 0 to 4) with the response categories having different anchors depending on the item. The total score for the measure can range of score from 0 to 20, with higher scores indicating greater severity of repetitive thoughts and behaviors. The clinician is asked to review the score of each item on the measure during the clinical interview and indicate the raw score for each item in the section provided for "Clinician Use." The raw scores on the 5 items should be summed to obtain a total raw score. If the individual has a score of 8 or higher, you may want to consider a more detailed assessment for an obsessive compulsive disorder. In addition, the clinician is asked to calculate and use the **average total score**. **The average total score** reduces the overall score to a 5-point scale, which allows the clinician to think of the individual's repetitive thoughts and behavior in terms of none (0), mild (1), moderate (2), severe (3), or extreme (4). The use of the average total score was found to be reliable, easy to use, and clinically useful to the clinicians in the DSM-5 Field Trials. The **average total score** is calculated by dividing the raw total score by number of items in the measure (i.e., 5).

Note: If 2 or more items are left unanswered on the measure (i.e., more than 25% of the total items are missing), the total scores should not be calculated. Therefore, the individual (or informant) should be encouraged to complete all of the items on the measure. If only 4 of the 5 items on the measure are answered, you are asked to prorate the raw score by first summing the scores of items that were answered to get a **partial raw score**. Next, multiply the partial raw score by the total number of items on the measure (i.e., 5). Finally, divide the value by the number of items that were actually answered (i.e., 4) to obtain the prorated total raw score.

Prorated Score =   (Partial Raw Score x number of items on the measure)
                     Number of items that were actually answered

If the result is a fraction, round to the nearest whole number.

Frequency of Use

To track change in the severity of the individual's repetitive thoughts and behavior over time, the measure may be completed at regular intervals as clinically indicated, depending on the stability of the individual's symptoms and treatment status. For individuals of impaired capacity, it is preferred that completion of the measure at follow-up appointments is by the same knowledgeable informant. Consistently high scores on the measure may indicate significant and problematic areas for the individual that might warrant further assessment, treatment, and follow-up. Your clinical judgment should guide your decision.

CHAPTER 2

Obsessive-Compulsive Disorder

Mayumi Okuda, M.D.
H. Blair Simpson, M.D., Ph.D.

Obsessive-compulsive disorder (OCD) is an often-disabling condition. In epidemiological samples, nearly two-thirds of individuals with OCD report severe role impairment (Ruscio et al. 2010). Among neuropsychiatric conditions, OCD is a leading cause of health-related disability in the world (World Health Organization 2008).

In DSM classifications prior to DSM-5, OCD was grouped with the anxiety disorders. In the new diagnostic classification, DSM-5, OCD is in a separate chapter on obsessive-compulsive and related disorders (OCRDs). In this chapter, we describe changes in the OCD diagnosis for DSM-5 (American Psychiatric Association 2013), provide an overview of OCD, and review recent treatment advances.

Diagnostic Criteria and Symptomatology

Changes made to the OCD diagnostic criteria for DSM-5 are outlined in this section (see Box 2–1 for the criteria). As in DSM-IV (American Psychiatric

Association 1994), Criterion A describes the characteristic symptoms of OCD: obsessions and compulsions. *Obsessions* are repetitive and persistent thoughts (e.g., of contamination), urges (e.g., to hurt someone), or images (e.g., of violent scenes). The DSM-IV definition of obsessions included the word *impulse,* which has been replaced with *urge* in DSM-5 to avoid confusion with impulse-control disorders. Importantly, obsessions are not experienced as pleasurable or voluntary. They are intrusive and unwanted and cause marked distress or anxiety. Experiences of anxiety or distress help differentiate the obsessions of OCD from the recurrent thoughts or images that are present in other disorders (e.g., intrusive sexual images in paraphilic disorders). Although the vast majority of individuals report that their obsessions generate at least moderate anxiety or distress (Leckman et al. 2010), a small subset do not report more than mild anxiety or distress. This is reflected in the new definition of obsessions, which now states that at some time during the disturbance, obsessions cause marked anxiety or distress in *most individuals.* Given that different cultures may have different definitions of what is inappropriate, obsessions are no longer described as "inappropriate" but as "unwanted" (Leckman et al. 2010). In DSM-5, two features about obsessions that help to distinguish OCD from generalized anxiety disorder and psychotic disorders were removed from the DSM-IV definition of obsessions in Criterion A and incorporated instead into the expanded list of differential diagnoses in Criterion D.

BOX 2–1. DSM-5 Diagnostic Criteria for Obsessive-Compulsive Disorder

---

A. Presence of obsessions, compulsions, or both:

Obsessions are defined by (1) and (2):

1. Recurrent and persistent thoughts, urges, or images that are experienced, at some time during the disturbance, as intrusive and unwanted, and that in most individuals cause marked anxiety or distress.

2. The individual attempts to ignore or suppress such thoughts, urges, or images, or to neutralize them with some other thought or action (i.e., by performing a compulsion).

Compulsions are defined by (1) and (2):

1. Repetitive behaviors (e.g., hand washing, ordering, checking) or mental acts (e.g., praying, counting, repeating words silently) that the individual feels driven to perform in response to an obsession or according to rules that must be applied rigidly.

2. The behaviors or mental acts are aimed at preventing or reducing anxiety or distress, or preventing some dreaded event or situation; however, these behaviors or mental acts are not connected in a realistic way with what they are designed to neutralize or prevent, or are clearly excessive.

Note: Young children may not be able to articulate the aims of these behaviors or mental acts.

B. The obsessions or compulsions are time-consuming (e.g., take more than 1 hour per day) or cause clinically significant distress or impairment in social, occupational, or other important areas of functioning.

C. The obsessive-compulsive symptoms are not attributable to the physiological effects of a substance (e.g., a drug of abuse, a medication) or another medical condition.

D. The disturbance is not better explained by the symptoms of another mental disorder (e.g., excessive worries, as in generalized anxiety disorder; preoccupation with appearance, as in body dysmorphic disorder; difficulty discarding or parting with possessions, as in hoarding disorder; hair pulling, as in trichotillomania [hair-pulling disorder]; skin picking, as in excoriation [skin-picking] disorder; stereotypies, as in stereotypic movement disorder; ritualized eating behavior, as in eating disorders; preoccupation with substances or gambling, as in substance-related and addictive disorders; preoccupation with having an illness, as in illness anxiety disorder; sexual urges or fantasies, as in paraphilic disorders; impulses, as in disruptive, impulse-control, and conduct disorders; guilty ruminations, as in major depressive disorder; thought insertion or delusional preoccupations, as in schizophrenia spectrum and other psychotic disorders; or repetitive patterns of behavior, as in autism spectrum disorder).

Specify if:

With good or fair insight: The individual recognizes that obsessive-compulsive disorder beliefs are definitely or probably not true or that they may or may not be true.

With poor insight: The individual thinks obsessive-compulsive disorder beliefs are probably true.

With absent insight/delusional beliefs: The individual is completely convinced that obsessive-compulsive disorder beliefs are true.

Specify if:

Tic-related: The individual has a current or past history of a tic disorder.

Individuals attempt to ignore or suppress these obsessions (e.g., using thought suppression) or to neutralize them with another thought or action (e.g., performing a compulsion). *Compulsions* (or rituals) are repetitive behaviors (e.g., washing, checking) or mental acts (e.g., counting) aimed at reducing the distress triggered by obsessions, according to rules that must be applied rigidly, or preventing a feared event (e.g., contracting an illness). Compulsions are not pleasurable, although some individuals experience relief from anxiety or distress. Compulsions are not connected in a realistic way to the feared event (e.g., arranging items symmetrically to prevent harm to a loved one) or are clearly excessive.

DSM-5 removed the need for individuals to recognize obsessions and/or compulsions as *excessive* or *unreasonable* (previously Criterion B). Children in particular tend to be less insightful. Given that insight varies in individuals with OCD, there is now a broader range of insight options described as specifiers (good or fair insight, poor insight, and absent insight/delusional OCD beliefs; these are discussed later).

Criterion B emphasizes that obsessions and compulsions must be time consuming or cause significant distress or impairment. The frequency and severity of obsessions and compulsions vary across individuals with OCD. Whereas some individuals have mild to moderate symptoms, others have nearly constant intrusive thoughts or compulsions that can be incapacitating. This criterion helps to distinguish the disorder from the occasional intrusive thoughts or repetitive behaviors that have been found in up to half of healthy control subjects (e.g., double-checking that a door is locked) (Leckman et al. 2010). DSM-5 reworded the criterion so that "take more than 1 hour a day" is now an example, emphasizing that this is merely a guideline and that obsessing for 55 minutes a day, for example, can still be diagnosed as OCD if other diagnostic criteria are met.

Regarding Criterion C, factors such as a stroke in cortico-striato-thalamo-cortical (CSTC) circuits exclude a diagnosis of OCD, and a diagnosis of OCRD due to another medical condition should be made (Leckman et al. 2010). However, if OCD co-occurs with a tic disorder in the context of a streptococcal infection, both OCD and the tic disorder are diagnosed, because the association between the streptococcal infection and the development of OCD remains unclear (see subsection "Environmental Factors" later in the chapter).

Criterion D identifies other psychiatric disorders that need to be differentiated from OCD. In DSM-5, this list was expanded (see Box 2–1), to remind clinicians that disorders other than OCD can be characterized by intrusive thoughts or repetitive behaviors.

The new insight specifier resulted in the elimination of OCD's delusional variant from the psychosis section of DSM. This change has clinical implications: An individual with OCD who has poor or absent insight or delusional OCD beliefs should be diagnosed with, and receive treatment for, OCD—that is, serotonin reuptake inhibitors (SRIs) rather than antipsychotics as the first line of treatment. In the DSM-IV field trial, there was a range of insight in OCD patients; most patients had good or fair insight (e.g., recognizing that their OCD beliefs were definitely or probably not true or might or might not be true), but 26% had poor insight (mostly certain their feared consequences *would* occur), and 4% had delusional OCD beliefs (completely certain that their feared consequence would occur) (Leckman et al. 2010). More recent studies similarly report a range of insight in OCD.

Additionally, DSM-5 includes tic-related OCD as a new specifier. This subgroup differs from those without a history of tic disorders in several clinically important ways. OCD with a comorbid tic disorder is more often characterized by early onset and male predominance, a higher frequency of symmetry obsessions and ordering compulsions, higher likelihood of remission as seen in longitudinal cohort studies, and higher rates of familial transmission (Leckman et al. 2010). Some data suggest that tic-related OCD is more likely to respond to SRI augmentation with an antipsychotic (Bloch et al. 2006).

The content of obsessions and compulsions is heterogeneous. Grouped into different so-called symptom dimensions, these include cleaning (contamination obsessions, cleaning compulsions), symmetry (symmetry obsessions, repeating/ordering/counting compulsions), forbidden or taboo thoughts (e.g., sexual/religious obsessions and related compulsions), and harm (e.g., fears of harm to self or others, checking compulsions). Individuals with OCD may also have difficulties discarding or accumulating objects (hoarding) as a result of OCD obsessions (e.g., fears of harm). (Hoarding behavior that is not triggered by OCD obsessions and that meets other diagnostic criteria for hoarding disorder should be diagnosed as hoarding disorder, not as OCD.) Individuals with OCD may exhibit symptoms in more than one dimension. Avoidance of triggers of obsessions and compulsions is also frequently found in individuals with OCD (Table 2–1).

TABLE 2–1. Screening questions for obsessive-compulsive disorder

Do you have unpleasant thoughts you can't get rid of?

Do you worry that you might impulsively harm someone?

Do you have to count things, wash your hands, or check things over and over?

Do you worry a lot about whether you performed religious rituals correctly or have been immoral?

Do you have troubling thoughts about sexual matters?

Do you need things arranged symmetrically or in a very exact order?

Do these worries and behaviors interfere with your functioning at work, with your family, or with social activities?

Do you spend a lot of time thinking or acting on these thoughts?

Do these thoughts or behaviors trouble you?

Source. Adapted from American Psychiatric Association 2007b.

Case Example: Samantha

Samantha, a 28-year-old African American woman who works at a post office, was referred for a psychiatric evaluation by her dermatologist. Upon presentation, she reported feeling very anxious and afraid of "going crazy." She could not stop worrying about contracting a sexually transmitted disease by touching objects that could infect her. Constantly vigilant for potentially contaminated objects, she avoided touching most things in daily life. Her fears led her to wash her hands with antibacterial soap up to 50 times a day, spending hours a day on this routine. Unable to stop excessive hand washing, she had developed a contact dermatitis. She became increasingly afraid of any type of physical contact with people and had started to wear latex gloves when she left her apartment, which resulted in social isolation. At work, she often left her desk to wash her hands, and it took her many hours to sort through mail that she considered potentially contaminated. She was worried that she would lose her job because her supervisors had given her several warnings about her decreased productivity.

Case Example: Anthony

Anthony, a 10-year-old child, was referred to a child psychiatrist by his pediatrician. During the past year, Anthony had been doing poorly at school and at home. He was unable to concentrate in class, being consumed by thoughts and sequences he had to complete in his head. He had to repeat to himself conversations he had heard at home to confirm he had not heard words that he considered inappropriate. After repeatedly doing this, he had to think of words that started with the letter *M*. He was frequently bullied by his classmates, who saw him arranging items and often called him a "freak." In addition to having to think about things in a certain sequence, Anthony had to brush his teeth and tie and untie his shoes a specific number of times. His toys had to be arranged in a particular way, which led to frequent arguments with his parents. He feared his mother would die if he did not complete these rituals, and he could not be reassured that this would not happen. He threw tantrums if prevented from completing his rituals, and if interrupted, he had to start all over again. Desperate, his parents allowed him to complete them, and he often was late for school or missed classes as a result. Anthony had no friends and spent most of his time by himself in fear that he would be interrupted or made fun of.

Epidemiology

In the United States, the 12-month prevalence of OCD has been reported as 1.2%, with approximately one-third of cases in the severe category. Similar prevalence rates have been reported in different countries, ranging from 1.1% (Korea and New Zealand) to 1.8% (Puerto Rico). The lifetime prevalence of OCD has been reported to range from 0.7% (in Taiwan) to 2.3% (in the United States) and 2.5% (in Puerto Rico) (Ruscio et al. 2010).

Comorbidity

The vast majority of individuals with OCD (90%) in the general population meet diagnostic criteria for another psychiatric disorder at some point in their lives (Ruscio et al. 2010). Using DSM-IV criteria, the largest epidemiological sample to include individuals with OCD found that the most common comorbid lifetime conditions are anxiety and mood disorders (76% and 63%, respectively) (Ruscio et al. 2010). Obsessive-compulsive personality disorder (25%) is also frequently comorbid with OCD (American Psychiatric Association 2007a, 2013). According to different studies, 10%–40% of individuals with early-onset OCD have a history of Tourette's syndrome or chronic tic disorder (Leckman et al. 2010). Children with tic-related OCD have higher rates of disruptive behavior disorders (attention-deficit/hyperactivity disorder and oppositional defiant disorder) and trichotillomania (hair-pulling disorder) as well as other pervasive developmental disorders (Leckman et al. 2010). Conversely, approximately one-third to one-half of individuals with Tourette's syndrome or chronic tic disorders have a lifetime diagnosis of OCD (Pallanti et al. 2011).

Disorders that are not common in individuals with OCD but occur more frequently than in those without OCD include body dysmorphic disorder (BDD), trichotillomania (hair-pulling disorder), and excoriation (skin-picking) disorder (Bienvenu et al. 2012). In addition, lifetime rates of OCD are elevated among individuals with psychotic disorders, bipolar disorder, and eating disorders (Pallanti et al. 2011).

Course and Prognosis

The median age at onset of OCD was 19 years in the largest epidemiological sample to include individuals with OCD (Ruscio et al. 2010). Approximately one-quarter of cases begin by age 10 years. Onset after age 30 is rare. The onset of symptoms is typically gradual; acute presentations have been associated with infectious etiologies (Leckman et al. 2010). Individuals with childhood-onset OCD appear to have a more favorable prognosis; in 44% of cases, symptoms remit by early adulthood (Koran and Simpson 2013).

Only half of individuals with OCD seek treatment. Treatment rates are higher for severe cases, but only a minority receive specific treatment for OCD (Ruscio et al. 2010). If untreated, OCD tends to have a fluctuating and often chronic course. The longest naturalistic follow-up study conducted to date (more than 40 years) consisted of a sample of 144 individuals with OCD who during most of the follow-up period did not receive effective treatment. Approximately half of the sample continued to experience clinically significant symptoms decades later, and a third continued to have symptoms that met the full criteria for OCD (Skoog and Skoog 1999).

Psychosocial Impairment and Suicidality

OCD is associated with reduced quality of life that is comparable to that in schizophrenia and depressive disorders. Studies that directly compared patients with OCD with patients with panic disorder, social anxiety disorder, heroin dependence, hemodialysis, and renal transplantation have reported a greater impact on quality of life in individuals with OCD than in these other patients (Macy et al. 2013). Greater psychosocial impairment is associated with greater OCD symptom severity and the presence of comorbid conditions, particularly major depression.

Studies suggest that the incidence of suicide attempts is higher in individuals with OCD compared with the general population. Most available information comes from a few studies (Alonso et al. 2010; Torres et al. 2011). In clinical samples, rates of suicide attempts have been reported from 10% to 27% (Torres et al. 2011). Individuals attempting or committing suicide are more likely to be unmarried, endorse symmetry/ordering obsessions and compulsions, and have greater OCD severity, avoidant personality disorder, a history of a comorbid mood disorder, and a history of prior suicide attempts (Alonso et al. 2010). In the largest clinical sample examining the prevalence and correlates of suicidality in OCD, 36% (210) of 582 outpatients had had suicidal thoughts at some point in their lives, 20% (117) had made suicide plans, 11% (64) had attempted suicide at some point, and 10% (58) had current suicidal thoughts. The following were associated with suicidal behaviors (thoughts, plans, or attempts): OCD symptoms of the sexual/religious dimension, a history of major depressive disorder and posttraumatic stress disorder, a comorbid substance use disorder (with suicidal thoughts and suicide plans), and comorbid impulse-control disorders (Torres et al. 2011). Information on completed suicide is scarce.

Developmental Considerations

Early-onset OCD is usually associated with significant disruption in social, familial, academic, and vocational functioning. OCD symptoms may adversely affect the trajectory of normal childhood and adolescent development, which can lead to impairments in adult life. For example, contamination fears may result in school absenteeism if the child fears exploring different environments. Counting rituals and intrusive thoughts can affect concentration and interfere with cognitive and language milestones, adversely impacting school performance and educational attainment. Symptoms can also result in difficulties socializing with peers. Adolescents may struggle to build intimate relationships and to become independently functioning adults (Piacentini et al. 2003).

Individuals' symptoms may result in family members' modifications of routines and roles (e.g., limiting visitors for fear of contamination). Accommodation, the process by which family members assist or participate in patient rituals, has been linked to poorer treatment outcomes. Accommodation has been reported in as many as 75% of families of children and adolescents with OCD. It has been associated with higher family burden, poorer quality of life, symptom persistence, and reinforcement of fear and avoidance behaviors, which may affect the effectiveness of exposure-based treatments (Piacentini et al. 2003).

Gender-Related Issues

Males typically have an earlier age at onset of OCD than females. Males constitute the majority of very early onset cases, with nearly one-quarter of males having onset of the disorder before age 10. For females, the highest peak of onset occurs during adolescence (Ruscio et al. 2010). Early-onset OCD with a history of a tic disorder is also more common in males.

Gender differences in symptom dimensions have also been reported. Females are more likely to report contamination obsessions and cleaning/washing compulsions, whereas a greater proportion of males report sexual/religious obsessions (Leckman et al. 2010). Reports of exacerbation of OCD during the premenstrual period have suggested a role for hormonally related fluctuations in OCD symptoms. The prevalence of these exacerbations remains unclear, given that most data come from retrospective studies (Abramowitz et al. 2003; Labad et al. 2005). Although few studies have focused on the peripartum period, some have suggested that pregnancy and the puerperium may precipitate or exacerbate OCD (American Psychiatric Association 2007a; Russell et al. 2013). A recent meta-analysis ($N=6,922$) suggested that pregnant and postpartum women are approximately 1.5–2 times more likely to experience OCD compared with women in the general population (Russell et al. 2013).

Cultural Aspects of Phenomenology

OCD demographics (e.g., gender distribution, age at onset) and core symptoms seem largely independent of culture, ethnicity, and geographic location (Lewis-Fernández et al. 2010; Matsunaga and Seedat 2007). For instance, four- or five-factor models of symptoms (e.g., contamination/cleaning, forbidden thoughts/checking, symmetry/ordering, and harm/hoarding) have been replicated in different countries (Leckman et al. 2010). Furthermore, worldwide, contamination/cleaning obsessions and compulsions and forbidden thoughts/checking obsessions and compulsions are the most frequently occurring symptoms (Matsunaga and Seedat 2007). There are also similarities across cultures in course and comorbidity patterns (Leckman et al. 2010).

Nonetheless, cultural context may shape the specific content of obsessions and compulsions. For example, some studies have suggested that in countries where religion has a markedly influential role in society, individuals with religious obsessions/compulsions may be more likely to remain undiagnosed, have greater illness severity, and have longer delays in treatment seeking.

Assessment and Differential Diagnosis

In assessing the patient's symptoms with the objective of establishing an OCD diagnosis using DSM-5 criteria, it is important to differentiate the obsessions and compulsions of OCD from similar symptoms found in other disorders. Disorders to be considered in the differential diagnosis of OCD include those described below (see also Table 2–2).

Other Obsessive-Compulsive and Related Disorders

Obsessive preoccupation and/or repetitive behaviors are symptoms of other OCRDs. When the focus of obsessions and compulsions is on perceived defects in physical appearance, BDD should be diagnosed rather than OCD. In trichotillomania (hair-pulling disorder), the compulsive behavior is limited to hair pulling in the absence of obsessions. Hoarding disorder symptoms focus on the excessive accumulation of objects, persistent difficulty discarding possessions, and distress associated with discarding items. However, when an individual has obsessions that are typical of OCD (e.g., concerns about incompleteness or harm), and these lead to compulsive hoarding behaviors (e.g., not discarding old newspapers because they may contain information that could prevent harm), a diagnosis of OCD should be given instead.

Anxiety Disorders

The anxious ruminations that are present in generalized anxiety disorder are typically about real-life concerns. In contrast, OCD obsessions often involve content that is odd, irrational, or of a seemingly magical nature. Moreover, obsessions in OCD are commonly linked to compulsions. Individuals with specific phobia have a fear reaction to specific objects or situations, but the objects/situations are usually more circumscribed, and compulsions are not present. In social anxiety disorder, feared situations are limited to social scenarios, and avoidance is aimed at reducing social anxiety.

TABLE 2–2. Differential diagnosis of obsessive-compulsive disorder (obsessive-compulsive disorder)

Differential diagnosis	Symptoms	
	Obsessions	Compulsions
Body dysmorphic disorder	Focused on concerns about perceived defects or flaws in physical appearance	Behaviors done in response to appearance concerns (e.g., mirror checking, skin picking, excessive grooming)
Trichotillomania (hair-pulling disorder)	Not present	Behavior limited to hair pulling
Hoarding disorder	Not typical OCD obsessions (e.g., concerns about incompleteness, harm)	Accumulation of objects not done in response to an obsession
Generalized anxiety disorder	About real life concerns; not odd, irrational, or of a seemingly magical nature	Not present
Specific phobia	Not present	Not present
Social anxiety disorder	Not present; fear limited to social situations	Reassurance seeking aimed at reducing social anxiety
Major depressive disorder	Mood-congruent ruminations in the context of depressed mood; not necessarily experienced as intrusive or distressing	Not present

TABLE 2–2. Differential diagnosis of obsessive-compulsive disorder (obsessive-compulsive disorder) *(continued)*

Differential diagnosis	Symptoms	
	Obsessions	Compulsions
Manic episode	Hyperreligious preoccupations associated with elevated mood and other symptoms of mania	Not a compensatory behavior in response to obsessions
Paraphilias	Limited to sexual content	Limited to sexual behaviors
		Pleasurable; wishes to resist in response to negative consequences of behavior
Gambling disorder	Limited to gambling content	Limited to gambling behaviors
		Pleasurable; wishes to resist in response to negative consequences of behavior
Substance use disorder	Limited to substance use	Limited to substance use or substance use–related behaviors
		Pleasurable; wishes to resist in response to negative consequences of behavior
Eating disorder	Limited to concerns about weight and food	Limited to behaviors that will decrease weight or food intake (e.g., excessive exercise)

TABLE 2–2. Differential diagnosis of obsessive-compulsive disorder (obsessive-compulsive disorder) *(continued)*

Differential diagnosis	Symptoms	
	Obsessions	Compulsions
Tic disorder	Not present	Movements less complex than compulsions—sudden, rapid, recurrent, and nonrhythmic
Stereotypic movement disorder	Not present	Movements less complex than compulsions—repetitive, seemingly driven, and apparently purposeless
Psychotic disorders	Psychotic beliefs not limited to OCD beliefs; other psychotic symptoms present (e.g., hallucinations, thought disorder)	Not present
Obsessive-compulsive personality disorder	Not present; instead, long-standing pattern of excessive perfectionism and rigid control	Not present

Depressive Disorders and Bipolar and Related Disorders

OCD obsessions can be confused with ruminations of major depressive disorder. However, depressive ruminations are usually mood congruent and not necessarily experienced as intrusive or distressing. Moreover, ruminations are not linked to compulsions. In the case of manic episodes, if hyperreligious preoccupations have an obsessive quality, these are associated with elevated mood and other manic symptoms not found in OCD. As noted earlier, mood disorders (i.e., depressive and bipolar disorders, which were grouped together in DSM-IV) frequently occur in individuals with OCD. Both diagnoses should be given when these co-occur.

Paraphilic Disorders and Substance-Related and Addictive Disorders

Although certain behaviors may be described as *compulsive*, including sexual behaviors (e.g., paraphilias), gambling (e.g., gambling disorder), and substance use (e.g., substance use disorder), these behaviors differ from OCD compulsions in that they are usually experienced as pleasurable, and wishes to resist them typically reflect the behaviors' deleterious consequences.

Feeding and Eating Disorders

OCD can be distinguished from the eating disorders in that the obsessions and compulsions of the OCD patient are not limited to concerns about weight, food, or exercise.

Neurodevelopmental Disorders

Both OCD compulsions and tics can be preceded by sensory phenomena or premonitory sensory urges (e.g., musculoskeletal sensations, "just right" perceptions) (Leckman et al. 2010). Stereotypic behaviors in stereotypic movement disorder, on the other hand, are not associated with premonitory urges, preceding sensations, or an urge to perform them. Tics and stereotypic movements are typically less complex than compulsions and are not aimed at preventing or reducing the anxiety triggered by obsessions, or performed according to certain rules. OCD and tic disorders often co-occur. In these instances, both diagnoses should be given, and the OCD tic-related specifier should be used.

Schizophrenia Spectrum and Other Psychotic Disorders

Although individuals with OCD may have no insight (delusional beliefs), the delusional beliefs are related to OCD. A psychotic disorder diagnosis is not given unless the individual has other features of a psychotic disorder (e.g., hallucinations or formal thought disorder).

Obsessive-Compulsive Personality Disorder

Obsessive-compulsive personality disorder is not characterized by intrusive thoughts, urges, or images or by repetitive behaviors that are performed in response to intrusions. Instead, it involves an enduring and pervasive maladaptive pattern of excessive perfectionism, rigid control, and other personality characteristics.

Etiology and Pathophysiology

Environmental Factors

Several environmental factors have been implicated in OCD. For example, some cases of childhood-onset OCD and tic disorders manifest abruptly in susceptible individuals and may be due to an autoimmune process following infection with Group A β-hemolytic *Streptococcus*. This syndrome was originally called *pediatric autoimmune neuropsychiatric disorder associated with streptococcal infections* (PANDAS) (Leckman et al. 2010). However, streptococcal infection may be only one of many causes for abrupt onset of OCD. As a result, this syndrome is now called *pediatric acute-onset neuropsychiatric syndrome* or *childhood acute neuropsychiatric symptoms*.

Exacerbations of OCD in the premenstrual and postpartum period suggest that hormonal fluctuations may play a role in the etiology of OCD (Labad et al. 2005).

Genetic Factors

Twin and family studies suggest that there is genetic susceptibility to OCD. Studies have reported findings indicating a greater genetic influence in childhood-onset OCD (45%–65% in childhood vs. 27%–47% in adult-onset OCD). Serotonin (5-HT) and glutamate genes are the most consistently implicated in OCD (Pauls 2010; Wu et al. 2012).

Neurocircuitry

Evidence for the role of CSTC circuits in the pathophysiology of OCD comes from imaging studies that examined the neuroanatomy, circuit function, and neurochemistry of OCD. Findings vary across structural studies of subjects with OCD compared with healthy control subjects. The most consistently reported structural abnormalities in OCD involve the basal ganglia, orbitofrontal cortex, anterior cingulate cortex, and striatum (Milad and Rauch 2012; Pittenger et al. 2011).

Positron emission tomography and functional magnetic resonance imaging studies have also implicated the CSTC circuits. As an example, studies in individuals with OCD in resting state or with symptom provocation have reported hyperactivity in the orbitofrontal cortex, caudate, anterior cingulate cortex, and thalamus.

In addition to the CSTC circuits, other studies have suggested dysfunctions in the amygdalo-cortical circuitry (Milad and Rauch 2012). For example, functional neuroimaging studies have reported significantly reduced activation in the ventromedial prefrontal cortex, caudate, and hippocampus during fear conditioning, as well as in the cerebellum, posterior cingulate cortex, and putamen during extinction recall, in individuals with OCD (Milad et al. 2013).

Neurochemistry

Abnormalities in 5-HT, dopamine, and glutamate systems have been hypothesized to play a role in OCD. Evidence is still inconclusive, and more research is needed. Studies of peripheral markers of 5-HT function and those examining the distribution of serotonin transporters (5-HTT) and 5-HT_{2A} receptors have reported inconsistent findings (Koo et al. 2010; Matsumoto et al. 2010; Simpson et al. 2003, 2011). Fewer studies have examined the dopamine system but have suggested dopamine transporter binding alterations in the basal ganglia (Koo et al. 2010).

Increased glutamatergic signaling in CSTC circuits has also been proposed (Wu et al. 2012). More recently, a study suggested decreased γ-aminobutyric (GABA) acid levels in individuals with OCD compared with control subjects (Simpson et al. 2012).

Summary

The relative contribution of environmental and genetic factors in the development of OCD is still under investigation. It is likely that abnormalities in multiple neurotransmitter systems are related to OCD symptoms. Dysfunction in different circuitries is believed to contribute to the pathophysiology of OCD; the CSTC circuit is the most widely studied. Other circuits, including the amygdalo-cortical circuitry, have been implicated as well.

Treatment

General Approaches to Treatment and Special Considerations

First-line treatments for OCD are SRIs (i.e., clomipramine and the selective serotonin reuptake inhibitors [SSRIs]), cognitive-behavioral therapy (CBT) using exposure and response prevention (ERP), or their combination. In terms of pharmacotherapy, all of the SRIs have been found to be efficacious in randomized controlled trials. SSRIs are also effective treatment for several depressive and anxiety disorders that are frequently comorbid with OCD. Although SSRIs continue to be the recommended first-line medication treatment for OCD, approximately 25%–60% of patients do not respond adequately to initial treatment (Van Ameringen et al. 2014). Strong evidence for the use of serotonin-norepinephrine reuptake inhibitors (SNRIs) is lacking.

First-Line Treatments: Serotonin Reuptake Inhibitors and Cognitive-Behavioral Therapy

Serotonin Reuptake Inhibitors

Selective serotonin reuptake inhibitors.   SSRIs have been shown to be efficacious for OCD in several large, multisite randomized trials. A meta-analysis of 17 randomized trials ($N = 3,097$) with OCD patients found SSRIs to be more effective than placebo in reducing OCD symptoms (Bloch et al. 2010). None of the individual SSRIs have shown superiority over the others (Bloch et al. 2010). Thus, the choice among the SSRIs can be made on the basis of prior treatment response, side-effect profile, acceptability to the patient, and potential for drug interactions. Currently, all of the SSRIs except for citalopram and escitalopram have been approved for the treatment of OCD in adults by the U.S. Food and Drug Administration (FDA). Fluoxetine, fluvoxamine, and sertraline are the only FDA-approved SSRIs in children. SSRIs are generally safe and well tolerated. Most common side effects include gastrointestinal problems, agitation, sleep disturbances, and sexual side effects. If an adequate trial of the SSRI results in no response, the patient should be given another trial of monotherapy with either a second SSRI or clomipramine. Fewer than half of patients benefit from switching from one SSRI to another, and the likelihood of response diminishes as the number of failed adequate trials increases.

Clomipramine.   Clomipramine, a tricyclic antidepressant that is a potent SRI, is FDA approved for treatment of OCD in adults and children. A meta-analysis of seven randomized trials ($N = 392$) found clomipramine to be superior to placebo in reducing OCD symptoms. Some meta-analyses of randomized trials have suggested that clomipramine has a greater effect size than SSRIs, although direct comparisons find no significant differences between clomipramine and several SSRIs (American Psychiatric Association 2007a). In addition to the side effects related to its serotonergic action, clomipramine can cause anticholinergic effects (e.g., dry mouth, constipation, delayed urination), antihistaminergic effects (e.g., sedation, weight gain), antiadrenergic effects (e.g., orthostatic hypotension), and cardiac conduction delay or seizures. Thus, SSRIs are usually tried prior to clomipramine.

Course and duration of serotonin reuptake inhibitor treatment.   Higher doses of SSRIs than are usually recommended in depression are associated with improved efficacy in OCD (Bloch et al. 2010). The medication should be started at a low dosage to enhance tolerability (e.g., fluoxetine 10 or 20 mg/ day), and the dosage should be titrated as tolerated (recommended dosing is provided in Table 2–3). To prevent early discontinuation, it is important to remind patients that there is typically a 4- to 6-week delay in drug response. Higher-than-FDA-recommended dosing of SSRIs may help some patients with OCD (e.g., fluoxetine 120 mg/day) (Koran and Simpson 2013).

An adequate trial has been defined as 8–12 total weeks of an SRI (4–6 weeks at maximum tolerable dose; American Psychiatric Association 2007a). Patients who continue medication have a lower rate of relapse than patients receiving placebo (American Psychiatric Association 2007a). Patients who respond to an adequate trial of an SRI should continue taking the medication for at least 1–2 years. If the medication is discontinued, it should be tapered slowly (e.g., 10%–25% every 1–2 months) (American Psychiatric Association 2007a).

Cognitive-Behavioral Therapy

CBT is the recommended first-line treatment for OCD. CBT may be more effective than SRIs for OCD without comorbidity. The type of CBT with the strongest empirical evidence is ERP (Koran and Simpson 2013; American Psychiatric Association 2007a). In clinical trials, dropout rates for CBT with ERP are similar to those for medication (Foa et al. 2005).

ERP involves in vivo exposures to feared situations, imaginal exposures to feared consequences, and ritual prevention, in which patients contract to refrain from engaging in compulsions. Exposure assignments are tailored to the different obsessive fears of the patient (e.g., fear of contamination) and are typically conducted gradually, with situations provoking moderate distress confronted before ones generating more severe distress. Imaginal exposures consist of elaborating detailed image scripts and then listening to or reading these scripts repeatedly until they are experienced as less anxiety provoking. In order to be effective, exposure practices are routinely assigned for completion between sessions, and patients are coached to refrain from rituals to the extent possible. Several manuals are available for therapists and patients (see "Recommended Readings" at the end of this chapter).

When delivered expertly to patients who adhere to the treatment, ERP can be highly effective, with 74%–80% achieving some reduction in symp-

TABLE 2–3. Suggested serotonin reuptake inhibitor dosage ranges for obsessive-compulsive disorder

Drug class	Medication	Starting dosage, mg/day[a]	Usual target dosage, mg/day	Usual maximum dosage, mg/day	Occasionally prescribed maximum dosage, mg/day[b]
Selective serotonin reuptake inhibitor	Fluoxetine	20	40–60	80	120
	Fluvoxamine	50	200	300	450
	Paroxetine	20	40–60	60	100
	Sertraline[c]	50	200	200	400
	Escitalopram	10	20	40	60
	Citalopram	20	40	d	d
Tricyclic antidepressants	Clomipramine	25	100–250	250	e

[a]Some patients may need to start at half this dosage or less to minimize undesired side effects such as nausea or to accommodate anxiety about taking medications.

[b]These dosages are sometimes used for rapid metabolizers or for patients with no or mild side effects and inadequate therapeutic response after 8 weeks or more at the usual maximum dosage.

[c]Sertraline, alone among the selective serotonin reuptake inhibitors, is better absorbed with food.

[d]Citalopram should no longer be used at dosages greater than 40 mg/day, or 20 mg/day in individuals older than 60 years (U.S. Food and Drug Administration 2012). Please consult the FDA communication for other details.

[e]Combined plasma levels of clomipramine plus desmethylclomipramine 12 hours after the dose should be kept below 500 ng/mL to minimize risk of seizures and cardiac conduction delay.

Source. Adapted from American Psychiatric Association 2007a.

toms (e.g., response rates to 25%) and 33%–43% achieving minimal symptoms after 17 sessions (Foa et al. 2005; Simpson et al. 2006, 2008, 2013). At the same time, good outcome relies upon patient adherence (Koran and Simpson 2013). One issue for ERP is how accessible this treatment is outside urban or specialty academic centers. Several research groups are studying whether technology (e.g., Internet-based ERP with therapist support by e-mail) can solve this problem (Andersson et al. 2012). Many questions remain, including how acceptable these programs will be to patients and for which patients they will be most effective (Andersson et al. 2012).

Second-Line Treatments: Serotonin-Norepinephrine Reuptake Inhibitors and Other Medications as Monotherapy

Serotonin-Norepinephrine Reuptake Inhibitors

Evidence from randomized controlled trials examining the use of SNRIs in OCD is either limited (i.e., venlafaxine) or nonexistent (i.e., duloxetine). These medications are not FDA approved for treatment of OCD.

Other Medications as Monotherapy

Few studies are available on other medications as monotherapy for OCD. Small randomized controlled trials have suggested possible benefits of several other agents, including mirtazapine and D-amphetamine (American Psychiatric Association 2007a). These agents are typically tried only after all first-line treatments fail.

Augmentation Strategies

When an SRI trial results in a partial response, SRI augmentation is recommended. Common augmentation strategies include the addition of CBT, antipsychotics, a low dose of clomipramine (added to an SSRI), or D-amphetamine.

Augmenting Serotonin Reuptake Inhibitors With Other Medications

Augmentation with antipsychotics.   Several randomized controlled trials of augmenting SRIs with haloperidol, risperidone, quetiapine, and olanzapine in OCD have been conducted. A few smaller randomized controlled trials have been conducted with aripiprazole and paliperidone. Whereas some individual studies have supported antipsychotic augmentation, other individual studies have failed to show benefits.

Two meta-analyses examining augmentation of SRIs with a first- or second-generation antipsychotic for patients with treatment-refractory OCD have been conducted (Bloch et al. 2006; Van Ameringen et al. 2014). Overall, data are strongest for risperidone and haloperidol; data supporting quetiapine and olanzapine remain inconclusive. Response was more robust for patients with comorbid tics. Since these meta-analyses were done, additional trials of quetiapine and olanzapine have been completed, but results continue to be mixed (Koran and Simpson 2013).

A few open-label trials and two small randomized controlled studies examining aripiprazole (5–20 mg/day) have suggested benefits in some patients. Larger randomized trials are needed (Koran and Simpson 2013; American Psychiatric Association 2007a; Sayyah et al. 2012). One available randomized controlled study examined the use of paliperidone in individuals whose OCD had not responded to two or more adequate SRI trials. The study found significant baseline-to-posttreatment symptom reduction in the group receiving paliperidone compared with those receiving placebo. However, there were no significant between-group differences (Storch et al. 2013).

Antipsychotic augmentation is associated with greater weight gain and/ or sedation than is SSRI or clomipramine monotherapy. Side effects of antipsychotic drugs include extrapyramidal symptoms, metabolic syndrome, and neuroleptic malignant syndrome. Antipsychotic medication should be added only after the patient has not responded to SRI monotherapy. Low antipsychotic dosages appear effective (e.g., 0.5–3 mg/day of risperidone or the equivalent). To prevent long-term adverse effects, it is recommended that antipsychotics be discontinued if there is no clear evidence of improvement after 4 weeks of treatment. One retrospective study suggested a high risk of relapse when the antipsychotic was discontinued; 13 of 15 patients had a return of OCD symptoms when their antipsychotic was stopped (American Psychiatric Association 2007a).

Serotonin reuptake inhibitor augmentation with clomipramine. Although not systematically studied, another SRI augmentation strategy includes the use of low doses of clomipramine (≤75 mg/day, typically between 10 and 50 mg/ day) to augment SSRIs in patients who have a partial response to an SSRI. However, SSRIs can result in markedly increased levels of clomipramine and should ideally be used in conjunction with monitoring of electrocardiography, pulse, blood pressure, and serum levels of the drug and its metabolites (desmethylclomipramine) (American Psychiatric Association 2007a). A screening electrocardiogram may be advisable in those with heart disease or for individuals older than 40 years.

Other serotonin reuptake inhibitor augmentation strategies. Other agents that have shown possible benefits in either open pilot trials or small randomized controlled trials include D-amphetamine, topiramate, lamotrigine, pregabalin, N-acetylcysteine, morphine sulfate, celecoxib, granisetron, and amisulpride (Askari et al. 2012; Koran and Simpson 2013; American Psychiatric Association 2007a; Metin et al. 2003; see Figure 2–1). However, given the modest evidence for augmentation with some of these agents, their use should be reevaluated in the future, when results from larger controlled trials become available.

Small randomized studies have not shown clear benefits for lithium, buspirone, clonazepam, pindolol, L-triiodothyronine, desipramine, glycine, and naltrexone; results from a large randomized study of ondansetron were also negative (Koran and Simpson 2013).

Augmenting Serotonin Reuptake Inhibitors With CBT Using Exposure and Response Prevention

Several randomized controlled trials now strongly support augmenting SRIs with ERP after an inadequate or incomplete response to the SRI alone. A recent study suggested that CBT may be more effective than antipsychotic augmentation of an SRI (Simpson et al. 2013).

Several trials have compared SRI nonresponders who received continued medication treatment alone versus continued medication plus ERP. Results indicate that ERP augmentation significantly increases rates of treatment response or remission, compared with continued medication alone (American Psychiatric Association 2007a; Simpson et al. 2008). One trial also reported that in individuals who continued an SRI, addition of ERP was significantly superior to risperidone and to placebo in terms of response rates, symptom reduction, improvement in insight, level of functioning, and quality of life (Simpson et al. 2013).

Augmenting Cognitive–Behavioral Therapy With D-Cycloserine

D-Cycloserine, a partial agonist at the N-methyl-D-aspartate (NMDA) receptor, enhances fear extinction in animal models and has thus been proposed to enhance extinction learning in ERP. To date, three small randomized trials have compared ERP alone with ERP augmented with D-cycloserine. Two of the studies showed a faster time to response but did not show an increased response by the end of the trial (Koran and Simpson 2013). D-Cycloserine is not yet recommended in routine practice.

Treatment in Children and Adolescents

Most experts recommend either CBT alone or the combination of CBT and an SRI as first-line treatment in children and adolescents. This recommendation is supported by the Pediatric OCD Treatment Study (POTS; $N=112$, ages 7–17 years), which compared CBT alone (including cognitive training

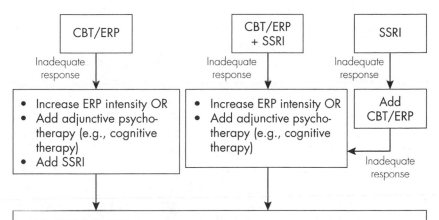

No SSRI response:
- Switch SSRI (repeat for more than one SSRI trial)
- Switch to clomipramine or venlafaxine or mirtazapine
- Augment with antipsychotic (discontinue if no response in 1 month)

Partial SSRI response:
- Augment with antipsychotic (discontinue if no response in 1 month)
- Augment with clomipramine if patient is taking SSRI
- Augment with other agents (e.g., D-amphetamine, memantine, pregabalin, topiramate, lamotrigine, N-acetylcysteine)

Try several of these alternatives, if no response, consider experimental treatments (e.g., TMS)

If OCD is treatment refractory and criteria for neurosurgical interventions are met, consider DBS or ablative procedures.

Criteria for treatment-refractory OCD:
- Three adequate trials with an SRI (SSRI or clomipramine) AND
- Augmentation of at least one of the previous drugs for 1 month with at least two of the following medications: antipsychotic, lithium, benzodiazepine, or buspirone AND
- Adequate CBT with at least 20 hours of ERP

FIGURE 2–1. Suggested treatment algorithm for obsessive-compulsive disorder (OCD).

CBT = cognitive-behavioral therapy; DBS = deep brain stimulation; ERP = exposure and response prevention; SRI = serotonin reuptake inhibitor; SSRI = selective serotonin reuptake inhibitor; TMS = transcranial magnetic stimulation.

and ERP), SRI (sertraline) alone, their combination, and placebo (Pediatric OCD Treatment Study Team 2004). Participants in the study fell within the moderate to moderately severe range of illness. Combined treatment was significantly more effective than the other three conditions, and both CBT with ERP and sertraline alone were significantly more effective than placebo. Remission rates for combined treatment did not significantly differ from those for CBT alone but did differ from sertraline alone and placebo. CBT alone did not statistically differ from sertraline but did differ from placebo. Remission rates for sertraline did not statistically differ from those for placebo.

A meta-analysis of eight randomized or quasi-randomized controlled trials including 343 individuals with OCD age 18 years or younger (age range, 4–18 years) compared CBT with varying degrees of ERP alone or in combination with a wait list, family-based relaxation training, pill placebo, and an SRI. All of the protocols included ERP to varying degrees (ranging between 12 and 20 sessions). The meta-analysis found lower OCD severity and lower symptom persistence rates in the groups receiving CBT compared with the placebo or wait-list comparison groups. There were no significant differences in terms of severity or persistence between CBT alone and medication alone. Combined CBT and medication was superior to medication alone but not to CBT alone (O'Kearney et al. 2006).

Similarly, another meta-analysis, which included randomized controlled trials of patients 19 years or younger (13 studies, $N = 1,117$), found both CBT and SRIs to be superior to control conditions. The effect size of CBT was large (1.45; 95% confidence interval [CI], 0.68–2.22), whereas the medication effect size was medium (0.48; 95% CI, 0.36–0.61). Among SRIs, clomipramine had the largest effect size (Watson and Rees 2008). However, clomipramine's advantages were offset by other significant advantages of SSRIs, including improved tolerability and safety.

In 2004, the FDA placed a black box warning on all antidepressant medications, publicizing a twofold increased risk for suicidal thinking or behavior in children and adolescents taking these medications (2% vs. 4%). On the other hand, a recent analysis of data from published and unpublished studies (12 adult, 4 geriatric, and 4 youth randomized controlled trials of fluoxetine and venlafaxine) found no evidence of increased suicide risk among youths receiving active medication; instead, severity of depression improved with medication and was significantly related to suicidal ideation or behavior (Gibbons et al. 2012). Clinicians and families have to weigh the risks of treating versus not treating disabling illnesses such as OCD.

Augmentation Strategies in Children and Adolescents

Children and adolescents whose symptoms remain significant despite an initial trial of either CBT with ERP or an SRI may be considered for augmentation. Paralleling findings in adults, studies have reported that the addition of CBT to medication continuation compared with medication continuation alone results in significantly greater response rates (Franklin et al. 2011).

Augmentation with an antipsychotic is often used, despite the fact that there are no data from randomized controlled trials in pediatric OCD and only some data from retrospective reports, case reports, and open-label studies (Masi et al. 2013). Therefore, clinicians should proceed with caution, because this group may be particularly vulnerable to the long-term effects of these medications. Some reports have suggested that children and adolescents may be more likely to develop antipsychotic-induced weight gain and antipsychotic-associated diabetes compared with adults.

Novel Medications: Glutamate Modulators

Several medications thought to modulate the glutamate system have shown some promise for refractory OCD. Two small, double-blind, randomized controlled trials testing memantine (a noncompetitive NMDA receptor antagonist) as an augmentation agent have been conducted so far, with positive results; larger trials are needed (Koran and Simpson 2013).

A single 40-minute, 0.5 mg/kg intravenous infusion of ketamine (another noncompetitive NMDA glutamate receptor antagonist) was tested in a small randomized, double-blind, placebo-controlled trial that included individuals with OCD and near-constant obsessions (Rodriguez et al. 2013). The study authors reported significant improvement in obsessions during the infusion and maintenance of gains 1 week post-infusion. Intravenous ketamine remains an experimental treatment.

Neurosurgery and Neuromodulation

Up to 10% of patients have *treatment-refractory OCD,* defined as having at least three failed adequate SRI trials, augmentation of at least one of the previous medications with at least two agents (lithium, buspirone, an antipsychotic, or a benzodiazepine), and adequate CBT with at least one ERP trial performed in combination with medication. Clinicians should determine whether these criteria have been met before considering patients as potential candidates for neurosurgery and other interventions described in the following sections (see Figure 2–1). Clinicians must also consider whether prior CBT trials have been "adequate" in terms of therapist training and experience with CBT, number of sessions, and completion of homework assignments.

Neurosurgery: Guided Lesions and Deep Brain Stimulation

Surgery.   Neurosurgical studies have shown symptom reduction after interventions that disrupt connections between frontocortical and subcortical areas. Lesions in the anterior limb of the internal capsule, the anterior cingulate, and/or the subcaudate region appear to be beneficial in cases of highly refractory OCD. These lesions can be generated using either traditional magnetic resonance imaging–guided stereotactic neurosurgery or radiosurgery, which does not require a craniotomy. In one of the few long-term follow-up studies of neurosurgery, 48% of patients (12 of 25) with severe, treatment-refractory OCD responded to unilateral or bilateral capsulotomy. Reported postoperative side effects include seizures, significant problems with executive functioning, memory difficulties, apathy, and disinhibition (Koran and Simpson 2013).

Deep brain stimulation.   Deep brain stimulation (DBS) is currently being investigated as a neurosurgical alternative for treatment-resistant OCD (Koran and Simpson 2013) and is FDA approved under the Humanitarian Device Exemption program. DBS is an invasive procedure that requires craniotomy to implant stimulating electrodes in specific brain targets. The FDA has approved targeting of the ventral striatum/ventral capsule.

Studies have reported clinically significant symptom reductions and functional improvement in approximately one-third to two-thirds of patients undergoing DBS (Blomstedt et al. 2013; Koran and Simpson 2013). Stimulation-related complications are usually reversible by adjusting the stimulation. Side effects include infection, hemorrhage, confusion, and seizures. Severe adverse effects are uncommon, and the mortality rate has been estimated at 0.6%.

Neuromodulation: Transcranial Magnetic Stimulation and Electroconvulsive Therapy

Transcranial magnetic stimulation.   Transcranial magnetic stimulation (TMS) is a neurophysiological technique that permits noninvasive stimulation of the cerebral cortex. Studies conducted in treatment-resistant OCD vary in terms of the nature of the stimulation (high vs. low frequency) as well as the specific brain target. In several randomized controlled trials using high-frequency repetitive TMS (rTMS) over the right dorsolateral prefrontal cortex, no effects were found. On the other hand, in two small randomized trials using low-frequency rTMS targeting the supplemental motor area, there were significantly greater response rates in individuals undergoing TMS compared with those who were receiving sham TMS (Koran and Simpson 2013).

Electroconvulsive therapy.   The few studies investigating the use of electroconvulsive therapy have not demonstrated efficacy in the treatment of OCD.

Summary

We recommend that adults with OCD start treatment with CBT with ERP, an SSRI, or both (Figure 2–1). CBT with ERP is often recommended first for pediatric OCD. An SSRI could be considered first in patients with a severe comorbid disorder that may interfere with CBT and that responds to SSRI treatment. SSRIs could also be considered first in patients who had a previous good response to medication or prefer medication, or when CBT with ERP is not available.

Although a substantial proportion of patients respond to first-line treatments, many will exhibit clinically significant ongoing OCD symptoms. For patients with a partial response to an SSRI, augmenting with CBT is an effective strategy. Other options include switching to another SSRI or to clomipramine; and augmenting the SSRI with another medication (e.g., an antipsychotic, clomipramine, or D-amphetamine). Which strategy to pursue needs to be tailored based on individual clinical characteristics (e.g., D-amphetamine in comorbid attention-deficit/hyperactivity disorder) and patient preference. Newer pharmacological strategies for SSRI augmentation remain limited, with glutamatergic agents (e.g., memantine) showing some promise. Ongoing work on the various brain mechanisms that lead to the symptoms of obsessions and compulsions in individuals and thereby to a diagnosis of OCD will hopefully be the basis for novel, personalized therapeutic alternatives.

Key Points

- Worldwide, the lifetime prevalence of obsessive-compulsive disorder (OCD) has been reported to be from 0.7% to 2.5%. The 12-month prevalence is 1.1%–1.8%.

- OCD is frequently comorbid with other psychiatric disorders, particularly anxiety disorders, depressive disorders, and bipolar and related disorders.

- The median age at onset of OCD is 19 years, with one-quarter of male cases starting by age 10; onset after the third decade is rare.

- If untreated, OCD tends to have a fluctuating course with periods of improvement, although in a substantial proportion of patients, clinically significant symptoms persist.

- OCD is associated with significant impairment and higher rates of suicide attempts than are found in the general population.

- Several environmental factors have been implicated in OCD, including group A β-hemolytic streptococcal infection and hormonal influences.

- Twin and family studies suggest a genetic contribution to OCD, with greater genetic influences in pediatric-onset OCD.

- Patients with OCD should be treated with cognitive-behavioral therapy (CBT) with exposure and response prevention (ERP), a selective serotonin reuptake inhibitor (SSRI), or both. CBT with ERP should be considered first-line treatment for noncomorbid OCD, especially in pediatric OCD. In patients with a severe comorbid disorder that may interfere with CBT and that responds to SSRI treatment, an SSRI should be considered first, followed by CBT augmentation as necessary. SSRIs can be used first either in patients who prefer medication to CBT with ERP or when the latter is not available.

- In adults, clomipramine and all of the SSRIs except for citalopram and escitalopram have been approved by the U.S. Food and Drug Administration (FDA). In children, clomipramine, fluoxetine, fluvoxamine, and sertraline have been approved by the FDA. High dosages are often most effective.

- An *adequate trial* is defined as keeping serotonin reuptake inhibitors (SRIs) within the therapeutic range at the maximal tolerable dose for at least 4–6 weeks (8–12 total weeks of SRI). If an adequate trial of an SSRI results in no response, clinicians may switch to another SSRI or clomipramine. With partial response to an SSRI, augmentation with CBT with ERP should be tried prior to other augmentation strategies.

- If SRI augmentation with antipsychotic medications is tried, the antipsychotic should be stopped if there is no response within 4 weeks.

- Deep brain stimulation is an experimental alternative for patients with treatment-refractory OCD. It is FDA approved under the Humanitarian Device Exemption program.

- Glutamate modulators have shown some promise in small randomized trials.

References

Abramowitz JS, Schwartz SA, Moore KM, et al: Obsessive-compulsive symptoms in pregnancy and the puerperium: a review of the literature. J Anxiety Disord 17(4):461–478, 2003 12826092

Alonso P, Segalàs C, Real E, et al: Suicide in patients treated for obsessive-compulsive disorder: a prospective follow-up study. J Affect Disord 124(3):300–308, 2010 20060171

American Psychiatric Association: Diagnostic and Statistical Manual of Mental Disorders, 4th Edition. Washington, DC, American Psychiatric Association, 1994

American Psychiatric Association: Practice Guideline for the Treatment of Patients With Obsessive-Compulsive Disorder. Arlington, VA, American Psychiatric Association, 2007a. Available at: http://psychiatryonline.org/pb/assets/raw/sitewide/practice_guidelines/guidelines/ocd.pdf. Accessed December 22, 2014.

American Psychiatric Association: Treating Obsessive-Compulsive Disorder: A Quick Reference Guide. Arlington, VA, American Psychiatric Association, 2007b. Available at: http://psychiatryonline.org/pb/assets/raw/sitewide/practice_guidelines/guidelines/ocd-guide.pdf. Accessed December 22, 2014.

American Psychiatric Association: Diagnostic and Statistical Manual of Mental Disorders, 5th Edition. Arlington, VA, American Psychiatric Association, 2013

Andersson E, Enander J, Andrén P, et al: Internet-based cognitive behaviour therapy for obsessive-compulsive disorder: a randomized controlled trial. Psychol Med 42(10):2193–2203, 2012 22348650

Askari N, Moin M, Sanati M, et al: Granisetron adjunct to fluvoxamine for moderate to severe obsessive-compulsive disorder: a randomized, double-blind, placebo-controlled trial. CNS Drugs 26(10):883–892, 2012 22873680

Bienvenu OJ, Samuels JF, Wuyek LA, et al: Is obsessive-compulsive disorder an anxiety disorder, and what, if any, are spectrum conditions? A family study perspective. Psychol Med 42(1):1–13, 2012 21733222

Bloch MH, Landeros-Weisenberger A, Kelmendi B, et al: A systematic review: antipsychotic augmentation with treatment refractory obsessive-compulsive disorder. Mol Psychiatry 11(7):622–632, 2006 16585942

Bloch MH, McGuire J, Landeros-Weisenberger A, et al: Meta-analysis of the dose-response relationship of SSRI in obsessive-compulsive disorder. Mol Psychiatry 15(8):850–855, 2010 19468281

Blomstedt P, Sjöberg RL, Hansson M, et al: Deep brain stimulation in the treatment of obsessive-compulsive disorder. World Neurosurg 80(6):e245–e253, 2013 23044000

Foa EB, Liebowitz MR, Kozak MJ, et al: Randomized, placebo-controlled trial of exposure and ritual prevention, clomipramine, and their combination in the treatment of obsessive-compulsive disorder. Am J Psychiatry 162(1):151–161, 2005 15625214

Franklin ME, Sapyta J, Freeman JB, et al: Cognitive behavior therapy augmentation of pharmacotherapy in pediatric obsessive-compulsive disorder: the Pediatric OCD Treatment Study II (POTS II) randomized controlled trial. JAMA 306(11):1224–1232, 2011 21934055

Gibbons RD, Brown CH, Hur K, et al: Suicidal thoughts and behavior with antidepressant treatment: reanalysis of the randomized placebo-controlled studies of fluoxetine and venlafaxine. Arch Gen Psychiatry 69(6):580–587, 2012 22309973

Koo MS, Kim EJ, Roh D, et al: Role of dopamine in the pathophysiology and treatment of obsessive-compulsive disorder. Expert Rev Neurother 10(2):275–290, 2010 20136383

Koran LM, Simpson HB: Guideline Watch (March 2013): Practice Guideline for the Treatment of Patients With Obsessive-Compulsive Disorder. Washington, DC, American Psychiatric Association, 2013. Available at: http://psychiatryonline.org/pb/assets/raw/sitewide/practice_guidelines/guidelines/ocd-watch.pdf. Accessed December 22, 2014.

Labad J, Menchón JM, Alonso P, et al: Female reproductive cycle and obsessive-compulsive disorder. J Clin Psychiatry 66(4):428–435, quiz 546, 2005 15816784

Leckman JF, Denys D, Simpson HB, et al: Obsessive-compulsive disorder: a review of the diagnostic criteria and possible subtypes and dimensional specifiers for DSM-V. Depress Anxiety 27(6):507–527, 2010 20217853

Lewis-Fernández R, Hinton DE, Laria AJ, et al: Culture and the anxiety disorders: recommendations for DSM-V. Depress Anxiety 27(2):212–229, 2010 20037918

Macy AS, Theo JN, Kaufmann SCV, et al: Quality of life in obsessive compulsive disorder. CNS Spectr 18(1):21–33, 2013 23279901

Masi G, Pfanner C, Brovedani P: Antipsychotic augmentation of selective serotonin reuptake inhibitors in resistant tic-related obsessive-compulsive disorder in children and adolescents: a naturalistic comparative study. J Psychiatr Res 47(8):1007–1012, 2013 23664673

Matsumoto R, Ichise M, Ito H, et al: Reduced serotonin transporter binding in the insular cortex in patients with obsessive-compulsive disorder: a [11C]DASB PET study. Neuroimage 49(1):121–126, 2010 19660554

Matsunaga H, Seedat S: Obsessive-compulsive spectrum disorders: cross-national and ethnic issues. CNS Spectr 12(5):392–400, 2007 17514083

Metin O, Yazici K, Tot S, et al: Amisulpride augmentation in treatment resistant obsessive-compulsive disorder: an open trial. Hum Psychopharmacol 18(6):463–467, 2003 12923825

Milad MR, Rauch SL: Obsessive-compulsive disorder: beyond segregated cortico-striatal pathways. Trends Cogn Sci 16(1):43–51, 2012 22138231

Milad MR, Furtak SC, Greenberg JL, et al: Deficits in conditioned fear extinction in obsessive-compulsive disorder and neurobiological changes in the fear circuit. JAMA Psychiatry 70(6):608–618, quiz 554, 2013 23740049

O'Kearney RT, Anstey KJ, von Sanden C: Behavioural and cognitive behavioural therapy for obsessive compulsive disorder in children and adolescents. Cochrane Database Syst Rev (4):CD004856, 2006 17054218

Pallanti S, Grassi G, Sarrecchia ED, et al: Obsessive-compulsive disorder comorbidity: clinical assessment and therapeutic implications. Front Psychiatry 2:70, 2011 22203806

Pauls DL: The genetics of obsessive-compulsive disorder: a review. Dialogues Clin Neurosci 12(2):149–163, 2010 20623920

Pediatric OCD Treatment Study Team: Cognitive-behavior therapy, sertraline, and their combination for children and adolescents with obsessive-compulsive disorder: the Pediatric OCD Treatment Study (POTS) randomized controlled trial. JAMA 292(16):1969–1976, 2004 15507582

Piacentini J, Bergman RL, Keller M, et al: Functional impairment in children and adolescents with obsessive-compulsive disorder. J Child Adolesc Psychopharmacol 13 (suppl 1):S61–S69, 2003 12880501

Pittenger C, Bloch MH, Williams K: Glutamate abnormalities in obsessive compulsive disorder: neurobiology, pathophysiology, and treatment. Pharmacol Ther 132(3):314–332, 2011 21963369

Rodriguez CI, Kegeles LS, Levinson A, et al: Randomized controlled crossover trial of ketamine in obsessive-compulsive disorder: proof-of-concept. Neuropsychopharmacology 38(12):2475–2483, 2013 23783065

Ruscio AM, Stein DJ, Chiu WT, et al: The epidemiology of obsessive-compulsive disorder in the National Comorbidity Survey Replication. Mol Psychiatry 15(1):53–63, 2010 18725912

Russell EJ, Fawcett JM, Mazmanian D: Risk of obsessive-compulsive disorder in pregnant and postpartum women: a meta-analysis. J Clin Psychiatry 74(4):377–385, 2013 23656845

Sayyah M, Sayyah M, Boostani H, et al: Effects of aripiprazole augmentation in treatment-resistant obsessive-compulsive disorder (a double blind clinical trial). Depress Anxiety 29(10):850–854, 2012 22933237

Simpson HB, Lombardo I, Slifstein M, et al: Serotonin transporters in obsessive-compulsive disorder: a positron emission tomography study with [(11)C]McN 5652. Biol Psychiatry 54(12):1414–1421, 2003 14675806

Simpson HB, Huppert JD, Petkova E, et al: Response versus remission in obsessive-compulsive disorder. J Clin Psychiatry 67(2):269–276, 2006 16566623

Simpson HB, Foa EB, Liebowitz MR, et al: A randomized, controlled trial of cognitive-behavioral therapy for augmenting pharmacotherapy in obsessive-compulsive disorder. Am J Psychiatry 165(5):621–630, 2008 18316422

Simpson HB, Slifstein M, Bender J Jr, et al: Serotonin 2A receptors in obsessive-compulsive disorder: a positron emission tomography study with [11C]MDL 100907. Biol Psychiatry 70(9):897–904, 2011 21855857

Simpson HB, Shungu DC, Bender J Jr, et al: Investigation of cortical glutamate-glutamine and γ-aminobutyric acid in obsessive-compulsive disorder by proton magnetic resonance spectroscopy. Neuropsychopharmacology 37(12): 2684–2692, 2012 22850733

Simpson HB, Foa EB, Liebowitz MR, et al: Cognitive-behavioral therapy vs risperidone for augmenting serotonin reuptake inhibitors in obsessive-compulsive disorder: a randomized clinical trial. JAMA Psychiatry 70(11):1190–1199, 2013 24026523

Skoog G, Skoog I: A 40-year follow-up of patients with obsessive-compulsive disorder [see comments]. Arch Gen Psychiatry 56(2):121–127, 1999 10025435

Storch EA, Goddard AW, Grant JE, et al: Double-blind, placebo-controlled, pilot trial of paliperidone augmentation in serotonin reuptake inhibitor-resistant obsessive-compulsive disorder. J Clin Psychiatry 74(6):e527–e532, 2013 23842022

Torres AR, Ramos-Cerqueira AT, Ferrão YA, et al: Suicidality in obsessive-compulsive disorder: prevalence and relation to symptom dimensions and comorbid conditions. J Clin Psychiatry 72(1):17–26, quiz 119–120, 2011 21272513

U.S. Food and Drug Administration: FDA Drug Safety Communication: Revised recommendations for Celexa (citalopram hydrobromide) related to a potential risk of abnormal heart rhythms with high doses, 2012. Available at: http://www.fda.gov/drugs/drugsafety/ucm297391.htm. Accessed December 22, 2014.

Van Ameringen M, Simpson W, Patterson B, et al: Pharmacological treatment strategies in obsessive compulsive disorder: a cross-sectional view in nine international OCD centers. J Psychopharmacol 28(6):596–602, 2014 24429223

Watson HJ, Rees CS: Meta-analysis of randomized, controlled treatment trials for pediatric obsessive-compulsive disorder. J Child Psychol Psychiatry 49(5):489–498, 2008 18400058

World Health Organization: The Global Burden of Disease: 2004 Update. Geneva, Switzerland, World Health Organization, 2008

Wu K, Hanna GL, Rosenberg DR, et al: The role of glutamate signaling in the pathogenesis and treatment of obsessive-compulsive disorder. Pharmacol Biochem Behav 100(4):726–735, 2012 22024159

Recommended Readings

Abramowitz JS: Getting Over OCD: A 10-Step Workbook for Taking Back Your Life. New York, Guilford, 2009

American Academy of Child and Adolescent Psychiatry: Facts for Families: Obsessive-Compulsive Disorder in Children and Adolescents. No. 60, Updated July 2013.

Available at: http://www.aacap.org/AACAP/Families_and_Youth/Facts_for_
Families/Facts_for_Families_Pages/Obsessive_Compulsive_Disorder_In_Children_
And_Adolescents_60.aspx. Accessed December 22, 2014.

Anxiety and Depression Association of America: http://www.adaa.org/

Foa EB, Yadin E, Lichner TK: Exposure and Response (Ritual) Prevention for Obsessive-Compulsive Disorder, Therapist Guide, 2nd Edition. New York, Oxford
University Press, 2012

International OCD Foundation: http://iocdf.org

Koran LM, Simpson HB: Guideline Watch (March 2013): Practice Guideline for the
Treatment of Patients With Obsessive-Compulsive Disorder. Washington, DC,
American Psychiatric Association, 2013. Available at: http://psychiatryon-
line.org/pb/assets/raw/sitewide/practice_guidelines/guidelines/ocd-watch.pdf.
Accessed December 22, 2014.

Koran LM, Hanna GL, Hollander E, et al: Practice guideline for the treatment of patients with obsessive-compulsive disorder. Am J Psychiatry 164(7 suppl):5–53,
2007

Leckman JF, Denys D, Simpson HB, et al: Obsessive-compulsive disorder: a review of
the diagnostic criteria and possible subtypes and dimensional specifiers for
DSM-V. Depress Anxiety 27(6):507–527, 2010

Yadin E, Foa EB, Lichner TK: Treating Your OCD With Exposure and Response
(Ritual) Prevention: Workbook (Treatments That Work). New York, Oxford University Press, 2012

CHAPTER 3

Body Dysmorphic Disorder

Katharine A. Phillips, M.D.

Body dysmorphic disorder (BDD) is a common yet very underrecognized disorder. Because patients are typically ashamed of and embarrassed by their symptoms, they usually do not reveal them to clinicians unless specifically asked. It is important to screen patients for BDD and to identify this disorder when present, because it usually causes tremendous suffering and substantial impairment in psychosocial functioning. In addition, rates of suicidal ideation, suicide attempts, and completed suicide appear markedly high.

BDD has many similarities to obsessive-compulsive disorder (OCD), as noted by Pierre Janet more than a century ago (Phillips 1991). Since then, numerous studies that have directly compared BDD to OCD have elucidated their many similarities, and BDD is widely considered one of the disorders that is most closely related to OCD. Thus, BDD's inclusion in DSM-5's new chapter of obsessive-compulsive and related disorders (OCRDs) is well supported (American Psychiatric Association 2013). Nonetheless, BDD and OCD have some important differences; for example, BDD is characterized by poorer insight, more comorbid major depressive disorder and perhaps substance use disorders, and higher rates of suicidality, and it requires a different cognitive-behavioral therapy (CBT) approach. In addition, in a prospective longitudinal study, BDD symptoms persisted in a sizable proportion of participants whose comorbid OCD remitted, suggesting BDD is not simply a symptom of OCD. Thus, it is important to recognize BDD's and OCD's similarities while also differentiating them in clinical settings.

BDD has received far less investigation than OCD; systematic research has been conducted only during the past few decades. Yet recently, research on BDD has dramatically increased. It is worth noting that as the research literature on BDD increases, constructs that are not the same as BDD but may overlap with it are sometimes equated with BDD. These include "dysmorphic concern" and "BDD symptoms"; the latter appears to often reflect subclinical BDD or body image dissatisfaction. Studies that use these constructs are generally not included in this chapter. Regarding research on BDD (this chapter's focus), the substantial increase in this area of investigation has yielded many new and important findings—on course of illness, neuroimaging, visual processing abnormalities, information processing abnormalities, and other areas. Importantly, recent advances in the development and testing of effective CBT approaches, along with the availability of effective medication options, offer great hope to patients with this often-debilitating disorder.

Diagnostic Criteria and Symptomatology

Before it was included in the classification system for the first time as a separate disorder, in DSM-III-R in 1987 (American Psychiatric Association 1987), BDD was known as "dysmorphophobia." This term, coined in the 1800s by the Italian psychiatrist Enrico Morselli, comes from the Greek word *dysmorphia*, which refers to "misshapenness" or "ugliness" (Phillips 1991). Individuals with BDD are preoccupied with one or more perceived defects or flaws in their appearance that are not observable or appear only slight to others (see Criterion A in Box 3–1; American Psychiatric Association 2013). In other words, patients incorrectly perceive themselves as looking ugly, deformed, unattractive, or even grotesque or monstrous when they actually look normal. Examples of these preoccupations are "I look hideous," "I look ugly, and everyone is staring at me," or "My face is horribly red and looks disgusting." Often, the physical "defects" that the patient perceives are not visible to others. If appearance defects or flaws *are* present, they are only slight. In this case, others do not notice the "defects" unless the patient points them out, and even then they are minimal and within the normal range. For DSM-5, only minor wording changes were made to Criterion A. For example, the word *imagined,* which DSM-IV (American Psychiatric Association 1994) used to describe the physical defects, is no longer used because it was confusing for some patients, especially those with poor or absent insight. Preoccupation with appearance defects that are clearly noticeable and observable by others (e.g., at conversational distance) is diagnosed as "other specified OCRD," not as BDD (see Chapter 7, "Other Obsessive-Compulsive and Related Disorders in DSM-5").

BOX 3–1. DSM-5 Diagnostic Criteria for Body Dysmorphic Disorder

A. Preoccupation with one or more perceived defects or flaws in physical appearance that are not observable or appear slight to others.

B. At some point during the course of the disorder, the individual has performed repetitive behaviors (e.g., mirror checking, excessive grooming, skin picking, reassurance seeking) or mental acts (e.g., comparing his or her appearance with that of others) in response to the appearance concerns.

C. The preoccupation causes clinically significant distress or impairment in social, occupational, or other important areas of functioning.

D. The appearance preoccupation is not better explained by concerns with body fat or weight in an individual whose symptoms meet diagnostic criteria for an eating disorder.

Specify if:

With muscle dysmorphia: The individual is preoccupied with the idea that his or her body build is too small or insufficiently muscular. This specifier is used even if the individual is preoccupied with other body areas, which is often the case.

Specify if:

Indicate degree of insight regarding body dysmorphic disorder beliefs (e.g., "I look ugly" or "I look deformed").

With good or fair insight: The individual recognizes that the body dysmorphic disorder beliefs are definitely or probably not true or that they may or may not be true.

With poor insight: The individual thinks that the body dysmorphic disorder beliefs are probably true.

With absent insight/delusional beliefs: The individual is completely convinced that the body dysmorphic disorder beliefs are true.

Reprinted from American Psychiatric Association: *Diagnostic and Statistical Manual of Mental Disorders*, 5th Edition. Arlington, VA, American Psychiatric Association. Copyright 2013, American Psychiatric Association. Used with permission.

Most commonly, disliked areas involve the face and head; more specifically, they most often focus on the skin (e.g., perceived acne, scarring, color, wrinkles), nose (e.g., too large or misshapen), and hair (e.g., too little head hair or too much facial or body hair) (Phillips and Diaz 1997; Phillips et al. 2005b). However, any body part can be the focus of preoccupation (e.g., eyes, teeth, jaw, ears, head size or shape, breasts, thighs, stomach, hands, body build). A common misconception is that BDD can be diagnosed only if the patient is preoccupied with just one body area, such as a large and mis-shapen nose. However, areas of preoccupation may range from just one area to virtually every aspect of the person's appearance; on average, patients are preoccupied with five to seven body areas over the course of their illness (Phillips et al. 2005b). More than 25% of patients with BDD have at least one concern that involves symmetry (e.g., asymmetrical eyebrows or uneven hair) (Hart and Phillips 2013). Symmetry concerns that involve physical appearance should be diagnosed as BDD, not as OCD.

The appearance preoccupations are intrusive and time consuming. To be diagnosed as BDD, these preoccupations should occur for about 1 hour a day or more (as for OCD obsessions). On average, patients are preoccupied with their perceived appearance defects for 3–8 hours a day, and some are preoccupied for the entire day. The appearance preoccupations are unwanted and not pleasurable; they usually cause substantial, and sometimes extreme, distress. BDD preoccupations are also usually difficult to resist and control (Phillips 2009).

The appearance preoccupations usually trigger intense dysphoria, distress, anxiety, depressed mood, shame, and other painful emotions (Phillips 2009; Phillips et al. 2010b). These distressing emotions in turn drive patients to perform repetitive compulsive behaviors that typically focus on checking, fixing, or hiding the perceived flaws and are intended to alleviate emotional distress. These behaviors are not pleasurable, and they often do not decrease—and may even increase—distress (Phillips 2009). All individuals with BDD, at some time during the course of the disorder, perform such repetitive behaviors in response to the appearance concerns, as reflected in a new criterion (Criterion B) in DSM-5 (see Box 3–1; Phillips et al. 2010b). These behaviors have many similarities to OCD compulsions, and thus they are often referred to as *compulsions* or *rituals*; a possible difference, however, is that BDD compulsions may be less likely to reduce anxiety and distress.

Criterion B was added to DSM-5 to provide a fuller description of BDD's key clinical features; these behaviors (e.g., comparing and mirror checking) are usually a prominent and problematic aspect of the clinical presentation. The addition of Criterion B also helps clinicians differentiate BDD from major depressive disorder, social anxiety disorder, and other disorders with which it may be confused. Furthermore, when a patient with BDD is being treated with CBT, these behaviors need to be targeted with ritual prevention. The very small number of individuals who meet all diagnostic criteria for BDD *except* Criterion B should be diagnosed with "other specified OCRD" rather than BDD.

Common repetitive behaviors, which must be excessive, and lifetime rates of these behaviors are as follows (Phillips and Diaz 1997; Phillips et al. 2005b):

- Comparing disliked body parts with the same areas on others: 88%
- Checking disliked body parts in mirrors or other reflecting surfaces: 87%
- Grooming (e.g., applying makeup; cutting, styling, shaving, or removing head hair, facial hair, or body hair): 59%
- Seeking reassurance about the perceived defects or questioning others about how they look (e.g., "Do I look okay?"): 54%
- Touching the disliked areas to check their appearance: 52%
- Changing clothes (e.g., to more effectively camouflage disliked areas or to find a flattering outfit that distracts others from the "defects"): 46%
- Dieting (e.g., to make a "wide" face narrower): 39%
- Skin picking to improve perceived skin flaws: 38%
- Tanning (e.g., to darken "pale" skin): 25%
- Exercising: 21%
- Lifting weights: 18%

Additional repetitive behaviors include compulsive hair plucking/pulling (e.g., to make "crooked" eyebrows more symmetrical) and excessive shopping (e.g., for makeup, skin or hair products, or clothes to minimize the perceived flaws). Although most behaviors are observable by others, some repetitive acts—such as comparing oneself with others—may be mental, as noted by Criterion B. Camouflaging one's perceived flaws (e.g., with a hat, makeup, sunglasses, hair, clothes, body position), which more than 90% of patients with BDD do, has some features of a safety-seeking behavior (the goal of which is to avoid or escape unpleasant feelings or to prevent a feared event, such as being ridiculed by others); however, camouflaging can also be done repeatedly (e.g., reapplying makeup 30 times a day) and thus may fulfill Criterion B (Phillips 2009). The repetitive behaviors that patients may engage in are unlimited. For example, they may tie their calves tightly with rope to try to make them smaller, develop complex counting rituals to track loss of individual hairs, or make and repeatedly watch videos to track the perceived worsening of hair loss, acne, or wrinkles.

Some of these repetitive behaviors can be risky and harm patients. For example, skin picking can occur for hours a day and involve use of sharp implements such as pins, needles, or razor blades; thus it can cause considerable skin damage, which may require sutures or surgery. Picking through and damaging major blood vessels, such as the carotid artery, can be life threatening (Phillips 2009). Compulsive mirror checking can cause car accidents (e.g., if the rearview mirror is checked while driving) or dangerous falls (e.g., if a reflecting mirror is checked while on a ladder). Tanning may increase the risk of skin cancer. Most patients with BDD seek cosmetic procedures for BDD concerns, some repeatedly, which involve anesthesia risks. In addition, some dissatisfied patients sue or physically attack or even murder the treating physician (Sarwer and Crerand 2008).

It should be noted that skin picking as a symptom of BDD occurs in response to a preoccupation with perceived skin defects; the picking intends to fix or improve a perceived skin flaw. In contrast, picking that occurs in excoriation (skin-picking) disorder is not triggered by thoughts about appearance. Similarly, hair plucking/pulling as a symptom of BDD is triggered by preoccupation with perceived defects in the hair's appearance (e.g., asymmetry), which the pulling/plucking attempts to improve. In contrast, hair pulling that occurs in trichotillomania (hair-pulling disorder) is not triggered by appearance preoccupations.

For DSM-5 criteria for BDD to be met, the appearance preoccupations and resulting repetitive behaviors must cause clinically significant distress or impairment in social, occupational, or other important areas of functioning (Criterion C). In addition, if the patient's only appearance concerns involve excessive body fat or weight, and these concerns meet diagnostic criteria for an eating disorder, they should be diagnosed as an eating disorder rather than BDD (Criterion D). However, eating disorders and BDD (involving preoccupations with other body areas) often co-occur (Phillips et al. 2005b).

DSM-5 has two new specifiers that should be considered after ascertaining that a patient's symptoms meet all diagnostic criteria for BDD.

1. *With muscle dysmorphia:* This specifier identifies individuals, most of whom are men, who are preoccupied with the idea that their body build is too small or not muscular enough. These patients may describe themselves as looking "puny," "tiny," or "too small." Most actually look normal, although some are unusually muscular as a result of excessive weight lifting or use of potentially dangerous anabolic steroids, which can increase muscle mass. Some, but not all, patients with muscle dysmorphia have abnormal eating behavior (e.g., eating large amounts of food or high-protein meals). In samples of men ascertained for BDD, most of those with muscle dysmorphia also have other more typical BDD concerns (e.g., involving skin or facial features). Compared with other forms of BDD, muscle dysmorphia appears to be associated with higher rates of suicidality, substance-related disorders, and anabolic steroid use as well as poorer quality of life (Phillips 2009; Phillips et al. 2010b).

2. *Insight:* An insight specifier has been added to BDD, OCD, and hoarding disorder in DSM-5. The specifier for BDD indicates insight regarding BDD beliefs (e.g., "I look ugly"). Levels of insight are as follows:

   • *"With good or fair insight":* Patients recognize that their beliefs about their appearance are definitely or probably not true or that they may or may not be true.

- • *"With poor insight"*: Patients think their BDD beliefs probably are true.
- • *"With absent insight/delusional beliefs"*: Patients are completely convinced that their BDD beliefs are true.

Insight regarding the perceived appearance defects (e.g., "I look ugly") is usually absent or poor; most individuals are completely or mostly convinced that their view of their perceived deformities is accurate (Eisen et al. 2004; Phillips et al. 2012). This is one important way in which BDD differs from OCD. In OCD, only about 2%–4% of patients have delusional OCD beliefs; about 85% have excellent, good, or fair insight into the beliefs that underlie their obsessions (e.g., whether the house really will burn down if they do not check the stove 30 times). In contrast, about one-third of patients have delusional BDD beliefs, and only about one-quarter have excellent, good, or fair insight (Phillips et al. 2012). The poorer insight that is typically characteristic of BDD may largely explain why those with BDD tend to be more reluctant to accept and engage in mental health treatment than those with OCD. Research evidence indicates that delusional and nondelusional BDD (i.e., BDD characterized by good, fair, or poor insight) are the same disorder, with insight spanning a spectrum from good to absent, as reflected in the new specifier (Phillips et al. 2014). Individuals with the delusional form of BDD tend to have greater morbidity than those with some insight, but this difference appears accounted for by their tendency to have more severe BDD symptoms (Phillips et al. 2014).

DSM-5's new insight specifier is important for several reasons (Phillips et al. 2014):

1. It clarifies that individuals who are completely convinced that their BDD belief is true should be diagnosed with "BDD with absent insight/delusional beliefs" rather than a psychotic disorder, as was done in DSM-IV.
2. It implies that delusional and nondelusional BDD should be treated similarly; indeed, both delusional and nondelusional BDD respond to serotonin reuptake inhibitor (SRI) monotherapy and to CBT.
3. Specifying level of insight allows clinicians to identify patients with poor or absent insight who may be more reluctant to accept the idea that they have a mental disorder (BDD) rather than actual physical deformities; such patients may require more motivational interviewing and attention to the therapeutic alliance in order to engage and retain them in mental health treatment.

Nearly 30% of patients with BDD experience panic attacks that are triggered by BDD symptoms (e.g., when looking at perceived defects in the mirror or feeling that others are scrutinizing them, or when under bright lights). Such panic attacks are not diagnosed as panic disorder because they do not "come out of the blue." The DSM-5-wide panic attack specifier may be used in such cases.

A majority of patients with BDD have ideas or delusions of reference, falsely believing that others take special notice of them in a negative way because of how they look (e.g., mock, talk about, or stare at them) (Phillips et al. 2005b, 2012). Referential thinking, which is more common in BDD than in OCD, may contribute to social avoidance. BDD is associated with high levels of social anxiety and avoidance, anxiety, depressed mood, neuroticism, and rejection sensitivity as well as low self-esteem (Phillips 2009). Many patients are ashamed of how they look and the fact that they worry so much about their appearance; they may conceal their concerns because they do not want to be considered vain. It is also worth mentioning BDD by proxy, a form of BDD in which an individual is preoccupied with perceived flaws in another person's appearance (e.g., a spouse or child) and meets diagnostic criteria for BDD.

Case Example: Scott

Scott, a 21-year-old single white male, had been obsessed since age 13 with perceived acne, a "big" head, and his "small" body build. When he presented for treatment, his chief complaint was "I keep thinking about how ugly I look, and it's ruining my life." Although other people told him that he was handsome and did not have the defects he perceived, Scott was convinced that he looked "ugly and disgusting," stating, "I know what I see when I look in the mirror." He thought about his perceived defects for 6–8 hours a day, which caused severe distress. He believed that when people looked at him they thought he looked repulsive and that others singled him out of the crowd because he looked so strange. Scott spent 5–6 hours a day performing repetitive behaviors, such as comparing his skin, head size, and body build with those of other people and with celebrities online, checking mirrors, asking his parents if he looked okay (while never accepting their reassurance), repeatedly washing and scrubbing his face, and picking his skin to remove tiny blemishes. Scott also lifted weights for several hours a day and took five types of supplements to increase his muscle mass. He spent several hours a day obtaining information about supplements and anabolic steroids online.

As a result of his appearance concerns, Scott became depressed, anxious, and socially withdrawn. He stopped dating because he thought he was so ugly that no one would want to be with him. He missed many classes because his symptoms made it difficult to focus on schoolwork, he did not want others to see him, and he believed his classmates ridiculed him because of how he looked. For these reasons, he dropped out of high school during his senior year. He subsequently spent most of his time alone in his bedroom, despite his family's efforts to persuade him to attend school, participate in family events, and see his friends. He had considered suicide many times and had attempted suicide once because he thought that life wasn't worth living if he looked like a "freak."

Epidemiology

The point (current) prevalence of DSM-IV BDD in nationwide epidemiological studies of adults is 2.4% in the United States and 1.7%–1.8% in Germany (Buhlmann et al. 2010; Koran et al. 2008; Rief et al. 2006). Thus, although BDD used to be considered rare, it appears to be about twice as common as anorexia nervosa, schizophrenia, and OCD. In epidemiological samples, those with BDD are less likely to be living with a partner or employed and more likely to report suicidal ideation and suicide attempts due to appearance concerns (Rief et al. 2006). Although epidemiological data are not available in youths, a study of 566 U.S. high school students found a current prevalence of DSM-IV BDD of 2.2% (Mayville et al. 1999).

Two U.S. studies found a prevalence of 13% and 16% among general adult psychiatric inpatients (Conroy et al. 2008; Grant et al. 2001). In one study, BDD was more common than many other disorders, including schizophrenia, OCD, posttraumatic stress disorder, and eating disorders; patients with BDD had significantly lower scores on the Global Assessment of Functioning Scale and twice the lifetime rate of suicide attempts as patients without BDD (Grant et al. 2001). In the other inpatient study, a high proportion of patients reported that their BDD symptoms were a major reason or "somewhat of a reason" for their suicidal thinking (50% of subjects), suicide attempts (33%), or substance use (42%) (Conroy et al. 2008). In studies of adolescent psychiatric inpatients, 6.7%–14.3% of subjects had current BDD (Dyl et al. 2006; Grant et al. 2001). BDD also appears fairly common among adults in dermatology settings (9%–15%), cosmetic surgery settings (7%–15% in most studies), and orthodontia settings (8%) and among patients presenting for oral or maxillofacial surgery (10%) (Phillips 2009).

In epidemiological samples, BDD is slightly more common in females than in males (Buhlmann et al. 2010; Koran et al. 2008; Rief et al. 2006). In clinical samples of individuals ascertained for BDD, the gender ratio has differed somewhat, possibly reflecting different ascertainment methods. The largest samples contained an equal proportion of males and females or a slight preponderance of females (Phillips and Diaz 1997; Phillips et al. 2005b).

Comorbidity

Major depressive disorder is the most common comorbid disorder, with a lifetime rate of about 75% (Phillips and Diaz 1997; Phillips et al. 2005b). BDD usually has its onset before major depressive disorder, and many patients attribute their depressive symptoms to the distress caused by BDD symptoms (Phillips 2009). Other commonly co-occurring disorders are social anxiety disorder (social phobia), which affects nearly 40% of patients (lifetime), and

OCD, which affects about one-third of patients with BDD (lifetime) (Phillips and Diaz 1997; Phillips et al. 2005b).

Lifetime substance use disorders are also common, occurring in about 30%–50% of those with BDD (Grant et al. 2005; Phillips and Diaz 1997). Alcohol and marijuana use are most common. In one study, nearly 70% of individuals with a comorbid substance use disorder attributed their substance use, at least in part, to the distress caused by BDD symptoms; 30% cited BDD as the main reason or a major reason for their substance use disorder (Grant et al. 2005). Many patients appear to use substances to self-medicate in an effort to diminish social anxiety or emotional pain caused by BDD symptoms.

About 20% of men with muscle dysmorphia abuse potentially dangerous anabolic steroids in an attempt to become more muscular (Phillips et al. 2010b). These drugs may cause abuse or dependence, and they carry a risk of adverse physical and psychiatric effects, which include depressive symptoms when discontinuing use as well as aggressive behavior ("roid rage").

Course and Prognosis

BDD usually has its onset in early adolescence. The most common age at onset is 12 or 13 years, and two-thirds of individuals have onset of BDD before age 18 (Bjornsson et al. 2013). The mean age at BDD onset is 16 or 17 (Bjornsson et al. 2013). Subclinical BDD symptoms (mean onset at age 12– 13 years) often precede onset of the full disorder (Phillips et al. 2006a). Earlier age at BDD onset may be associated with greater morbidity (see "Developmental Considerations" later in this chapter). In one study, subjects with onset before age 18 were more likely to have been psychiatrically hospitalized (Bjornsson et al. 2010). In two studies, those with BDD onset before age 18 had more comorbidity and were more likely to have attempted suicide (Bjornsson et al. 2013).

The only prospective naturalistic study of the course of BDD found that BDD tended to be chronic (Phillips et al. 2013a). In this 4-year follow-up study of a broadly ascertained sample of individuals with BDD, the cumulative probability was only 0.20 for full remission and 0.55 for full *or* partial remission from BDD (remission required as little as 8 consecutive weeks of minimal or no BDD symptoms for full remission and less than DSM-IV criteria for partial remission). A lower likelihood of full or partial remission was predicted by more severe BDD symptoms at intake into the study, a longer lifetime duration of BDD, and being an adult. Among subjects whose BDD partially or fully remitted at some point during the follow-up period, the cumulative probability of subsequent full relapse was 0.42; for subsequent full *or* partial relapse, it was 0.63. More severe BDD at intake and earlier age at BDD onset predicted full or partial relapse. It should be noted that although most study subjects received treatment in the community, relatively few received what is considered adequate treatment; BDD usually improves when evidence-based treatments are implemented (see "Treatment" section later in this chapter).

Psychosocial Impairment and Suicidality

BDD is associated with markedly poor psychosocial functioning and mental health-related quality of life across a broad range of domains (Phillips et al. 2005c). On standardized measures, differences between individuals with BDD and norms are very large and typically several standard deviation units below normative scores (Phillips et al. 2005c). Scores on the Short Form Health Survey (SF-36; Ware 1993) mental health subscales are 0.4–0.7 standard deviation units poorer than for depression. Impairment in functioning can range from moderate to extreme. A patient with moderate functional impairment due to BDD may, for example, avoid dating and some but not all social events; she may be able to attend school but be late and miss some classes. A patient with extreme and incapacitating BDD may quit his job, avoid all social contact, and stay in his bedroom at all times. More severe BDD symptoms are associated with poorer functioning and quality of life (Phillips et al. 2005c). Males tend to have somewhat greater functional impairment than females (Phillips et al. 2005c).

Among individuals with BDD that is moderate in severity, nearly one-third have been completely housebound for at least 1 week because of BDD symptoms; some have been housebound for years because they feel too ugly to be seen. Nearly 40% have been psychiatrically hospitalized, and more than one-quarter attribute at least one psychiatric hospitalization primarily to BDD (Phillips and Diaz 1997; Phillips et al. 2005b).

Perhaps the most concerning aspect of BDD is the high rate of suicidality. From a clinical perspective, reasons for suicidality may include hopelessness about being "deformed"; feeling angry and hopeless because rituals do not improve the "defects"; feeling rejected by others because of being "ugly"; social isolation (which overlaps with the concept of "thwarted belongingness"); ideas/delusions of reference, which may increase social isolation; negative core beliefs (e.g., unlovability, worthlessness); a high prevalence of comorbid major depressive disorder; and a belief that a cosmetic procedure made the patient look even worse.

Rates of suicidal ideation and suicide attempts are high in both clinical and epidemiological samples and in adults as well as youth (Buhlmann et al. 2010; Phillips and Diaz 1997; Phillips et al. 2005a). In samples of convenience or in clinical samples of individuals ascertained for BDD, about 80% have experienced suicidal ideation, and 24%–28% have attempted suicide (Phillips and Diaz 1997; Phillips et al. 2005a; Veale et al. 1996a). In a study of psychiatric inpatients, the suicide attempt rate among those with BDD was double the rate among inpatients without BDD (Grant et al. 2001), and among inpatients with anorexia nervosa, those who had BDD in addition to anorexia had triple the number of suicide attempts compared with those without BDD (Grant et al. 2002). In a retrospective study in two dermatology practices over 20 years, most of the patients who committed suicide had had acne or BDD (Cotterill and Cunliffe 1997). Individuals with BDD appear more likely to experience suicidality than those with OCD (Phillips et al. 2007).

Suicidality rates also appear markedly elevated in epidemiological samples, where rates might be expected to be lower. In an epidemiological study from Germany, 31% of subjects with BDD reported thoughts about committing suicide specifically due to appearance concerns, and 22% had actually attempted suicide due to appearance concerns (Buhlmann et al. 2010).

Greater BDD severity independently predicts suicidal ideation and suicide attempts (Phillips et al. 2005a). In addition, suicidal ideation is associated with lifetime comorbid major depressive disorder, and suicide attempts are associated with lifetime comorbid substance use disorder and posttraumatic stress disorder (Phillips et al. 2005a).

There are only limited data on completed suicide, but the rate appears markedly elevated compared with the general population and perhaps even higher than in disorders with high suicide rates, such as bipolar disorder and major depressive disorder (Phillips and Menard 2006).

Developmental Considerations

A clinically important and underrecognized aspect of BDD is that it is a disorder of childhood and adolescence. As noted earlier, a majority of cases have their onset before age 18. Available data, although limited, suggest that many of BDD's clinical features appear largely similar in youths and adults (Albertini and Phillips 1999; Phillips et al. 2006a). However, youths may be even more severely ill than adults: they appear to have poorer insight regarding their appearance, and they are more likely than adults to have delusional BDD beliefs (59% vs. 33%; Phillips et al. 2006a). Their poorer insight may possibly reflect adolescents' poorer metacognitive skills, which may mediate poor insight in some psychiatric disorders. At a trend level, youths are more likely than adults to have more severe BDD and to have been psychiatrically hospitalized (43% vs. 24%). Of note, youths are significantly more likely than adults to have attempted suicide (44% vs. 24%) (Phillips et al. 2006a). A study in a psychiatric adolescent inpatient setting found that compared with youths with no significant body image concerns, those with BDD had significantly higher levels of anxiety and depression and significantly higher scores on a standardized measure of suicide risk (Dyl et al. 2006). These findings are consistent with data indicating that greater body image dissatisfaction more generally in adolescents is associated with higher suicide risk.

School refusal and dropout are particularly concerning consequences of BDD in youths. In one study, 18% of youths with BDD had dropped out of school primarily because of BDD symptoms (Albertini and Phillips 1999). In another study, 22% of youths had dropped out of school primarily because of psychopathology, and 29% more had not attended school for at least a week in the past month because of psychopathology (for most, BDD was the primary diagnosis) (Phillips et al. 2006a). Thus, youths who refuse to attend school should be carefully assessed for BDD.

BDD typically has profound and detrimental effects on family functioning. BDD in youths, especially when untreated, often adversely affects the development trajectory, impeding completion of developmental transitions and tasks, such as completing school, dating, and developing social competence. Not uncommonly, these deficits persist well into adulthood and may even be lifelong.

Case Example: Maria

Maria, a 16-year-old Hispanic high school student, presented with a chief complaint of "I look really ugly, and everyone at school is laughing at me because I look so bad." Maria thought that she had "horrible" acne and facial scarring and that her hair looked "ridiculous and hideous." She also believed that her stomach "stuck out too much." Maria thought about her appearance for 3–4 hours a day, and she spent about 3 hours a day styling her hair to make it look "presentable," checking mirrors, asking her parents if she looked okay, shopping for makeup and hair products, and sucking in her stomach to make it look flatter. When possible, she covered her stomach with her hand and turned "the really bad" side of her face away from people when talking with them. Maria was "pretty certain" that she really did look ugly.

As a result of these concerns, Maria sometimes avoided being with her friends, and she turned down social opportunities. She was often late for school because she got "stuck" in the mirror styling her hair and coating her skin with makeup to cover her perceived scars. She often left class to check her appearance and groom in the bathroom mirror. She avoided dating and talking with boys because this made her feel especially self-conscious about how she looked.

Gender–Related Issues

BDD appears to have largely similar features in females and males, including similar demographic characteristics, disliked body areas, types of compulsive BDD behaviors, BDD severity, suicidality, and comorbidity. Both genders appear equally likely to seek and receive cosmetic treatment for their BDD concerns (Phillips and Diaz 1997; Phillips et al. 2006b).

Some gender differences are apparent; however, many may reflect cultural preferences and concerns regarding appearance in men and women (Phillips and Diaz 1997; Phillips et al. 2006b). Men are more likely to be preoccupied with supposedly thinning hair, genitals (usually focusing on "small" penis size), and small body build (muscle dysmorphia), which affects men nearly exclusively. In contrast, women appear more likely to be preoccupied with weight (usually thinking that they weigh too much), breasts, hips, legs, and excessive body hair. Women are more likely than men to camouflage their bodies to hide disliked areas, check mirrors, and pick their skin. They are also more likely to have a comorbid eating disorder, and men are more likely to have a comorbid substance use disorder, consistent with gender-related findings in the general population. Men may be more likely to be single, and they may experience somewhat greater impairment in psychosocial functioning (e.g., unemployed and receiving disability payments).

Cultural Aspects of Phenomenology

Although most studies of BDD have focused on patients in Western settings, an increasing number have been done around the world. No studies have directly compared BDD's clinical features across different countries or cultures, but a qualitative descriptive comparison of case reports and case series from around the world suggested more similarities than differences in terms of demographic and clinical features (Phillips 2005). Thus, BDD may be largely invariant across cultures.

However, this comparison also suggested that cultural values and preferences may influence and shape BDD symptoms to some degree. For example, concerns about eyelids and having a small, rather than a large, nose may be more common in Asian countries than in Western countries. Indeed, culturally related concerns about physical appearance and the importance of physical appearance might influence or amplify preoccupations with perceived physical deformities. Nonetheless, there is a growing literature on the universality of certain concepts of beauty, and the extent to which cultural factors impact BDD's pathogenesis or clinical expression remains unclear.

Taijin kyofusho, or *anthropophobia* (fear of people), literally meaning a fear of interpersonal relations, is a construct in the Japanese diagnostic system that includes a BDD-like variant known as *shubo-kyofu* ("phobia of a deformed body"). However, *shubo-kyofu* appears more prominently focused on a fear that one's ugliness will offend other people.

Assessment and Differential Diagnosis

Assessment

Screening for and Diagnosing Body Dysmorphic Disorder

In clinical settings, BDD usually goes undiagnosed (Conroy et al. 2008; Grant et al. 2001; Phillips 2009). Patients usually do not spontaneously reveal their appearance concerns to a mental health clinician or family members because they are too embarrassed, fear they will be negatively judged (e.g., considered vain), worry that their concerns will not be understood, or do not know that their symptoms are treatable by a mental health clinician (Conroy et al. 2008). However, most patients want clinicians to ask about them (Conroy et al. 2008). Thus, to detect BDD, clinicians should ask patients about BDD symptoms, especially patients with another OCRD, major depressive disorder, or social anxiety disorder. Questions are provided in Table 3–1.

It is important to consider the following when screening patients for and diagnosing BDD:

- Express empathy and do not trivialize the patient's concerns. Keep in mind that patients usually suffer tremendously because of their symptoms; it is best not to minimize their concerns or express surprise or skepticism about their symptoms.
- Do not use the word "imagined": DSM-IV used this term, but it has been removed in DSM-5 because many patients consider their flaws to be real, not imagined.
- Avoid using words such as "defect" or "deformity" when initially asking about BDD symptoms. Although terms such as these are very fitting for some patients' concerns, they may be too harsh for others to initially endorse. Terms such as "appearance concerns" may be more acceptable to patients.
- Do not simply ask patients if they think there is something wrong with their bodies; this question may be interpreted to refer to bodily functioning, and it may miss BDD.
- Do not require that the patient have sought medical advice about the perceived defects; some patients do not do this because they are too embarrassed to reveal their concerns to anyone. Also, not all individuals have access to health care.
- Do not argue with patients about how they actually look. Because patients typically have poor or absent insight, this approach is usually unsuccessful, and providing reassurance about their appearance may actually reinforce the ritual of reassurance seeking.

TABLE 3–1.   Questions to diagnose body dysmorphic disorder

Criterion A: Preoccupation

Ask "Are you very worried about your appearance in any way?" or "Are you unhappy with how you look?"

If yes, invite the patient to describe his or her concern by asking, "What don't you like about how you look?" or "Can you tell me about your concern?"

Ask if there are other disliked body areas—for example, "Are you unhappy with any other aspects of your appearance, such as your face, skin, hair, nose, or the shape or size of any other body area?"

Ascertain that the patient is preoccupied with these perceived flaws by asking, "How much time would you estimate that you spend each day thinking about your appearance, if you add up all the time you spend?" or "Do these concerns preoccupy you?"

Criterion B: Repetitive behaviors

Ask "Is there anything you feel an urge to do over and over again in response to your appearance concerns?" Give examples of repetitive behaviors.

Criterion C: Clinically significant distress or impairment in functioning

Ask "How much distress do these concerns cause you?" Ask specifically about resulting anxiety, social anxiety, depression, feelings of panic, and suicidal thinking.

Ask about effects of the appearance preoccupations on the patient's life—for example, "Do these concerns interfere with your life or cause problems for you in any way?" Ask specifically about effects on work, school, other aspects of role functioning (e.g., caring for children), relationships, intimacy, family and social activities, household tasks, and other types of interference.

Criterion D: Concerns not better explained by an eating disorder

Ask diagnostic questions for anorexia nervosa, bulimia nervosa, and binge-eating disorder.

Muscle dysmorphia specifier

Ask "Are you preoccupied with the idea that your body build is too small or that you're not muscular enough?"

Insight specifier

Elicit a global belief about the perceived defect(s): "What word would you use to describe how bad your [fill in disliked areas] look?" *Optional:* "Some people use words like 'unattractive,' 'ugly,' 'deformed,' 'hideous.' The global belief must be inaccurate. Do not use beliefs that are true, such as "I don't look perfect" or "I want to be prettier."

Ask "How convinced are you that these body areas look [fill in patient's global descriptor]?"

Screening, Diagnostic, Severity, and Insight Measures

Scales that can be used for clinical or research purposes are provided in Table 3–2 and are freely available at www.bodyimageprogram.com (Eisen et al. 1998; Phillips 2005; Phillips et al. 1997).

Differential Diagnosis

Other Psychiatric Disorders

Table 3–3 summarizes key mental disorders to consider in the differential diagnosis and approaches to accurately diagnosing BDD. Regarding the OCRDs, as previously discussed, BDD has both similarities to and differences from OCD. If preoccupations/obsessions focus on appearance concerns, including symmetry concerns, BDD should be diagnosed rather than OCD. If skin picking or hair plucking/pulling is done in response to appearance concerns and is intended to improve perceived appearance flaws, BDD should be diagnosed rather than excoriation (skin-picking) disorder or trichotillomania (hair-pulling disorder).

Perhaps the most difficult differential diagnosis is between certain presentations of BDD and an eating disorder. Studies that have directly compared BDD to eating disorders indicate that those with BDD are concerned with more body areas (typically not weight) and have more negative self-evaluation and self-worth, more avoidance of activities, and poorer functioning and quality of life due to appearance concerns (Hrabosky et al. 2009; Rosen and Ramirez 1998).

Although it is easy to differentiate an eating disorder from BDD when BDD concerns focus on non–weight and non–body shape concerns (e.g., hair or nose), the differential diagnosis is more difficult when BDD concerns do focus on weight or body shape. As indicated by BDD Criterion D, if appearance concerns focus on being too fat or thoughts that parts of the body (e.g., stomach, arms, and thighs) are too fat, and these concerns qualify for a diagnosis of anorexia nervosa, bulimia nervosa, or binge-eating disorder, then BDD is not diagnosed. However, when eating disorder symptoms are present but do not meet full diagnostic criteria for one of these disorders, it may be difficult to determine whether such a presentation should be diagnosed as "other specified eating disorder" or as BDD. In such cases, careful patient questioning and clinical judgment are needed to make the correct diagnosis. From a treatment perspective, it is important to address abnormal eating behavior that may jeopardize one's physical health; psychosocial treatments for BDD do not address such behaviors.

TABLE 3–2. Screening, diagnostic, severity, and insight measures for body dysmorphic disorder (BDD)

Body Dysmorphic Disorder Questionnaire (BDDQ; Phillips 2005)

Screens for the presence of BDD. (The BDDQ is not meant to diagnose BDD. An in-person evaluation is recommended for diagnosis.)

Brief self-report questionnaire that maps onto DSM-IV diagnostic criteria for BDD. (The current version does not include repetitive behaviors as required by DSM-5 diagnostic criteria, but it is expected to have adequate sensitivity and specificity for DSM-5 BDD.)

Adolescent and adult versions are available.

Takes 1–5 minutes to administer.

Scoring: Visit www.bodyimageprogram.com or see Phillips 2005.

Measure has good sensitivity and specificity.

BDD Diagnostic Module (Phillips 2005)

Diagnoses BDD. (The Structured Clinical Interview for DSM [SCID] can also be used to diagnose BDD; it is probably preferable to use the SCID for DSM-5 when it becomes available, as it will include DSM-5's new Criterion B.)

Rater-administered, semistructured instrument modeled after the format used in the SCID. Maps onto DSM-IV diagnostic criteria for BDD.

Adolescent and adult versions are available.

Takes 10–15 minutes to administer.

Scoring: BDD is present if diagnostic criteria are met.

Measure has good interrater reliability.

TABLE 3–2. Screening, diagnostic, severity, and insight measures for body dysmorphic disorder (BDD) *(continued)*

Measure	Description
Yale-Brown Obsessive Compulsive Scale Modified for Body Dysmorphic Disorder (BDD-YBOCS; Phillips 2005; Phillips et al. 1997)	Rates current (past week) severity of BDD; should *not* be used as a diagnostic measure and should not be used in individuals who have not been diagnosed with BDD. Rater-administered, 12-item, semistructured instrument modeled after the Yale-Brown Obsessive Compulsive Scale for obsessive-compulsive disorder (OCD). Adolescent and adult versions are available. Takes 15 minutes to administer. Scoring: Scores range from 0 to 48, with higher scores indicating more severe BDD. A score of 20 or higher is the cut point for a diagnosis of BDD. Scores lower than 20 reflect subclinical, or subthreshold, BDD. Measure has good interrater and test-retest reliability, strong internal consistency, and good convergent and discriminant validity, and is sensitive to change.
Brown Assessment of Beliefs Scale (BABS; Eisen et al. 1998; Phillips et al. 2013b)	Assesses current (past week) insight/delusionality of inaccurate beliefs. Can be used to assess inaccurate beliefs in a variety of disorders, such as OCD, psychotic depression, eating disorders, olfactory reference syndrome, and schizophrenia. In BDD, the BABS assesses the person's insight regarding his or her beliefs about the perceived appearance flaws—for example, "I look ugly."

TABLE 3–2. Screening, diagnostic, severity, and insight measures for body dysmorphic disorder (BDD) *(continued)*

Brown Assessment of Beliefs Scale *(continued)*

Seven-item, rater-administered, semistructured scale.

Adolescent and adult versions are available.

Takes 10 minutes to administer.

Scoring: Provides a dimensional score that ranges from 0 to 24, with higher scores reflecting poorer insight/greater delusionality; also categorizes beliefs according to different levels of insight/delusionality:

Score of 4 on item 1 (conviction) plus a total score of 18 or higher on items 1–6 equals *absent insight/delusional beliefs*.

Total score of 13–17 on items 1–6 equals *poor insight* (a total score of 18 or higher plus a score of 0–3 on item 1 also equals poor insight).

Total score of 8–12 on items 1–6 equals *fair insight*.

Total score of 4–7 on items 1–6 equals *good insight*.

Total score of 0–3 on items 1–6 equals *excellent insight*.

Item 7 is NOT included when scoring this scale.

Measure has good interrater and test-retest reliability, strong internal consistency, and good convergent and discriminant validity, and is sensitive to change.

TABLE 3–3. Considerations in the differential diagnosis of body dysmorphic disorder (BDD)

Disorder in differential	Why BDD may be misdiagnosed	When BDD should be diagnosed
Obsessive-compulsive disorder	Both disorders are characterized by obsessions, preoccupations, and repetitive behaviors.	Obsessions (preoccupations) and behaviors focus on appearance.
Eating disorders	Both involve dissatisfaction with one's appearance and distorted body image.	If appearance concerns focus only on being too fat or on body shape (being fat) and qualify for an eating disorder diagnosis, then BDD is not diagnosed. However, eating disorders and BDD commonly co-occur (with BDD symptoms typically focusing on non-weight concerns), in which case both disorders should be diagnosed.
Social anxiety disorder (social phobia)	Fear of rejection and humiliation, social anxiety, and social avoidance are very common symptoms of BDD	In BDD, these symptoms are due to embarrassment and shame about perceived appearance flaws; if diagnostic criteria for BDD are met, BDD should be diagnosed rather than social anxiety disorder.
Agoraphobia	Some people with BDD avoid going out of the house or to public places because they think they are too ugly to be seen.	Diagnose BDD if avoidance is due to feeling too ugly to be seen or worry that other people will stare at or mock the patient because of how he or she looks.
Generalized anxiety disorder (GAD)	Excessive anxiety and worry—core features of GAD—are often seen in BDD.	Diagnose BDD if anxiety and worry are caused by concerns about perceived defects in one's appearance.

TABLE 3–3.   Considerations in the differential diagnosis of body dysmorphic disorder (BDD) *(continued)*

Disorder in differential	Why BDD may be misdiagnosed	When BDD should be diagnosed
Major depressive disorder	Many patients with BDD have depressive symptoms, which often appear to be secondary to the distress and impairment that BDD causes. Often, depressive symptoms that coexist with BDD are diagnosed, but BDD is missed, or BDD symptoms are considered a symptom of depression, and BDD is not diagnosed.	BDD is characterized by prominent preoccupation with one's appearance and compulsive repetitive behaviors. BDD should be diagnosed in depressed individuals if diagnostic criteria for BDD are met.
Psychotic disorders	BDD may be characterized by delusional appearance beliefs and BDD-related delusions of reference.	Patients whose symptoms meet diagnostic criteria for BDD and whose only psychotic symptoms consist of delusional appearance beliefs or related delusions of reference should receive a diagnosis of BDD with absent insight/delusional beliefs. BDD is not characterized by other psychotic symptoms, disorganized speech or behavior, or negative symptoms.
Gender dysphoria	Disliking and wishing to get rid of sex characteristics often involves their appearance.	BDD should not be diagnosed if the patient is preoccupied with only his or her genitals and/or secondary sex characteristics and the patient's symptoms meet other diagnostic criteria for gender dysphoria.

TABLE 3–3. Considerations in the differential diagnosis of body dysmorphic disorder (BDD) *(continued)*

Disorder in differential	Why BDD may be misdiagnosed	When BDD should be diagnosed
Excoriation (skin-picking) disorder	Skin picking is a common symptom of BDD.	If skin picking is triggered by a preoccupation with perceived skin flaws and is intended to improve the skin's appearance, BDD should be diagnosed.
Trichotillomania (hair-pulling disorder)	Some patients with BDD remove their hair (body, facial, head) to try to improve their appearance.	If hair pulling is triggered by a preoccupation with hair that is considered ugly or abnormal in appearance and the hair pulling is intended to improve appearance, BDD should be diagnosed.
Olfactory reference syndrome (ORS)	Both BDD and ORS involve bodily preoccupation.	If the preoccupation focuses on body odor, ORS should be diagnosed. If it focuses on appearance, BDD should be diagnosed.
Panic disorder	Patients with BDD can have panic attacks that are cued by BDD concerns or behaviors (e.g., mirror checking, feeling scrutinized by others, bright lights).	For panic disorder to be diagnosed, panic attacks must "come out of the blue." If a BDD thought or behavior triggers the attack, BDD should be diagnosed; the DSM-5-wide panic attack specifier may be used.

Normal Appearance Concerns

Unlike normal appearance concerns, BDD is characterized by time-consuming and excessive appearance-related preoccupations (Criterion A) and excessive repetitive behaviors (Criterion B). BDD must also cause clinically significant distress or impairment in functioning (Criterion C). Body image dissatisfaction or other subclinical appearance concerns should not be considered equivalent to BDD.

Clearly Noticeable Physical Defects

Preoccupation with appearance defects or flaws that are clearly noticeable or observable (e.g., at conversational distance) is not diagnosed as BDD. If such defects cause preoccupation as well as clinically significant distress or impairment in functioning, they may be diagnosed as "other specified OCRD." BDD-related skin picking, which is triggered by appearance concerns, can cause noticeable skin lesions and scarring; BDD should nonetheless be diagnosed in such cases.

Etiology and Pathophysiology

BDD's etiology and pathophysiology are likely multifactorial and complex. Like other psychiatric disorders, BDD likely results from a complex array of many distal genetic and environmental factors as well as many more-proximal factors (e.g., abnormalities in visual processing). Although emerging research in this area is exciting and is beginning to shed some light on possible underlying mechanisms, limitations include the fact that studies are few, some findings are inconsistent across studies, and few replication studies have been done. In addition, some studies have examined constructs that differ somewhat from BDD (e.g., dysmorphic concern and subclinical BDD). Furthermore, it is unclear whether some of the factors discussed in the following sections may contribute to, and increase the risk for, BDD's development or are a consequence of BDD. Nonetheless, these findings indicate that BDD is a neurobiologically based disorder and is not simply vanity.

Genetic Factors

Genes likely play a role in BDD's etiology, although they remain to be elucidated. Preliminary data indicate that the prevalence of BDD is higher in first-degree relatives of BDD probands than in the general population (Phillips 2005; Phillips et al. 2005b). In addition, BDD is more common in first-degree relatives of OCD probands than in control probands, suggesting shared etiology and pathophysiology (genetic and/or environmental; Bienvenu et al. 2012) with OCD. Several twin studies similarly suggest a genetic overlap between BDD and OCD (although they examined the broader concept of "dysmorphic concern" rather than the disorder BDD) (Monzani et al. 2012). These findings require replication.

Evolutionary Perspective

The application of evolutionary theory to disorders such as BDD is at a very preliminary stage. However, it might be argued that concerns with body appearance may in part have an evolutionary basis (i.e., a desire to attract mates or avoid social ostracism; Phillips 2009). Indeed, in animals, the absence of facial defects or greater symmetry of body parts, for example, may signal reproductive health and fitness or the absence of disease. Moreover, in the animal world, large body size confers some advantages. Certain abnormal behaviors in animals may be relevant to repetitive BDD behaviors—for example, compulsive grooming behaviors such as acral lick syndrome in dogs and compulsive feather plucking in birds.

Neurobiological Factors

What do patients with BDD actually see? There are currently no firm answers to this intriguing question. However, emerging findings from functional magnetic resonance imaging (fMRI) and other studies indicate that BDD is associated with abnormal visual processing. These abnormalities consist of a bias for encoding and analyzing details at the expense of holistic visual processing strategies (i.e., seeing "the big picture") (Feusner et al. 2010, 2011). Individuals with BDD appear to excessively focus on details of faces as well as non-face objects such as houses. These findings are consistent with clinical observations that people with BDD focus excessively on tiny details of their appearance while ignoring global aspects of how they look. Preliminary data also suggest abnormalities in executive functioning (e.g., Dunai et al. 2010), although findings differ somewhat across studies.

One structural magnetic resonance imaging study found no volumetric differences between BDD subjects and healthy control subjects; however, two studies found greater total white matter volume in BDD subjects (Phillips et al. 2010a). One of the latter two studies also found a leftward shift in caudate asymmetry, and the other found smaller orbitofrontal cortex and anterior cingulate and larger thalamic volumes (Phillips et al. 2010a). More recently, a small study found that BDD may be characterized by compromised white matter fibers (reduced organization) and inefficient connections—or poor integration of information—between different brain areas (Buchanan et al. 2013). Another study did not find this (although statistical power was somewhat limited) but did find a relationship between fiber disorganization and impairment in insight in tracts connecting visual with emotion/memory processing systems (Feusner et al. 2013). In addition, an fMRI study found relative hyperactivity in the left orbitofrontal cortex and bilateral head of the caudate when subjects viewed their own faces, which may possibly reflect obsessional preoccupation (Feusner et al. 2010). Although BDD subjects were not directly compared with OCD subjects, this activation pattern is also characteristic of OCD. Given the efficacy of SRIs for BDD (see "Treatment" later in the chapter), the neurotransmitter serotonin, as well as other neurotransmitters, may play an important role in BDD.

Emotion- and Information-Processing Biases

Individuals with BDD appear to have difficulty identifying emotional facial expressions and to have a bias toward interpreting neutral faces as contemptuous and angry (Buhlmann et al. 2006), consistent with their belief that others mock them because they look "deformed." Persons with BDD also have threatening interpretations of ambiguous scenarios; compared with individuals with OCD, they interpret ambiguous appearance-related and social information as more threatening (Buhlmann et al. 2002), which is also consistent with the frequent occurrence of ideas and delusions of reference in BDD.

Sociocultural and Environmental Factors

BDD appears to be associated with lower-than-average levels of parental care, a history of teasing, and childhood neglect or abuse (Buhlmann et al. 2007; Phillips 2009). In one study, patients with BDD reported higher rates of emotional and sexual abuse (but not physical abuse) than patients with OCD (Neziroglu et al. 2006). Regarding personality characteristics and temperament (which have both environmental and genetic determinants), BDD appears associated with very high levels of neuroticism and low levels of extroversion (Phillips 2005). Although all these factors are associated with other psychiatric disorders and are not specific to BDD, they are consistent with this disorder's clinical features. It is also likely that sociocultural factors focusing on the importance of appearance play a role in causing and maintaining BDD.

Treatment

General Approaches to Treatment and Special Considerations

Engaging and Retaining Patients in Treatment

One of the most challenging problems that clinicians face when treating patients with BDD is their poor BDD-related insight. Many believe not only that they truly are ugly or deformed, but also that their appearance concerns do not have a psychiatric or psychological cause, such as BDD (Phillips et al. 2012). As a result, many are reluctant to accept a diagnosis of BDD or psychiatric care, which they doubt can help them.

Thus, before clinicians discuss or offer treatment, it is important to lay some groundwork, such as the following, which may help patients to recognize that they have BDD and to accept psychiatric treatment:

- *Attend to the therapeutic alliance and instill hope.* Strive to build rapport and trust by expressing empathy for patients' suffering. Be nonjudgmental so patients do not feel that their concerns are trivial or that they are vain. Many patients, especially those who are more severely ill, feel hopeless and desperate about their symptoms; thus it is important to instill hope by conveying that most patients get better with the right treatment.
- *Avoid trying to talk patients out of their appearance beliefs or arguing with them about how they look.* Just as it is usually not helpful to try to talk a patient with schizophrenia out of a delusional belief, this approach also does not usually work with patients with BDD. Instead, the clinician might note that individuals with BDD see themselves very negatively and very differently from how others see them, for reasons that are not well understood; this mismatch in perception may involve abnormalities in visual perception and overfocusing on details, which may possibly be reinforced by BDD rituals such as mirror checking. It may not be helpful to say that the patient is pretty, beautiful, or handsome, because some patients negatively interpret positive words such as these.
- *Focus on the patients' suffering and the effect of BDD on their lives.* It is often helpful to discuss how the patients' concerns are causing them to suffer and are interfering with their functioning, which most patients can readily agree with.
- *Provide psychoeducation about BDD and its treatment.* Explain the disorder's clinical features and that it is a common and usually treatable disorder. Many patients are relieved to learn this. Patients may benefit from reading about BDD (e.g., Phillips 2009).

  - Provide information about recommended treatments and a rationale for these treatments.
  - Address any misconceptions about recommended treatments. For example, some patients are fearful of CBT exposures, worrying that the therapist will push them to do exposures they find too frightening. The clinician can explain that doable exposure exercises can be developed and that learning cognitive approaches first may make exposures easier to do. Fears or misconceptions about medication treatment should

also be addressed. For more reluctant patients, it can be helpful to frame a medication trial as an "experiment" in which patients can try the medication, assess its pros and cons after an optimal trial, and then make a decision, in collaboration with the physician, about whether to continue it.

• Focus on the potential benefits of psychiatric treatment.

• *Discourage patients from getting dermatological, surgical, dental, and other cosmetic treatments for BDD concerns.* Convey that such treatment is not recommended because available data indicate that it is almost never effective for BDD and can even make symptoms worse (Crerand et al. 2005; Phillips et al. 2001b; Sarwer and Crerand 2008). Encourage patients to try medication and/or CBT first, because such treatments appear to be helpful for a majority of patients.

• *Involve family members if appropriate and potentially helpful,* especially if they have brought the patient for treatment. They may be an important source of support for the patient and an ally for the clinician during the treatment process.

• *Consider use of motivational interviewing strategies that are modified for BDD.* These strategies may help to engage and retain reluctant patients in treatment.

Addressing Suicidality

Clinicians must carefully assess and monitor suicidal ideation. Suicidal patients should always receive an SRI trial that is adequate for BDD. SRIs often decrease suicidality and also protect against worsening of suicidality in patients with BDD (Phillips 2009; Phillips and Kelly 2009). Suicidal patients should also be strongly encouraged to participate in CBT for BDD, especially if suicidality appears largely BDD related. For more highly suicidal patients, clinicians should consider incorporating cognitive-behavioral approaches for suicidality into treatment (e.g., Wenzel et al. 2008). Higher-risk patients may need a higher level of care, although many refuse such care because they do not want other people to see them, in which case the clinician must determine whether commitment standards are met.

Using Body Dysmorphic Disorder–Specific Treatments

It is critically important to recognize that effective treatment for BDD—especially CBT for BDD—differs in some important ways from treatments for other disorders, such as OCD, social anxiety disorder, major depressive disorder, or schizophrenia. Because BDD differs from other disorders, it requires treatment that targets its unique symptoms. For example, compared with patients with OCD, those with BDD typically require more intensive strategies to engage them in treatment and ongoing motivational interventions. Cognitive interventions are more complex and intensive for BDD than for OCD, because many BDD patients have delusional beliefs and delusions of reference. Unlike with OCD, exposure exercises and behavioral experiments are needed to address prominent social avoidance in BDD. In addition, CBT for BDD includes a mindfulness/perceptual retraining intervention that targets visual processing abnormalities. Furthermore, treatment must target problematic behaviors that are unique to BDD, such as surgery seeking and skin picking or hair pulling due to appearance concerns.

Surgical, Dermatological, Dental, and Other Cosmetic Treatment

A majority of patients with BDD seek and receive cosmetic treatment. The surgery literature has referred to such patients as "polysurgery addicts." Studies from psychiatric settings indicate that about two-thirds of patients with BDD receive surgical, dermatological, dental, or other cosmetic treatment for their perceived appearance flaws (Crerand et al. 2005; Phillips et al. 2001b). Dermatological treatment is most often received (most often topical acne agents, but also treatments such as dermabrasion and isotretinoin [Accutane]), followed by surgery (most often rhinoplasty) (Crerand et al. 2005; Phillips et al. 2001b). The treatment outcome appears to usually be poor. One study ($N=50$) found that 81% of subjects were dissatisfied with past medical consultation or surgery (Veale et al. 1996a). In two other studies ($N=250$ and $N=200$), only 4%–7% of such treatments led to overall improvement in BDD (Crerand et al. 2005; Phillips et al. 2001b). BDD symptoms may be exacerbated by cosmetic treatment. Findings from these larger studies concur with those from a small prospective surgery study (Tignol et al. 2007) and with observations in the surgery and dermatology literature that patients with BDD may consult numerous physicians, pressure them to prescribe unsuitable treatments, and are often dissatisfied with the outcome (e.g., Sarwer and Crerand 2008). Such outcomes are perhaps not unexpected, given that individuals with BDD actually look normal but are prone to perceive "defects" where none actually exist and to become preoccupied with and distressed by them.

In a survey of cosmetic surgeons, 43% of respondents reported BDD patients were even more preoccupied with the treated "defects" and only 1% were free of their preoccupation after surgery (Sarwer 2002). In 39% of cases, the patient was free of his or her preoccupation but then focused on a different perceived defect. Of concern, 40% reported that a dissatisfied BDD patient had threatened them legally and/or physically. Occasional dissatisfied patients commit suicide or murder the physician (Phillips 1991, 2009). Thus, patients should be discouraged from seeking cosmetic treatment for BDD symptoms.

Pharmacotherapy

Serotonin Reuptake Inhibitors as First-Line Pharmacotherapy

SRIs are currently considered the medication of choice for BDD, including for patients with delusional BDD beliefs (Ipser et al. 2009; National Collaborating Centre for Mental Health 2006; Phillips 2009; Phillips and Hollander 2008). However, no medications are approved by the U.S. Food and Drug Administration (FDA) for the treatment of BDD because no pharmaceutical companies have sought this indication.

Prior to the 1990s, no treatment studies were done, and BDD was generally considered untreatable (Phillips 1991). However, early case series suggested that SRIs might have efficacy, consistent with BDD's similarities to OCD and the high co-occurrence of depressive symptoms (Phillips and Hollander 2008). Subsequently, four methodologically rigorous open-label SRI trials—two with fluvoxamine, one with citalopram, and one with escitalopram ($N=15$–30)—found that SRIs improved BDD and associated symptoms in 63%–83% of patients (intention-to-treat analyses; Phillips and Hollander 2008). In a clinical series of 33 children and adolescents with BDD, 53% of 19 subjects who received an SRI had improvement in BDD, whereas non-SRI medications were not efficacious for BDD (Albertini and Phillips 1999).

In a randomized, double-blind crossover study, 29 randomized subjects were treated for 8 weeks with the SRI tricyclic antidepressant clomipramine or the non-SRI tricyclic antidepressant desipramine (Hollander et al. 1999). Clomipramine was superior to desipramine for BDD symptoms and functional disability. These results suggested that SRIs may be preferentially efficacious for BDD, which is similarly the case with OCD and consistent with prior retrospective data on BDD (Phillips and Hollander 2008). Treatment efficacy was independent of the presence or severity of comorbid depression, OCD, or social anxiety disorder. In a subsequent 12-week randomized, double-blind, parallel-group study ($N=67$), fluoxetine was significantly more efficacious than placebo for BDD symptoms and psychosocial functioning (Phillips et al. 2002). The response rate to fluoxetine was 53%, versus 18% to placebo. In this study, too, efficacy of fluoxetine was independent of the presence of comorbid major depression or OCD.

Effective SRI treatment decreases BDD-related preoccupation, functional impairment, repetitive behaviors, and distress. Depressive symptoms, anxiety, anger-hostility, and mental health–related quality of life improved in all or most studies that examined these variables (Phillips and Hollander 2008).

No studies have directly compared the efficacy of different SRIs for BDD. However, a prospective series in a clinical practice ($N=90$) found similar response rates for each type of SRI (Phillips et al. 2001a).

Efficacy of serotonin reuptake inhibitor monotherapy for delusional body dysmorphic disorder.   Although it might be assumed that antipsychotics should be the mainstay of pharmacotherapy for delusional BDD, studies consistently indicate that delusional BDD is as responsive to SRI monotherapy as is nondelusional BDD (Phillips and Hollander 2008). Earlier clinical experience somewhat unexpectedly suggested that this might be the case, which was supported by subsequent findings in open-label trials and the previously noted placebo-controlled fluoxetine study, in which 50% of patients with delusional BDD responded to fluoxetine versus 55% with nondelusional BDD (Phillips and Hollander 2008). In the previously described crossover study, clomipramine monotherapy was even more efficacious for patients with delusional BDD than for those with nondelusional BDD. Thus, an SRI, rather than antipsychotic monotherapy, is recommended for BDD patients with the DSM-5 absent insight/delusional beliefs specifier.

Recommended dosing and trial duration.   Available data and clinical experience suggest that BDD often requires SRI dosages in the range typically recommended for OCD, which are higher than those typically used for depression and many other disorders (Phillips 2009); however, dosage finding studies have not been done in BDD. Some patients benefit from dosages that exceed the pharmaceutical company's maximum recommended dosage (this approach is not advised for clomipramine or citalopram, however).

The following are the mean daily dosages, as well as typical maximum dosages, used in the author's clinical practice: fluoxetine, 67 ± 24 mg (120 mg); clomipramine, 203 ± 53 mg (250 mg); fluvoxamine, 308 ± 49 mg (450 mg); sertraline, 202 ± 46 mg (400 mg); paroxetine, 55 ± 13 mg (90 mg); citalopram, 66 ± 36 mg (40 mg currently, per recent FDA recommendations); and escitalopram, 29 ± 12 mg (60 mg) (Phillips 2009). Citalopram is now a much less appealing option for BDD, given FDA dosing limits. Most patients, however, appear to receive relatively low SRI dosages, which is associated with poorer treatment response (Phillips et al. 2006c). It may be advisable to obtain an electrocardiogram if a higher escitalopram dosage is used.

The average time to response has ranged from 4–5 weeks for citalopram and escitalopram to 6–9 weeks for fluoxetine and fluvoxamine (Phillips and Hollander 2008). Even with fairly rapid SRI dose titration, however, many patients do not respond until the tenth or twelfth week of treatment. If SRI response is inadequate after 12–16 weeks of treatment, and the highest dosage tolerated by the patient or recommended by the manufacturer has been tried for at least 3–4 of those 12–16 weeks, a medication change should be made (by switching to another SRI or initiating SRI augmentation), because it does not appear that a nonresponder will convert to a responder after 12–16 weeks of treatment during which an adequate dose is reached (although research on this issue is needed) (Phillips 2009).

Based on clinical experience, patients who improve with an SRI should generally remain on it for at least several years, although many patients opt to continue an SRI for far longer. Lifelong treatment should be considered for patients with very severe BDD, those who have relapsed with prior discontinuation of SRIs, and those with multiple suicide attempts due to BDD (Phillips 2009).

Switching to another serotonin reuptake inhibitor versus augmenting. If response to an optimal 12- to 16-week SRI trial is only partial, a longer SRI trial can be considered to determine whether a partial response will further improve. Preliminary data suggest that about 40% of initial SRI responders further improve with continued SRI treatment for 6 more months (Phillips 2009). Alternatively, the SRI can be discontinued and another one tried. A report from a clinical practice found that of those patients who did not respond to an initial adequate SRI trial, 43% responded to at least one subsequent adequate SRI trial (Phillips et al. 2001a).

For partial SRI responders, however, it may be desirable to continue the SRI and augment it with another medication, especially if functioning or suicidality has notably improved with SRI treatment. SRI augmentation strategies may possibly be more effective for patients who have had a partial response, as opposed to no response, to an SRI (Phillips et al. 2001a). Buspirone is a good augmentation option. In a chart-review study, at a mean dosage of 57 ± 15 mg/day, buspirone effectively augmented SRIs in 33% ($n = 12$) of trials, with a large effect size (Phillips et al. 2001a). In the only controlled SRI augmentation study, the typical antipsychotic pimozide was not more efficacious than placebo in augmenting the SRI fluoxetine (response rate of 18% to both pimozide and placebo) (Phillips 2009). A small case series similarly suggested that olanzapine augmentation of SRIs was not efficacious for BDD (Phillips 2009). However, clinical experience suggests that adding an atypical antipsychotic such as ziprasidone or aripiprazole to an SRI is sometimes helpful, especially for associated agitation or severe anxiety.

Chart-review studies and clinical experience suggest that occasional patients improve with SRI augmentation with bupropion, lithium, methylphenidate, or venlafaxine (Phillips 2009). If clomipramine is combined with a selective serotonin reuptake inhibitor (SSRI), clomipramine levels must be closely monitored, given the SSRIs' potential to substantially raise the level of clomipramine and cause toxicity. Ideally, pulse, blood pressure, and drug and metabolite (desmethylclomipramine) serum levels should be monitored and electrocardiograms obtained. Clinicians can consider adding a benzodiaze-pine to an SRI to treat severe distress, agitation, or anxiety in patients for whom a benzodiazepine is not contraindicated.

Non–Serotonin Reuptake Inhibitor Medication as Monotherapy

If a number of adequate SRI trials have not been adequately helpful, non-SRIs may be considered, although efficacy data are very limited, and they are not currently recommended as first-line treatments for BDD. A small open-label venlafaxine trial (data reported for 11 completers) and an open-label trial of the antiepileptic levetiracetam ($n = 17$, intention-to treat sample) re-ported efficacy for BDD (Phillips and Hollander 2008). In a retrospective case series, monoamine oxidase inhibitors were efficacious in 30% ($n = 7$) of 23 cases (Phillips and Hollander 2008). The clomipramine/desipramine study noted earlier, case reports, and retrospective case series suggest that tricyclic antidepressants other than clomipramine are usually inefficacious (Phillips and Hollander 2008). Retrospective data suggest that antipsychotics are not effective as monotherapy for either delusional BDD or nondelusional BDD, although prospective studies are needed (Phillips and Hollander 2008), and these medications may have a role as SRI augmenters.

Other Somatic Treatments

Only case series data are available for electroconvulsive therapy, which sug-gests that it is usually ineffective for BDD (Phillips 2009), although its use may be considered for highly suicidal BDD patients with severe co-occurring depression. No studies or case series have reported on the efficacy of deep brain stimulation or transcranial magnetic stimulation for BDD.

Cognitive-Behavioral Therapy

Treatment Studies

CBT that is tailored to BDD's unique symptoms is the best-studied psycho-therapy for BDD and has been shown to be effective for a majority of pa-tients (Ipser et al. 2009; National Collaborating Centre for Mental Health 2006; Phillips 2009). Efficacy of individual and group CBT was reported in case series (Neziroglu and Yaryura-Tobias 1993; Wilhelm et al. 1999), and in a study of 10 patients who participated in an intensive behavioral therapy program, including a 6-month maintenance program, improvement was maintained at up to 2 years (McKay 1999).

Three published studies of CBT (an additional study used metacognitive therapy) have used a no-treatment wait-list control group. In a study that provided eight weekly 2-hour sessions of BDD-focused CBT in a group format, subjects in the CBT group improved more than those in the wait-list control group; BDD-focused CBT was efficacious for 77% (21) of the 27 women (Rosen et al. 1995). In a study of 19 patients, those treated with individual BDD-focused CBT improved significantly more than those on a no-treatment wait list, with 7 of 9 patients no longer meeting diagnostic criteria for BDD (Veale et al. 1996b).

More recently, a study that included a broader range of patients, including those with suicidal ideation and delusional BDD beliefs, randomly assigned 36 adults to 22 sessions of immediate manualized individual CBT for BDD over 24 weeks or to a 12-week wait list. By week 12, 50% (8 of 16) of participants receiving immediate CBT-BDD were responders, compared with 12% (2 of 17) of wait-listed participants ($P = 0.026$). By posttreatment (week 24), 81% (26 of 32) of participants in the combined ITT CBT-BDD sample, and 83% (24 of 29) of treatment completers, met the definition for response. CBT-BDD resulted in significant decreases in BDD severity; gains were maintained at 3- and 6-month follow-up. Depression, insight, and disability also significantly improved, and patient satisfaction was high (Wilhelm et al. 2014).

Despite their promising results, these studies used a wait-list control group and thus did not control for therapist time and attention, leaving open the question of whether nonspecific treatment factors such as these, rather than CBT itself, were responsible for improvement. A recent study (Veale et al. 2014), the first to control for these factors, found that BDD-focused CBT was more efficacious than anxiety management after 12 weeks of treatment. Outcomes improved even further after four additional CBT sessions, and gains were maintained at 1-month follow-up.

Components of CBT for Body Dysmorphic Disorder

CBT needs to be tailored specifically to BDD's unique symptoms. Because BDD, especially more severe BDD, is typically challenging to treat, and because BDD's treatment meaningfully differs from that of other disorders, use of a BDD-specific CBT manual is highly recommended. Two evidence-based CBT treatment manuals for adults are now available (Veale and Neziroglu 2010; Wilhelm et al. 2013). Therapists should have basic CBT training and some familiarity with BDD. If one manual is not adequately helpful, the other may be. An evidence-based manualized treatment manual is not currently available for children or adolescents with BDD.

The treatment described here is based on one of these treatment manuals (Wilhelm et al. 2013). First, the therapist must obtain a good understanding of the patient's BDD and other symptoms, provide psychoeducation about BDD, and build an individualized cognitive-behavioral model of the patient's illness, including hypothesized mechanisms that cause or maintain the patient's symptoms. This model is used to collaboratively develop a treatment plan and help the patient understand how CBT may be helpful. Treatment goals that involve enhancement of valued life activities should be set. It is often necessary to enhance motivation for treatment, using motivational interviewing strategies. The first three or four sessions should be used to lay this critically important foundation; if they are not, treatment may fail.

Once this foundation is set, treatment then focuses on the following core elements (Wilhelm et al. 2013):

- *Cognitive restructuring* helps patients learn to identify and evaluate their negative appearance-related thoughts and beliefs and to identify cognitive errors (e.g., mind reading, fortune telling, all-or-nothing thinking). Patients learn to develop more accurate and helpful appearance-related beliefs. Core beliefs (e.g., being unlovable, worthless, or inadequate) are addressed with more advanced cognitive techniques.
- *Response (ritual) prevention* helps patients cut down on repetitive compulsive behaviors (e.g., mirror checking, comparing).
- *Exposure* helps patients gradually face avoided situations (usually social situations). Exposure is combined with behavioral experiments in which patients design and carry out experiments to test the accuracy of their beliefs (e.g., going into a grocery store to test the hypothesis that 70% of people will move away from the patient with a look of horror within 5 seconds). Doing cognitive restructuring before and during exposures decreases distorted thinking and makes exposures easier to carry out.
- *Perceptual retraining,* which includes mindfulness skills, addresses patients' tendency to overfocus on tiny details of their appearance. It helps patients to develop a more holistic view of their appearance by looking at their entire face or body (not just disliked areas) when looking in the mirror, without performing BDD rituals, and to objectively (rather than negatively) describe their body.
- *Relapse prevention* at the end of treatment prepares patients to terminate formal treatment and to continue to implement learned strategies in their daily lives.
- *Structured daily homework* is a required treatment component that enables patients to practice and consolidate skills learned in session.

Additional approaches are recommended for patients with relevant symptoms (Wilhelm et al. 2013):

1. *Habit reversal* is used to treat BDD-related skin picking, hair plucking (e.g., to remove "excessive" body hair), and body touching.

2. *Activity scheduling* and *scheduling pleasant activities* are used for more severely depressed or inactive patients.
3. The problematic behaviors of *seeking and receiving cosmetic treatments* should be addressed.
4. *Body shape and weight concerns*, such as muscle dysmorphia, must also be addressed.
5. *Motivational interviewing* is used at any time during treatment when patients are ambivalent about initiating or continuing treatment.

For patients who are too severely ill or depressed to participate in CBT, medication may improve symptoms to the point where it is feasible for them to do CBT.

Approaches that are *not* recommended include staring in mirrors (this actually reinforces the ritual of mirror checking), listening to tapes that say the patient is ugly, and creating "flaws" such as painting bright red spots on their face or wearing strange hairdos and going out in public. In all of these circumstances, habituation seems unlikely to occur (perhaps because of patients' poor insight), and such approaches can make patients worse, even suicidal.

Frequency and Duration

The number of CBT sessions in studies has varied considerably, from 12 weekly sessions (Veale et al. 1996b) to 12 weeks of daily 90-minute sessions (Neziroglu and Yaryura-Tobias 1993). The optimal session frequency and treatment duration are unclear. Most experts would recommend weekly or more frequent sessions for about 6 months, plus daily homework (Wilhelm et al. 2013). More severely ill patients may require more intensive or longer treatment. After formal treatment ends, as-needed booster sessions should be used to reduce the risk of relapse, and patients should continue to practice CBT skills. Patients who have not worked or interacted with people for many years may benefit from skills training following CBT.

Approaches for Treatment-Refractory Body Dysmorphic Disorder

In my clinical experience, most BDD cases that appear treatment refractory are not. Most of these patients have not received adequate pharmacotherapy for BDD. Common problems include inadequately high SRI doses, too brief an SRI trial, and poor medication compliance. In addition, most patients have not been treated with an evidence-based manualized BDD-focused CBT treatment (Veale and Neziroglu 2010; Wilhelm et al. 2013), in part because these manuals have only recently been developed and tested. In some cases, poor homework compliance compromises the treatment outcome. Following recommended treatment strategies will likely convert many patients with apparently refractory illness into treatment responders. More severely ill patients should receive both medication and CBT, and more intensive treatment, such as partial hospital or residential treatment, that focuses on treatment of BDD can be considered.

Key Points

- Body dysmorphic disorder (BDD) is a common yet underrecognized disorder, with a point prevalence in nationwide epidemiological surveys of 1.7%–2.4%.

- BDD is associated with high rates of functional impairment and suicidality; clinicians should closely monitor BDD patients for suicidal ideation and behavior.

- Onset of BDD is usually during early adolescence; in two-thirds of cases, the onset is before age 18 years.

- BDD has similarities to obsessive-compulsive disorder but also some important differences, such as poorer insight, greater comorbidity with major depressive disorder and possibly also substance use disorders, and higher rates of suicidality—all of which have treatment implications.

- Clinicians should diagnose BDD when present and apply BDD-specific treatments; treatments (especially cognitive-behavioral therapy [CBT]) for other disorders are unlikely to be effective.

- Individuals with BDD may be difficult to engage and retain in treatment; various strategies, including motivational interviewing, may be needed.

- Serotonin reuptake inhibitors (SRIs), the first-line medications for BDD, are often effective for BDD and associated symptoms.

- Higher SRI dosages and a longer treatment trial than typically used for depression and most other disorders are often needed.

- CBT that is tailored to BDD's unique symptoms is the first-line psychosocial treatment approach.

- Because BDD can be challenging to treat with CBT, use of an evidence-based BDD-specific treatment manual is advised.

References

Albertini RS, Phillips KA: Thirty-three cases of body dysmorphic disorder in children and adolescents. J Am Acad Child Adolesc Psychiatry 38(4):453–459, 1999 10199118

American Psychiatric Association: Diagnostic and Statistical Manual of Mental Disorders, 3rd Edition Revised. Washington, DC, American Psychiatric Association, 1987

American Psychiatric Association: Diagnostic and Statistical Manual of Mental Disorders, 4th Edition. Washington, DC, American Psychiatric Association, 1994

American Psychiatric Association: Diagnostic and Statistical Manual of Mental Disorders, 5th Edition. Arlington, VA, American Psychiatric Association, 2013

Bienvenu OJ, Samuels JF, Wuyek LA, et al: Is obsessive-compulsive disorder an anxiety disorder, and what, if any, are spectrum conditions? A family study perspective. Psychol Med 42(1):1–13, 2012 21733222

Bjornsson AS, Didie ER, Grant JE, et al: Age at onset and clinical correlates in body dysmorphic disorder. Compr Psychiatry 54(7):893–903, 2013 23643073

Buchanan BG, Rossell SL, Maller JJ, et al: Brain connectivity in body dysmorphic disorder compared with controls: a diffusion tensor imaging study. Psychol Med 43(12):2513–2521, 2013 23473554

Buhlmann U, Wilhelm S, McNally RJ, et al: Interpretive biases for ambiguous information in body dysmorphic disorder. CNS Spectr 7(6):435–436, 441–443, 2002 15107765

Buhlmann U, Etcoff NL, Wilhelm S: Emotion recognition bias for contempt and anger in body dysmorphic disorder. J Psychiatr Res 40(2):105–111, 2006 15904932

Buhlmann U, Cook LM, Fama JM, et al: Perceived teasing experiences in body dysmorphic disorder. Body Image 4(4):381–385, 2007 18089284

Buhlmann U, Glaesmer H, Mewes R, et al: Updates on the prevalence of body dysmorphic disorder: a population-based survey. Psychiatry Res 178(1):171–175, 2010 20452057

Conroy M, Menard W, Fleming-Ives K, et al: Prevalence and clinical characteristics of body dysmorphic disorder in an adult inpatient setting. Gen Hosp Psychiatry 30(1):67–72, 2008 18164943

Cotterill JA, Cunliffe WJ: Suicide in dermatological patients. Br J Dermatol 137(2):246–250, 1997 9292074

Crerand CE, Phillips KA, Menard W, et al: Nonpsychiatric medical treatment of body dysmorphic disorder. Psychosomatics 46(6):549–555, 2005 16288134

Dunai J, Labuschagne I, Castle DJ, et al: Executive function in body dysmorphic disorder. Psychol Med 40(9):1541–1548, 2010 19951448

Dyl J, Kittler J, Phillips KA, et al: Body dysmorphic disorder and other clinically significant body image concerns in adolescent psychiatric inpatients: prevalence and clinical characteristics. Child Psychiatry Hum Dev 36(4):369–382, 2006 16741679

Eisen JL, Phillips KA, Baer L, et al: The Brown Assessment of Beliefs Scale: reliability and validity. Am J Psychiatry 155(1):102–108, 1998 9433346

Eisen JL, Phillips KA, Coles ME, et al: Insight in obsessive compulsive disorder and body dysmorphic disorder. Compr Psychiatry 45(1):10–15, 2004 14671731

Feusner JD, Moody T, Hembacher E, et al: Abnormalities of visual processing and frontostriatal systems in body dysmorphic disorder. Arch Gen Psychiatry 67(2):197–205, 2010 20124119

Feusner JD, Hembacher E, Moller H, et al: Abnormalities of object visual processing in body dysmorphic disorder. Psychol Med 41(11):2385–2397, 2011 21557897

Feusner JD, Arienzo D, Li W, et al: White matter microstructure in body dysmorphic disorder and its clinical correlates. Psychiatry Res 211(2):132–140, 2013 23375265

Grant JE, Kim SW, Crow SJ: Prevalence and clinical features of body dysmorphic disorder in adolescent and adult psychiatric inpatients. J Clin Psychiatry 62(7):517–522, 2001 11488361

Grant JE, Kim SW, Eckert ED: Body dysmorphic disorder in patients with anorexia nervosa: prevalence, clinical features, and delusionality of body image. Int J Eat Disord 32(3):291–300, 2002 12210643

Grant JE, Menard W, Pagano ME, et al: Substance use disorders in individuals with body dysmorphic disorder. J Clin Psychiatry 66(3):309–316, quiz 404–405, 2005 15766296

Hart AS, Phillips KA: Symmetry concerns as a symptom of body dysmorphic disorder. J Obsessive Compuls Relat Disord 2(3):292–298, 2013 24058899

Hollander E, Allen A, Kwon J, et al: Clomipramine vs desipramine crossover trial in body dysmorphic disorder: selective efficacy of a serotonin reuptake inhibitor in imagined ugliness. Arch Gen Psychiatry 56(11):1033–1039, 1999 10565503

Hrabosky JI, Cash TF, Veale D, et al: Multidimensional body image comparisons among patients with eating disorders, body dysmorphic disorder, and clinical controls: a multisite study. Body Image 6(3):155–163, 2009 19410528

Ipser JC, Sander C, Stein DJ: Pharmacotherapy and psychotherapy for body dysmorphic disorder. Cochrane Database Syst Rev (1):CD005332, 2009 19160252

Koran LM, Abujaoude E, Large MD, et al: The prevalence of body dysmorphic disorder in the United States adult population. CNS Spectr 13(4):316–322, 2008 18408651

Mayville S, Katz RC, Gipson MT, et al: Assessing the prevalence of body dysmorphic disorder in an ethnically diverse group of adolescents. J Child Fam Stud 8(3):357–362, 1999

McKay D: Two-year follow-up of behavioral treatment and maintenance for body dysmorphic disorder. Behav Modif 23(4):620–629, 1999 10533443

Monzani B, Rijsdijk F, Iervolino AC, et al: Evidence for a genetic overlap between body dysmorphic concerns and obsessive-compulsive symptoms in an adult female community twin sample. Am J Med Genet B Neuropsychiatr Genet 159B(4):376–382, 2012 22434544

National Collaborating Centre for Mental Health: Obsessive-Compulsive Disorder: Core Interventions in the Treatment of Obsessive-Compulsive Disorder and Body Dysmorphic Disorder (NICE Clinical Guidelines, No 31). Leicester, United Kingdom, British Psychological Society, 2006

Neziroglu FA, Yaryura-Tobias JA: Exposure, response prevention, and cognitive therapy in the treatment of body dysmorphic disorder. Behav Ther 24:431–438, 1993

Neziroglu F, Khemlani-Patel S, Yaryura-Tobias JA: Rates of abuse in body dysmorphic disorder and obsessive-compulsive disorder. Body Image 3(2):189–193, 2006 18089222

Phillips KA: Body dysmorphic disorder: the distress of imagined ugliness. Am J Psychiatry 148(9):1138–1149, 1991 1882990

Phillips KA: The Broken Mirror: Understanding and Treating Body Dysmorphic Disorder. New York, Oxford University Press, 2005

Phillips KA: Understanding Body Dysmorphic Disorder: An Essential Guide. New York, Oxford University Press, 2009

Phillips KA, Diaz S: Gender differences in body dysmorphic disorder. J Nerv Ment Dis 185:570–577, 1997

Phillips KA, Hollander E: Treating body dysmorphic disorder with medication: evidence, misconceptions, and a suggested approach. Body Image 5(1):13–27, 2008 18325859

Phillips KA, Kelly MM: Suicidality in a placebo-controlled fluoxetine study of body dysmorphic disorder. Int Clin Psychopharmacol 24(1):26–28, 2009 19060721

Phillips KA, Menard W: Suicidality in body dysmorphic disorder: a prospective study. Am J Psychiatry 163(7):1280–1282, 2006 16816236

Phillips KA, Hollander E, Rasmussen SA, et al: A severity rating scale for body dysmorphic disorder: development, reliability, and validity of a modified version of the Yale-Brown Obsessive Compulsive Scale. Psychopharmacol Bull 33(1):17–22, 1997 9133747

Phillips KA, Albertini RS, Siniscalchi JM, et al: Effectiveness of pharmacotherapy for body dysmorphic disorder: a chart-review study. J Clin Psychiatry 62(9):721–727, 2001a 11681769

Phillips KA, Grant J, Siniscalchi J, et al: Surgical and nonpsychiatric medical treatment of patients with body dysmorphic disorder. Psychosomatics 42(6):504–510, 2001b 11815686

Phillips KA, Albertini RS, Rasmussen SA: A randomized placebo-controlled trial of fluoxetine in body dysmorphic disorder. Arch Gen Psychiatry 59(4):381–388, 2002 11926939

Phillips KA, Coles ME, Menard W, et al: Suicidal ideation and suicide attempts in body dysmorphic disorder. J Clin Psychiatry 66(6):717–725, 2005a 15960564

Phillips KA, Menard W, Fay C, et al: Demographic characteristics, phenomenology, comorbidity, and family history in 200 individuals with body dysmorphic disorder. Psychosomatics 46(4):317–325, 2005b 16000674

Phillips KA, Menard W, Fay C, et al: Psychosocial functioning and quality of life in body dysmorphic disorder. Compr Psychiatry 46(4):254–260, 2005c 16175755

Phillips KA, Didie ER, Menard W, et al: Clinical features of body dysmorphic disorder in adolescents and adults. Psychiatry Res 141(3):305–314, 2006a 16499973

Phillips KA, Menard W, Fay C: Gender similarities and differences in 200 individuals with body dysmorphic disorder. Compr Psychiatry 47(2):77–87, 2006b 16490564

Phillips KA, Pagano ME, Menard W: Pharmacotherapy for body dysmorphic disorder: treatment received and illness severity. Ann Clin Psychiatry 18(4):251–257, 2006c 17162625

Phillips KA, Pinto A, Menard W, et al: Obsessive-compulsive disorder versus body dysmorphic disorder: a comparison study of two possibly related disorders. Depress Anxiety 24(6):399–409, 2007 17041935

Phillips KA, Stein DJ, Rauch SL, et al: Should an obsessive-compulsive spectrum grouping of disorders be included in DSM-V? Depress Anxiety 27(6):528–555, 2010a 20533367

Phillips KA, Wilhelm S, Koran LM, et al: Body dysmorphic disorder: some key issues for DSM-V. Depress Anxiety 27(6):573–591, 2010b 20533368

Phillips KA, Pinto A, Hart AS, et al: A comparison of insight in body dysmorphic disorder and obsessive-compulsive disorder. J Psychiatr Res 46(10):1293–1299, 2012 22819678

Phillips KA, Hart A, Menard W, et al: Psychometric evaluation of the Brown Assessment of Beliefs Scale in body dysmorphic disorder. J Nerv Ment Dis 201:640–643, 2013a 23817164

Phillips KA, Menard W, Quinn E, et al: A 4-year prospective observational follow-up study of course and predictors of course in body dysmorphic disorder. Psychol Med 43(5):1109–1117, 2013b 23171833

Phillips KA, Hart AS, Simpson HB, et al: Delusional versus nondelusional body dysmorphic disorder: recommendations for DSM-5. CNS Spectr 19(1):10–20, 2014 23659348

Rief W, Buhlmann U, Wilhelm S, et al: The prevalence of body dysmorphic disorder: a population-based survey. Psychol Med 36(6):877–885, 2006 16515733

Rosen JC, Ramirez E: A comparison of eating disorders and body dysmorphic disorder on body image and psychological adjustment. J Psychosom Res 44(3–4):441–449, 1998 9587886

Rosen JC, Reiter J, Orosan P: Cognitive-behavioral body image therapy for body dysmorphic disorder. J Consult Clin Psychol 63(2):263–269, 1995 7751487

Sarwer DB: Awareness and identification of body dysmorphic disorder by aesthetic surgeons: results of a survey of American Society for Aesthetic Plastic Surgery members. Aesthet Surg J 22(6):531–535, 2002 19332010

Sarwer DB, Crerand CE: Body dysmorphic disorder and appearance enhancing medical treatments. Body Image 5(1):50–58, 2008 18255365

Tignol J, Biraben-Gotzamanis L, Martin-Guehl C, et al: Body dysmorphic disorder and cosmetic surgery: evolution of 24 subjects with a minimal defect in appearance 5 years after their request for cosmetic surgery. Eur Psychiatry 22(8):520–524, 2007 17900876

Veale D, Neziroglu F: Body Dysmorphic Disorder: A Treatment Manual. Chichester, West Sussex, UK, Wiley-Blackwell, 2010

Veale D, Boocock A, Gournay K, et al: Body dysmorphic disorder. A survey of fifty cases. Br J Psychiatry 169(2):196–201, 1996a 8871796

Veale D, Gournay K, Dryden W, et al: Body dysmorphic disorder: a cognitive behavioural model and pilot randomised controlled trial. Behav Res Ther 34(9):717–729, 1996b 8936754

Veale D, Anson M, Miles S, et al: Efficacy of cognitive behaviour therapy versus anxiety management for body dysmorphic disorder: a randomised controlled trial. Psychother Psychosom 83(6):341–353, 2014

Ware JE Jr: SF-36 Health Survey Manual and Interpretation Guide. Boston, MA, The Health Institute, New England Medical Center, 1993

Wenzel A, Brown GK, Beck AT: Cognitive Therapy for Suicidal Patients: Scientific and Clinical Applications. Washington, DC, American Psychological Association, 2008

Wilhelm S, Otto MW, Lohr B, et al: Cognitive behavior group therapy for body dysmorphic disorder: a case series. Behav Res Ther 37(1):71–75, 1999 9922559

Wilhelm S, Phillips KA, Steketee G: Cognitive-Behavioral Therapy for Body Dysmorphic Disorder: A Treatment Manual. New York, Guilford, 2013

Wilhelm S, Phillips KA, Didie E, et al: Modular cognitive-behavioral therapy for body dysmorphic disorder: a randomized controlled trial. Behav Ther 45(3):314–327, 2014 24680228

Recommended Readings

International OCD Foundation: www.ocfoundation.org

Massachusetts General Hospital OCD and Related Disorders Program—Body Dysmorphic Disorder: www.massgeneral.org/bdd

Phillips KA: Understanding Body Dysmorphic Disorder: An Essential Guide. New York, Oxford University Press, 2009

Phillips KA, Hollander E: Treating body dysmorphic disorder with medication: evidence, misconceptions, and a suggested approach. Body Image 5(1):13–27, 2008

Rhode Island Hospital Body Dysmorphic Disorder Program: www.rhodeislandhospital.org/bdd

Veale D, Neziroglu F: Body Dysmorphic Disorder: A Treatment Manual. Chichester, West Sussex, UK, Wiley-Blackwell, 2010

Wilhelm S, Phillips KA, Steketee G: Cognitive-Behavioral Therapy for Body Dysmorphic Disorder: A Treatment Manual. New York, Guilford, 2013

CHAPTER 4

Hoarding Disorder

Ashley E. Nordsletten, Ph.D.
David Mataix-Cols, Ph.D.

Hoarding disorder (HD) is a newly recognized psychiatric diagnosis in DSM, formally debuting in the equally new "Obsessive-Compulsive and Related Disorders" chapter of DSM-5 (American Psychiatric Association 2013). As such, and despite the distress and impairment that typify its sufferers, HD remains a diagnostic entity that is unfamiliar to much of the psychiatric and general medical community. The aims of this chapter are, therefore, to acquaint clinicians with the diagnosis, epidemiology, clinical features, assessment, and known risk factors associated with HD. The concluding sections then offer guidelines for the clinical management of persons with HD.

Diagnostic Criteria and Symptomatology

Characterization of Hoarding Prior to DSM-5

Prior to DSM-5, hoarding was often conceptualized as a symptom of obsessive-compulsive disorder (OCD), despite not being directly mentioned either in DSM-IV-TR (American Psychiatric Association 2000) or in ICD-10 (World Health Organization 1992) as a typical symptom of OCD. Instead, "the inability to discard worn-out or worthless objects even when they have no sentimental value" was one of the eight criteria for obsessive-compulsive personality disorder (OCPD) in DSM-IV-TR (and remains so in DSM-5). By contrast, the equivalent diagnostic category in ICD-10 (called *anankastic personality disorder*) does not include such a criterion. When describing the differential diagnosis between OCPD and OCD, DSM-IV stated:

> Despite the similarity in names, obsessive-compulsive disorder is usually easily distinguished from obsessive-compulsive personality disorder by the presence of true obsessions and compulsions. A diagnosis of obsessive-compulsive disorder should be considered especially when hoarding is extreme (e.g., accumulated stacks of worthless objects present a fire hazard and make it difficult for others to walk through the house). When criteria for both disorders are met, both diagnoses should be recorded. (American Psychiatric Association 1994, pp. 671–672)

Of note, this clause was absent in editions of DSM prior to DSM-IV. Thus, although not explicitly stated in the OCD section, DSM-IV (and its text revision, DSM-IV-TR) assumed that when severe, hoarding *could* be a symptom of OCD. This allowed, for the first time, the assignment of an Axis I diagnosis to these individuals' condition, potentially enabling them to access treatment. However, it also created much confusion as clinicians struggled to decide whether a diagnosis of OCD was appropriate, particularly when hoarding appeared in the absence of other prototypical OCD symptoms (the majority of hoarding cases).

Indeed, a large volume of hoarding-specific work emerged that showed the vast majority of such cases did not meet diagnostic criteria for either OCD or OCPD (see Frost et al. 2011; Mataix-Cols et al. 2013; Pertusa et al. 2008, 2010b). Although it is clear that hoarding can emerge in the context of these conditions (e.g., retaining possessions due to fears of the items contaminating self or others), in most cases (>80%) hoarding symptoms appeared independent from such concerns. In addition, research noting important differences between hoarding and OCD regarding phenomenology, clinical course, cognitive-behavioral processes, neurocognitive correlates, and genetic profiles made evident the need to provide an alternative diagnostic category (for reviews, see Mataix-Cols et al. 2010; Pertusa et al. 2010a). Another important consideration was the fact that in many large OCD samples, hoarding consistently emerged as a predictor of poor treatment outcome (see Pertusa et al. 2010a for a review), suggesting that novel treatment approaches would be needed to handle hoarding cases and that splitting hoarding from OCD would lead to tighter diagnostic boundaries and better overall outcomes (Mataix-Cols et al. 2010).

These new insights, coupled with consideration of the obvious shortcomings of previous classification systems, ultimately led the DSM-5 Obsessive-

Compulsive Spectrum Sub-Work Group to propose the inclusion of HD in DSM-5 (Mataix-Cols et al. 2010). Extensive literature reviews on the topic were unanimous in their conclusion that HD fulfilled the definition of a "mental disorder" and that its inclusion as a new disorder offered more benefits (e.g., identifying a neglected majority of cases and enabling their access to care) than potential harms (Mataix-Cols and Pertusa 2012; Mataix-Cols et al. 2010; Nordsletten and Mataix-Cols 2012; see also Chapter 1, "Introduction and Major Changes for the Obsessive-Compulsive and Related Disorders in DSM-5," in this handbook). After extensive peer review, public consultation, and empirical validation of the proposed criteria, HD was finally approved for inclusion in DSM-5 in December 2012. To the best of our knowledge, ICD-11, which is still under development, is likely to follow suit and also include a similar diagnostic category.

The reasons for including HD in the chapter on obsessive-compulsive and related disorders (OCRDs) in DSM-5 are primarily historical, given the previous conceptualization of problematic hoarding as being a criterion of OCPD and/or a symptom of OCD. Although there are similarities between HD and other OCRDs (Phillips et al. 2010), it is also apparent that HD shares features with other emotional, impulse-control, and neurodevelopmental disorders, such as attention-deficit/hyperactivity disorder (Tolin and Villavicencio 2011). Predictably, forthcoming research will help further refine the most appropriate "neighborhood" for HD.

The DSM-5 subworkgroup also proposed the removal of the hoarding criterion of OCPD, a recommendation that was initially endorsed by the DSM-5 Personality and Personality Disorders Work Group (Mataix-Cols et al. 2010) but eventually not followed. Thus, in DSM-5, OCPD retains the "inability to discard objects" criterion, but clinicians are encouraged to consider the possibility of HD, rather than OCD, when the hoarding is "extreme" (American Psychiatric Association 2013, p. 681).

DSM-5 Hoarding Disorder

The diagnostic criteria for HD are provided in Box 4–1. As can be seen, the cardinal feature of the disorder involves a persistent and profound difficulty discarding or parting with one's possessions (Criterion A). The most commonly saved items are of a day-to-day type, such as newspapers, books, and old clothing, although the contents of a hoard may include possessions of any nature or value. Because of limited research, it is currently unclear whether accumulation of large numbers of animals in precarious veterinary conditions—a problematic behavior that is often referred to as "animal hoarding"—constitutes a special manifestation of HD or is underpinned in some cases by an alternative diagnosis (e.g., psychosis, dementia).

BOX 4–1. DSM-5 Diagnostic Criteria for Hoarding Disorder

A. Persistent difficulty discarding or parting with possessions, regardless of their actual value.

B. This difficulty is due to a perceived need to save the items and to distress associated with discarding them.

C. The difficulty discarding possessions results in the accumulation of possessions that congest and clutter active living areas and substantially compromises their intended use. If living areas are uncluttered, it is only because of the interventions of third parties (e.g., family members, cleaners, authorities).

D. The hoarding causes clinically significant distress or impairment in social, occupational, or other important areas of functioning (including maintaining a safe environment for self and others).

E. The hoarding is not attributable to another medical condition (e.g., brain injury, cerebrovascular disease, Prader-Willi syndrome).

F. The hoarding is not better explained by the symptoms of another mental disorder (e.g., obsessions in obsessive-compulsive disorder, decreased energy in major depressive disorder, delusions in schizophrenia or another psychotic disorder, cognitive deficits in major neurocognitive disorder, restricted interests in autism spectrum disorder).

Specify if:

> **With excessive acquisition:** If difficulty discarding possessions is accompanied by excessive acquisition of items that are not needed or for which there is no available space.

Specify if:

> **With good or fair insight:** The individual recognizes that hoarding-related beliefs and behaviors (pertaining to difficulty discarding items, clutter, or excessive acquisition) are problematic.

> **With poor insight:** The individual is mostly convinced that hoarding-related beliefs and behaviors (pertaining to difficulty discarding items, clutter, or excessive acquisition) are not problematic despite evidence to the contrary.

> **With absent insight/delusional beliefs:** The individual is completely convinced that hoarding-related beliefs and behaviors (pertaining to difficulty discarding items, clutter, or excessive acquisition) are not problematic despite evidence to the contrary.

Reprinted from American Psychiatric Association: *Diagnostic and Statistical Manual of Mental Disorders,* 5th Edition. Arlington, VA, American Psychiatric Association. Copyright 2013, American Psychiatric Association. Used with permission.

Regarding the reasons for difficulties discarding, patients typically cite the utilitarian value of their objects (e.g., "I'll use this in the future"), with strong sentimental attachment (e.g., "My mother gave me this") also emerging as a common factor. Alternative motives may include concerns about losing important information (e.g., "I am saving all these magazines to educate myself when I have more time to read them") and a desire to avoid being wasteful (e.g., "Discarding something that I see as usable means others won't be able to use it"). Individual patients are likely to report a combination of these underlying cognitions (see "Case Example: Fran" later in the chapter).

As a result of these concerns, individuals with HD experience marked distress when faced with the prospect of discarding their possessions (Criterion B). Avoidance of the discarding process, in turn, results in a buildup of items that clutter and congest the active living areas of a patient's home and substantially compromise their intended use (Criterion C). Those affected may be unable to sleep in their beds, sit in their living room, or cook in their kitchen. Extension of this clutter to space outside of the home is not uncommon, with gardens, vehicles, and even workplaces obstructed in some cases. Other patients pay for private storage spaces or ask family members to keep items in their home. In such cases, the hoarding activity is clearly problematic, but the home of the patient may appear relatively clutter free. It is for this reason that Criterion C may still be met in the presence of a usable environment, provided that this environment would be demonstrably cluttered and the item's use substantially compromised in the absence of "the interventions of third parties" (e.g., family members, housing authorities). The case example of Andrew, later in this chapter, illustrates such a scenario.

Patients' difficulties discarding and the obstruction caused by the associated clutter ultimately result in clinically significant distress and/or functional impairment (Criterion D). Functional impairment can take many forms, with patients reporting difficulties across social and occupational functioning. Health and safety issues, such as increased risk of falls or fires, are also widely reported and have been associated with increased rates of disability and mortality (e.g., due to "clutter avalanches"; Frost et al. 2000; Lucini et al. 2009; Tolin et al. 2008a). Quality of life is often notably impacted under such conditions and, as a consequence, family relationships are frequently strained (Drury et al. 2014). Resulting poor sanitation can pose broader health risks (e.g., respiratory diseases) and lead to legal proceedings ranging from forced clearings to evictions and, where relevant, the removal of dependents from the home (e.g., children, elderly charges; Frost et al. 2000). Despite these negative outcomes, individuals with HD may lack insight into the realities of their condition and deny the presence of the impairment that is evident to those in contact with them (Frost et al. 2010). In such cases, attempts to remove or discard the items will invariably generate conflict and distress on the part of the patient.

Criteria E and F address the importance of differential diagnosis in the process of diagnosing HD. Because hoarding symptoms can emerge in tandem with, or as a consequence of, a variety of medical and psychiatric con-

ditions, understanding whether the observed hoarding behavior is best characterized as HD is essential. This process is particularly important, given
that the condition at the root of the hoarding activity will have bearing on
the appropriate course of treatment. Thus, all non-HD causes of hoarding
behavior should be ruled out before a diagnosis of HD is settled upon (see
section "Differential Diagnosis" later in this chapter).

Other common associated features of HD are indecisiveness, perfectionism, avoidance, procrastination, difficulty planning and organizing tasks,
and distractibility (Frost and Hartl 1996; Frost et al. 2011; Steketee and Frost
2013), all of which are targeted in the cognitive-behavioral treatment of HD
(see section "Treatment").

Some individuals with HD (approximately 10%–20%) live in unsanitary
conditions, sometimes referred to as "domestic squalor" (Snowdon et al.
2012). The reasons for this are currently unclear. It is possible that patients
who have accumulated possessions for many decades may simply be unable
to reach and clean all areas of their homes, where dust, grime, dirt, and vermin may accumulate over time. In these cases, unsanitary living conditions
may be seen as a logical consequence of their condition. Another, not incompatible possibility is that impairment in executive functions may contribute to the inability to organize and keep a clean home environment. The
hypothesis that individuals with HD who live in unsanitary conditions have
more marked neuropsychological deficits, compared with patients who are
able to keep their homes clean, deserves empirical attention.

Specifiers

Once the diagnosis of HD has been established, clinicians should assess the
presence of two specifiers, which provide further clinically relevant information: 1) excessive acquisition and 2) level of insight (Box 4–1).

The "excessive acquisition" specifier is endorsed when an individual engages in the frequent and unnecessary acquisition of free or bought items.
Stealing of items is also covered under this specifier, although such behavior
is far less common than other forms of acquisition. Reducing excessive acquisition is one of the main goals when treating HD.

The "insight specifier" has three categories (good/fair, poor, absent/
delusional), which are intended to identify the degree to which individuals
recognize the problematic nature of their hoarding activity. When selecting
the appropriate level, clinicians should bear in mind that the definition of
insight for HD is somewhat different from that for OCD and body dysmorphic disorder. The evaluation of insight in HD requires the clinician to judge
the level of awareness patients have regarding the negative effects of their
symptoms (e.g., degree of functional impairment, risk to self and others, neg-

ative consequences for their families and neighbors). The presence of hoarding-related beliefs (e.g., a belief in the future utility of an object) is also relevant, although emphasized to a lesser degree in the HD conception of insight. Many patients with HD have limited insight into their difficulties and are reluctant to seek help (Tolin et al. 2010b). Increasing motivation for change is an integral part of the current psychological treatment for HD (Steketee and Frost 2013).

Case Example: Fran (A Typical Case of Hoarding Disorder With Excessive Acquisition)

For the past year, Fran has been living in a small corner of her large, two-bedroom apartment. Unable to access her bathroom or kitchen, she is reliant on public restroom facilities to bathe and must prepare and eat all of her meals outside of her home. Although she feels that she has "always" had difficulties discarding items, she reports that this behavior has worsened over time and become distinctly problematic in the years since her divorce, an event that resulted in her living independently for the first time. Currently, Fran's apartment is so overrun with possessions that she is unable to open her front door. Instead, she enters and exits the apartment through a heavily obstructed side door, which she can access only by crawling over the mounds of newspapers, books, and rubbish bags that occupy her floor space. In many areas, these piles of possessions reach the ceiling, making navigating the environment treacherous for Fran and anyone else who must access the apartment (e.g., building managers).

Regarding her reasons for saving items, Fran reports a strong belief in the utility of her possessions and expresses dismay at the ability of others to part with items that could be useful in the future. When prompted for an example, she relates how she recently watched someone throw away the lid of a yogurt cup in a public receptacle. Fran states that she "could not imagine doing something like this," and she promptly fished the item out of the garbage. This tendency to gather free or discarded items is typical for Fran, who finds it difficult to avoid the acquisition of any such items, particularly those that contain information (e.g., newspapers, flyers). In general, she enjoys her items and reports a strong attachment to the possessions she has amassed. She reports no ego-dystonic obsessions or compulsions that drive her saving and acquiring behaviors. However, she is increasingly distressed by her inability to use her home and states that she sometimes feels "homeless."

Her distress has been compounded recently, because the severity of her clutter has attracted the attention of the local housing authority, and Fran has subsequently begun receiving threats of eviction. She understands that to address these threats, she will need to discard items; however, the thought of starting to engage in this process makes her intolerably anxious. These threats, and her inability to address the issue, have prompted Fran to seek assistance from social services, who in turn referred her for psychiatric evaluation. A full psychiatric interview indicates that Fran endorses symptoms of depression and anxiety; however, these issues are not long-standing and appear linked to her current housing difficulties.

Case Example: Andrew (Hoarding Disorder With Clutter Obscured by Third-Party Intervention)

Andrew is a 40-year-old man who lives with his wife in a one-bedroom home. He reports difficulty discarding "always" and indicates particular problems parting with items he perceives as useful, such as books. Attempts to part with these items leave Andrew feeling intensely distressed, and as a result, he avoids the discarding process. In the past, this avoidance has resulted in extensive clutter throughout the pair's living environment. At its worst, Andrew and his wife were unable to use or access key areas of their home, including the living room and dining room. This arrangement has generated considerable discord in the family, and 2 years prior, Andrew's wife threatened to leave the marriage if he did not find a way to remove the items. Unable to face the prospect of discarding, he rented an additional apartment and external storage unit to house the obstructive items. Although these spaces were sufficient to accommodate his accumulation at the time, Andrew has continued acquiring items in the years since and can no longer confine his hoard to these additional properties. Unable to afford the rental of an additional space, he has now turned to family and friends, who have provided loft and garage space for the storage of various items.

As a result of this shuffling process, the level of clutter in Andrew's small home remains moderate, with key living spaces largely usable. However, the resources necessary to maintain the home's usable state have generated considerable distress. The financial burden of renting the extra storage space, for example, has been a continuous source of conflict between Andrew and his wife. In addition, relatives who thought they were offering him only short-term storage have become frustrated at the continued presence of possessions in their homes and have threatened to donate or discard these items. Despite these tensions, Andrew remains unwilling to part with any of the items and is currently looking for alternative means of storing them. Although he would prefer to bring all the items back into the home, he admits that this would be "impossible," because the proliferating items would "surely fill the home and then some."

Case Example: Scott (Hoarding in the Context of Obsessive-Compulsive Disorder)

Scott is a 30-year-old single man. Since the age of 19, he has experienced a persistent and troubling concern that he might contaminate and ultimately harm others. In response to this worry, he began spending several hours a day engaging in various cleaning rituals, centered on both himself (e.g., washing his hands, showering repeatedly) and his home environment. Several years later, he began to experience difficulties discarding items, as a result of a growing concern that individuals coming into contact with his discarded items might become contaminated. At present, he is unable to discard anything that has entered his home environment, including old food and general rubbish. Scott also reports feeling strongly compelled to acquire any item that he comes into contact with outside of the home—purchasing, for example, every orange he touches in the fruit bin at the grocery store or each newspaper in a stack of newspapers—because of concern that leaving any item he may have touched will put others at risk of infection. The influx of these items, and his inability to discard anything that enters the home, have left Scott unable to use his living space. At the time of assessment, he reports being unable to sleep in his bedroom, with the clutter extending throughout other key living areas and obstructing their use. When asked, he reports that he has no affection for or attachment to his items and would be very happy to part with them. However, his fears regarding contamination continue to preclude this action. This reality is highly distressing to Scott, who understands the irrationality of his thoughts and behaviors but remains paralyzed by the anxiety produced by his contamination concerns.

Epidemiology

Initial community surveys estimated the point prevalence of clinically significant hoarding to be 2%–6% in adults and 2% in adolescents (Fullana et al. 2010; Iervolino et al. 2009; Ivanov et al. 2013; Samuels et al. 2008). However, inconsistencies in the methods used to define hoarding in these studies—some relying on items from OCD measures, others using self-report scales of hoarding severity—made findings incomparable and conclusions difficult to draw.

In a more recent epidemiological study, the only study to date to define cases using the full DSM-5 criteria, the prevalence of HD was approximately 1.5% in adult men and women (Nordsletten et al. 2013a). This estimate, which was obtained principally through diagnostic interviews conducted face-to-face in the participants' homes (in 96% of cases), contrasts with some prior work (e.g., Iervolino et al. 2009; Samuels et al. 2009) in its suggestion that rates of HD are balanced across the genders. By contrast, help-seeking clinical samples are predominantly female, perhaps reflecting better insight and motivation for change (Pertusa et al. 2010b). Epidemiological studies are more consistent in their finding that the prevalence of HD seems to increase with advancing age (Nordsletten et al. 2013a; Samuels et al. 2008).

Consistent with the clinical observation of strained interpersonal relationships in hoarding cases (e.g., Drury et al. 2014), epidemiological investigations suggest that individuals with HD have lower rates of marriage and higher rates of divorce than their healthy counterparts (Nordsletten et al. 2013c; Timpano et al. 2011). In our epidemiological study (Nordsletten et al. 2013a), participants with HD were also significantly more likely to endorse a comorbid mental disorder and to feel that their hoarding difficulties impaired their social and occupational functioning. These findings accord with earlier studies suggesting that rates of other mental disorders (e.g., anxiety and DSM-IV mood disorders) are higher among individuals who endorse the hoarding dimension of an OCD screener (Fullana et al. 2010) as well as those who self-identify with hoarding difficulties (e.g., Frost et al. 2011).

Although such findings offer a working portrait of the HD population, it is crucial to bear in mind the limitations and barriers faced by such studies in recruiting individuals with HD. For example, while door-to-door recruitment is a standard recruitment strategy in epidemiological work, its utility for accessing the HD population is questionable given the concerns (e.g., eviction) and practical constraints (e.g., ability to move through the clutter) that may limit these individuals' willingness or ability to open their door. A lack of insight into the hoarding activity, or embarrassment regarding the state of the home, may further limit or bias participant samples. Future work will need to prioritize access to these challenging cases to ensure an accurate representation of this disorder's prevalence and characteristics.

Comorbidity

As noted in previous sections, before HD became a separate disorder in DSM-5, individuals with hoarding difficulties were often diagnosed as having OCD. Although the prevalence of comorbid OCD appears elevated in individuals with HD compared with the general population, with current estimates ranging from 5% to 24%, other comorbidities appear to be at least as common. The most common comorbid disorders are generalized anxiety disorder (31%–37%), major depressive disorder (26%–31%), panic disorder (17%), social anxiety disorder (14%), and posttraumatic stress disorder (14%) (Frost et al. 2011; Fullana et al. 2010; Mataix-Cols et al. 2013; Nordsletten et al. 2013c; Pertusa et al. 2010a). Symptoms typical of attention-deficit/hyperactivity disorder, particularly inattention, are also commonly reported (Tolin and Villavicencio 2011). These comorbidities, rather than the hoarding, may often be the main reason for clinical consultation. Although these additional symptoms may contribute to the overall impairment and disability of individuals with HD, the core symptoms of HD are, themselves, usually sufficient to cause clinically significant impairment.

General medical conditions may also be highly frequent in patients with HD, with epidemiological work indicating that the presence of HD is associated with both poorer perceived physical health and higher rates of disability (Nordsletten et al. 2013a). These limitations may be particularly evident in elderly individuals, who appear to have a disproportionally high rate of medical complications of HD, compared with age-matched control subjects (Ayers et al. 2014).

Course and Prognosis

Although prospective longitudinal studies are lacking, the course of HD appears to often be chronic and progressive. The inclusion of the word *persis-*

tent in the diagnostic criteria reflects this reality and is based on findings from retrospective studies that suggest hoarding symptoms are experienced constantly over time in the majority of cases (Mataix-Cols et al. 2010). In general, individuals with HD report that their hoarding behavior emerged in childhood or adolescence, although these individuals may not have met full HD diagnostic criteria at that time (Ayers et al. 2010; Grisham et al. 2006; Ivanov et al. 2013). Thereafter, a steady worsening of symptoms is typically reported over each decade of life (Ayers et al. 2010). Interference with everyday functioning generally emerges by the mid-20s, with clinically significant impairment developing a decade or so later (Grisham et al. 2006; Landau et al. 2011). Thus, based on retrospective report studies, many individuals may endorse full diagnostic criteria for HD by the mid-30s. Problems with acquisition, when they do emerge, appear to do so (or become more evident) earlier than problems with discarding (Grisham et al. 2006).

Emerging research also suggests that exposure to traumatic or emotionally distressing events, such as the death of a loved one, may precede the onset or exacerbation of symptoms in some cases, although further work is needed to establish any temporal or causal relationship (Landau et al. 2011). In such cases, addressing this trauma will be an additional challenge in the therapeutic process, just as the presence of medical complications are likely to present challenges for work in geriatric hoarding populations.

Psychosocial Impairment

Individuals with HD typically have a high degree of functional impairment. The presence of disorganized clutter throughout their living environment can preclude even basic activities, such as cooking or bathing, and puts patients at significantly higher risk for chronic illness (e.g., asthma, diabetes), fires, and injurious falls (Frost et al. 2000; Grisham et al. 2007; Lucini et al. 2009). These health and safety issues, which may also include unsanitary conditions or blocked exits, have been associated with increased disability and even mortality in this group (e.g., due to inability to navigate through the clutter during a fire) (Frost et al. 2000; Lucini et al. 2009). Legal repercussions, including the threat of eviction (6%) or the mandatory clearing of possessions, are also possible outcomes and have been associated, at least anecdotally, with marked rates of distress and instances of suicide among hoarding cases (Tolin et al. 2008a).

Beyond their physical impacts, the symptoms of HD can dramatically impair a person's quality of life, as well as the quality of life experienced by individuals in contact with him or her (Drury et al. 2014; Saxena 2011). Reduced rates of marriage and increased rates of divorce offer evidence of widespread domestic challenges (Mataix-Cols et al. 2013; Nordsletten et al.

2013c). In some extreme cases, the obstruction caused by the clutter is so pronounced that the needs of dependents (e.g., children, aging parents) can no longer be met, leading to the removal or relocation of these family members outside the home (Tolin et al. 2008b). Unsurprisingly, family relationships are highly strained in these contexts, with feelings of burden, distress, frustration, and rejection common among the adult relatives of those who hoard (Drury et al. 2014; Tolin et al. 2008b). Individuals with HD often report feelings of more pervasive social isolation and withdrawal (e.g., from work) as a result of their hoarding activity (Frost et al. 2000; Mataix-Cols et al. 2010; Pertusa et al. 2008). Dependence on caretakers and/or social services (e.g., unemployment benefits) also appears common in hoarding populations (Nordsletten et al. 2013a).

Developmental Considerations

Hoarding behaviors often emerge in the early years of life, with most patients retrospectively reporting a long-standing overattachment to possessions, often since childhood (Grisham et al. 2006; Ivanov et al. 2013). Despite these reports, research focused on the nature and prevalence of hoarding activity in young persons has only recently started to emerge (Ivanov et al. 2013).

The limited work in this area may be attributable, at least in part, to the inherent limitations of examining hoarding activity in this group; parental control of both acquisition and the home environment may, for instance, limit or eliminate evidence of hoarding activity in children and adolescents, and these parental interventions can be difficult to quantify. In addition, most children, at some stage, engage in collecting behavior that may resemble HD but that typically diminishes in intensity and disappears before adolescence. In the intervening years, adequate berth must be given for the passing of these developmentally appropriate saving activities. Recent work examining the prevalence of hoarding in adolescents (age 15 years) has acknowledged such considerations and tentatively estimated that 2% of the study population self-endorsed distressing or impairing hoarding symptoms (Ivanov et al. 2013), although it is unclear to what extent these symptoms reflect DSM-5 HD. Whether these difficulties represent early markers for the future development of HD therefore remains an important question for the future.

Patients who present to clinicians for treatment often do so late in life— an average age of 50 is typical for first-time treatment seekers—although the hoarding behavior, if it is part of HD, will often have been present for decades. In geriatric populations, HD may be particularly challenging, given the disproportionally high rate of medical complications, coupled with a reduced rate of health service utilization, compared with age-matched control subjects (Ayers et al. 2014). Furthermore, there is some suggestion in the literature that older adults with HD may be harder to engage in psychological treatment and tend to achieve poorer treatment outcomes (Ayers et al. 2011; Turner et al. 2010) compared with younger individuals, suggesting the need for early intervention in HD.

Gender–Related Issues

Because most early work focused on hoarding experienced in OCD populations, the relevance of these data for DSM-5 HD is questionable. In clinical, often self-referred, samples of individuals with hoarding difficulties, there is a clear predominance of female participants, perhaps reflecting better insight into their condition. In epidemiological samples, studies are split on whether hoarding activity is more common in one gender versus another. As noted previously, this research is characterized by considerable variation in operational definitions of "problematic hoarding," with early studies adapting OCD measures to evaluate and establish hoarding "caseness" (Ruscio et al. 2010) and later works employing hoarding-specific scales (Timpano et al. 2011) and clinical interviews (Nordsletten et al. 2013a). By changing the criteria for inclusion in the "case" population, these variant approaches have resulted in similarly variant descriptions of who constitutes this population. Although some epidemiological work suggests that severe hoarding is more common among men, the only epidemiological study to employ DSM-5 criteria found no gender differences in prevalence (Nordsletten et al. 2013a).

Small samples in studies specific to HD (as opposed to the broader concept of hoarding behavior) have limited the ability to carry out analyses by gender, leaving open the question of gender differences in regard to symptom phenomenology and comorbidity. In one rare example, Frost et al. (2011) found no gender differences in the endorsement of most common comorbid conditions (e.g., major depression, generalized anxiety, social phobia). The only exception concerned rates of OCD, which were higher among men (28%) than women (15%). Clearly, additional work is needed on this important issue.

Cultural Aspects of Phenomenology

Very little work has explored hoarding behavior through a cultural lens. Although it is well known that hoarding activity occurs outside of the Western world—with cases documented in Africa, Brazil, China, India, Iran, Japan, and Korea (Mataix-Cols et al. 2010)—these studies have shared the methodological limitations that characterize many of the hoarding investigations in the United States and Europe (e.g., focus on OCD measures and populations), making firm conclusions difficult to draw regarding the accuracy of prevalence estimates and their relevance for DSM-5 HD. Nonetheless, rates of problematic hoarding (as defined by self-report measures of hoarding severity) appear reasonably similar across cultures. Timpano et al. (2013), for example, have suggested similar rates of "clinically significant" hoarding activity among students in the United States (6%) and Germany (8%). Findings from a cross-European study, however, suggested variations in the prevalence of hoarding symptoms by country, with individuals in the Netherlands (odds ratio [OR]=0.21) significantly less likely than those in Belgium (OR = 1.85), France (OR=1.94), or Italy (OR=1.87) to endorse these behaviors (Fullana et al. 2010). Given the questionable validity of the measures and methods underlying these (and other) findings, additional work will be required to clarify current impressions.

Assessment and Differential Diagnosis

Assessment

Hoarding symptoms often need to be specifically asked about, because many patients may not spontaneously volunteer this information. The use of some simple screening questions, such as those offered in Table 4–1, may initiate a fruitful dialogue in such cases and can rapidly lead to a potential diagnosis.

TABLE 4–1.   Some quick screening questions for hoarding disorder

"Are the rooms of your home so full of items that it is hard for you to use these rooms normally?"

"Do you have difficulty discarding possessions?"

"Do you get upset if somebody suggests that you remove/throw away some of these items?"

A formal HD diagnosis requires an interview with a trained assessor, ideally in the person's home environment. The Structured Interview for Hoarding Disorder (SIHD; Nordsletten et al. 2014) is a freely available, validated, semistructured instrument that was designed to assist clinicians with the nuanced evaluation of this disorder (see Table 4–2). The content of this interview maps directly onto the DSM-5 criteria for HD, with questions relating to each diagnostic criterion and the specifiers. Its suitability for establishing the HD diagnosis has been demonstrated in several studies, including the London Field Trial for Hoarding Disorder, which showed that diagnoses determined using the instrument showed an excellent balance of sensitivity (0.98) and specificity (1.0) (Mataix-Cols et al. 2013).

TABLE 4–2. Commonly used clinician- and self-administered measures of hoarding and related symptoms

Measure	Description	Subscales	Score range	Clinical mean	Cutoff point
Structured Interview for Hoarding Disorder (Nordsletten et al. 2014)	Semistructured diagnostic interview developed alongside DSM-5 containing a core section to assess the presence of each DSM-5 HD criterion and associated specifiers; a differential diagnosis module to assist with parsing HD from OCD and ASD; and a risk assessment checklist	NA	NA	NA	NA
Saving Inventory—Revised (SI-R; Frost et al. 2004)	A 23-item questionnaire measuring the severity of hoarding symptoms across three core domains: excessive acquisition, saving and discarding behaviors and clutter; self-report	SI-R Total	0–92	62.00 (12.70)	41
		SI-R Acquisition	0–28	6.40 (3.60)	9
		SI-R Clutter	0–36	26.90 (6.60)	17
		SI-R Difficulty Discarding	0–28	9.20 (5.00)	14

TABLE 4–2. Commonly used clinician- and self-administered measures of hoarding and related symptoms *(continued)*

Measure	Description	Subscales	Score range	Clinical mean	Cutoff point
Clutter Image Rating (CIR; Frost et al. 2008)	Three-item, photograph-based instrument offering an objective reference point for the evaluation of "clinically significant clutter" in a hoarding environment; may be used as self-report or clinician report	CIR Average (average of rating for three rooms)	1–9	4.01 (1.80)	4
		CIR Total (sum of the ratings for three rooms)	3–27	NA	NA
Hoarding Rating Scale (HRS; Tolin et al. 2010a)	Five-item measure evaluating the severity of core hoarding symptoms and excessive acquisition; may be used as self-report (HRS-SR) or clinician-administered interview (HRS-I)	HRS Total	0–40	24.22 (5.67)	14
Hoarding Disorder Dimensional Scale (HD-D; American Psychiatric Association 2013)	Five-item dimensional measure developed for DSM-5; evaluates the severity of core hoarding symptoms and avoidance; based on the HRS; self-report	HD-D Total	0–20	12.6 (4.6)[a]	Not known

TABLE 4–2. Commonly used clinician- and self-administered measures of hoarding and related symptoms *(continued)*

Measure	Description	Subscales	Score range	Clinical mean	Cutoff point
UCLA Hoarding Severity Scale (UHSS; Saxena et al. 2007)	A 10-item semistructured scale assessing the presence and severity of the following hoarding-related components: clutter, urges to save items, excessive acquisition, difficulty discarding, social and occupational impairment, indecision and procrastination; scores reflect mean rate of occurrence for each symptom in the prior week; clinician administered	UHSS Total	0–40	26 (3.7)	Not known
Compulsive Acquisition Scale (CAS; Frost et al. 2002)	An 18-item questionnaire screening for the presence of excessive acquisition behaviors; acquisition of both free and bought items assessed; self-report	CAS Total	18–126	62.57 (19.30)[a]	48
		CAS Buy	12–84	NA	41
		CAS Free	6–42	NA	23

TABLE 4–2. Commonly used clinician- and self-administered measures of hoarding and related symptoms *(continued)*

Measure	Description	Subscales	Score range	Clinical mean	Cutoff point
Saving Cognitions Inventory (SCI; Steketee et al. 2003)	A 24-item questionnaire assessing the beliefs underlying a patient's saving behavior; self-report	SCI Total	24–168	104.00 (26.60)	NA
		SCI Control	3–21	16.30 (4.30)	NA
		SCI Emotional Attachment	10–70	40.00 (14.60)	NA
		SCI Memory	5–35	23.50 (6.20)	NA
		SCI Responsibility	6–42	24.70 (8.00)	NA

Note. ASD = autism spectrum disorder; HD = hoarding disorder; NA = not applicable; OCD = obsessive-compulsive disorder.
[a]Mataix-Cols et al. 2013.

Because the diagnosis of HD requires the presence of obstructive clutter (Criterion C), diagnostic assessments (such as the SIHD) are ideally done in the person's home environment. This approach enables the clinician to tangibly evaluate the scale of the clutter, assess the extent of the resulting obstruction/impairment, and determine the presence of health and safety risks (e.g., fire hazards, infestations, unsanitary living conditions) (Snowdon et al. 2012; Tolin et al. 2008a). To assist with this process, the SIHD also contains a risk assessment module.

When in-home assessments are not possible, clinicians can use photographs to assess the extent of clutter (Fernández de la Cruz et al. 2013). These photographs can be used in combination with the Clutter Image Rating (Frost et al. 2008), which consists of a series of photographs depicting increasingly obstructive levels of clutter across the bedroom, kitchen, and living room (see Table 4–2).

When patients with HD show limited or absent insight into their hoarding activity, a situation that may arise in a substantial proportion of hoarding cases, a multiple-informant approach (e.g., seeking both patient reports and information available from third parties) may be particularly helpful (Frost et al. 2010). Given that much of this population does not recognize their problem, clinicians may find that few of their hoarding patients are voluntarily presenting for assessment or treatment. Accordingly, during the assessment process, the clinician should be aware that conflicts may arise between the patients' accounts of their behavior and the portrait provided by third parties (e.g., patient records, social service reports, consultation with family members). Discrepancies should be tactfully addressed and clarification requested from all relevant sources. Should discrepancies persist, the clinician will need to exercise his or her clinical judgment in making a diagnostic determination.

Differential Diagnosis

As indicated by DSM-5 Criteria E and F, hoarding behavior can emerge as a consequence of a range of general medical and psychiatric conditions; in these cases, HD should not be diagnosed. Ruling out these alternative conditions is a crucial component of the diagnostic process, because determining the condition at the root of the hoarding behavior will have implications for treatment selection and response.

In accordance with Criterion E, HD should not be endorsed if the accumulation of objects can be attributed to a general medical condition, such as traumatic brain injury, brain tumor, cerebrovascular disease, infections of the central nervous system (e.g., herpes simplex encephalitis), or rare genetic conditions (e.g., Prader-Willi syndrome). For example, it is known that damage to the anterior ventromedial prefrontal and cingulate cortices is associated with the excessive, often indiscriminate, accumulation of objects (e.g., Anderson et al. 2005; Mataix-Cols et al. 2011). Among such individuals, the appearance of hoarding activity is inconsistent with their normal behavioral patterns and occurs suddenly following the traumatic event (Anderson et al. 2005). The nature of attachment to possessions is often unusual in these cases, with some individuals expressing little interest in their accumulated items and appearing indifferent to the discarding process (thus not fulfilling Criterion B), and others showing a strong reluctance to discard items that did not exist prior to the brain injury. In evaluating such cases, the focus of the clinician should be foremost on establishing the temporal relationship between the onset of the medical condition and onset of the hoarding activity. If, after the patient's history is taken, it is found that the hoarding activity predates the medical condition, the clinician will need to carefully consider the relevance of the remaining DSM-5 criteria before proceeding with an HD diagnosis (Mataix-Cols et al. 2011).

Likewise, a diagnosis of HD is inappropriate if the accumulation of objects is judged to be the consequence of a neurocognitive disorder, such as Alzheimer's disease or another degenerative condition (particularly those affecting the frontotemporal regions). In such cases, the hoarding behavior is likely to be accompanied by unusual features, such as severe self-neglect or domestic squalor, alongside other common neuropsychiatric symptoms, such as tics, disinhibition, gambling, ritualizing, and self-injurious activity (Snowdon et al. 2012).

HD should also not be diagnosed if the hoarding activity can be explained by the presence of a relevant neurodevelopmental disorder, such as autism spectrum disorder (ASD). Although research is sparse, it is known that individuals with ASD may engage in "restrictive repetitive behaviors and interests," which sometimes includes seeking or collecting objects. Thus, if problematic hoarding activity in a person with ASD appears confined to a single area of preoccupation (e.g., items are unified by a particular physical characteristic, such as texture [e.g., accumulating only shiny objects]), or the emphasis is on classifying objects rather than hoarding the objects, full DSM-5 HD criteria are not met, and the HD diagnosis should not be given (Pertusa et al. 2008).

Hoarding activity can also present as a symptom of several other psychiatric disorders, including schizophrenia (or other psychotic disorders), major depression, and OCD, in which case HD should not be diagnosed. For instance, when hoarding activity can be directly attributed to the delusions or negative symptoms of a schizophrenia spectrum disorder or the fatigue or loss of energy typifying a major depressive episode, a diagnosis of HD would be inappropriate. However, when the hoarding behavior occurs alongside these conditions but is judged independent of them (e.g., different onset and course, treatment response), a dual diagnosis (e.g., OCD and HD) may be considered appropriate.

In the context of OCD, hoarding behaviors most commonly emerge as a consequence of symmetry obsessions, feelings of incompleteness, or not "just right" perceptions (e.g., the compulsive urge to record and catalogue all possible life experiences in written or photographic form), in addition to more traditional concerns such as fears of harm or contamination (e.g., avoidance of discarding items for fear of contaminating or harming other people; see the case of Scott earlier in the chapter) (Pertusa et al. 2010b). Excessive accumulation of objects can also result from the avoidance that may be seen in typical OCD rituals. For example, a patient with OCD contamination obsessions may elect to stop discarding items such as garbage if doing so would necessitate endless washing or checking rituals. In these types of cases, in which the hoarding behavior is a symptom of OCD rather than HD, the behavior is generally experienced as unwanted. In contrast, in HD the person wishes to retain saved items and would be significantly distressed by the thought of discarding them.

Furthermore, rather than holding a strong emotional attachment to the involved items, those with OCD-based hoarding behavior usually perceive little to no sentimental or instrumental value in their obstructive possessions. Such individuals are furthermore unlikely to engage in the excessive acquisition that is common in HD; if present, items are usually acquired as a consequence of a specific obsession (e.g., the need to buy items that have been touched, in order to avoid contaminating others) rather than due to a genuine desire to possess them.

Further diagnostic assessment that is specific to the condition of concern (e.g., Autism Diagnostic Observation Schedule, Yale-Brown Obsessive Compulsive Scale) may be particularly valuable in complex cases. Clinicians may also find that clinical records, referral notes, or consultation with knowledgeable third parties (e.g., family members, social services) offers an informative complement to details divulged during the patient interview. In addition, examination of the clutter itself may offer diagnostic clues, because certain classes of items (e.g., body products, rotting vegetation) and patterns of disorganization (e.g., inappropriate storage of items, such as perishable food hidden in clothing) may evidence underlying neurological (e.g., dementia) or psychiatric (e.g., OCD, psychosis) conditions (Pertusa et al. 2010b). For a concise summary of considerations in the context of differential diagnosis, see Table 4–3.

It is also important to note the differences between HD and normative collecting, a common and benign human activity (Table 4–4). Both theoretical reviews (Nordsletten and Mataix-Cols 2012) and empirical work (Mataix-Cols et al. 2013; Nordsletten et al. 2013c) indicate that the vast ma-

TABLE 4–3. Some key features broadly differentiating hoarding disorder (HD) from alternative conditions

Feature	Expression in HD	Other conditions
Difficulties discarding	Essential for the diagnosis; attempts to discard or part with possessions result in considerable distress and anxiety.	May or may not be present. If the individual demonstrates indifference to the discarding process (e.g., little evident anxiety when items are removed by a family member or third party), alternative diagnostic options, such as organic brain damage, should be explored. In some cases, the buildup of possessions could be the product of, for example, lack of energy in major depression or negative symptoms in schizophrenia spectrum disorders. In other cases, the individual may experience great distress when discarding items (e.g., hoarding due to fears of contamination in OCD or special interests in ASD).
Reasons for acquiring/ saving	Items are sought and saved due to the patient's belief in their utility, strong emotional attachment to the items, not wanting to lose important information, or fear of being wasteful. Items are often imbued with intense meaning and viewed as comforting or valuable.	Items may be saved indiscriminately and for no apparent reason (e.g., in brain damage or dementia), accumulate passively (e.g., in depression), be saved because of an underlying obsession (e.g., "I and thus my items are contaminated"), or be saved because of a persecutory or paranoid delusion (e.g., "My items have personal information that will be used against me") and will generally not hold positive meaning for the individual. In ASD, the individual may have a strong and very focused interest in certain classes of objects.

TABLE 4–3. Some key features broadly differentiating hoarding disorder (HD) from alternative conditions *(continued)*

Feature	Expression in HD	Other conditions
Excessive acquisition	Present in most but not all cases; usually ego-syntonic in nature, at least initially.	May or may not be present. The accumulation of objects may be passive (e.g., in depression) or active (e.g., in brain damage or ASD). Excessive acquisition is rare in OCD, and when present, the behavior is largely ego-dystonic (driven by an unwanted urge or to prevent a feared consequence).
Symptom onset/ Clinical course	Usually gradual, chronic, and progressive; difficulties discarding emerge early in life and worsen with each decade of life.	May be sudden or gradual. A sudden onset of hoarding symptoms that are incongruous with previous activity may result from brain injury (e.g., damage to the frontal lobe). In neurodegenerative disorders (e.g., dementia), the onset may be more gradual. The rapid formation of severe clutter at a young age (e.g., prior to age 30), when no brain injury is present, may also suggest the presence of an alternative psychiatric condition such as ASD or OCD.

TABLE 4–3.   Some key features broadly differentiating hoarding disorder (HD) from alternative conditions *(continued)*

Feature	Expression in HD	Other conditions
Nature and treatment of objects	Any item can be saved, usually everyday objects like newspapers, books, or clothes. The clutter emerging in HD is typified by a high degree of disorganization, with items of varied value and function piled together across the living environment. It is this trademark disorganization that results in the functionally obstructed living quarters that, by definition, characterize HD environments. Although many individuals with HD save their items out of a belief they will "use them in the future," the disorganization ultimately results in the loss of this perceived utility as the items are lost or forgotten amid the hoard.	The saving of "bizarre" items, such as body products (e.g., feces, rotten food), is usually indicative of an alternative diagnosis (e.g., brain damage, schizophrenia, or dementia). Items may or may not be disorganized. In ASD, items are largely bound by a shared theme (i.e., special interest) or physical characteristic (e.g., material, texture or shape), and the individual regularly organizes or classifies his or her items.

TABLE 4–3. Some key features broadly differentiating hoarding disorder (HD) from alternative conditions *(continued)*

Feature	Expression in HD	Other conditions
Self-neglect and unhygienic (squalid) living conditions	Self-neglect and unhygienic or squalid living conditions are relatively rare in HD; HD is usually characterized by "clean clutter."	Self-neglect and severe domestic squalor are usually indicative of organic, neurodegenerative, or schizophrenia spectrum disorders.
Other features	No severe personality changes or other unusual behaviors that are incongruous with the person's premorbid behavior.	In "organic" cases, hoarding behavior may be accompanied by severe personality changes and other "out of character" behaviors, such as gambling, inappropriate sexual behavior, theft, stereotypies, or self-injurious behaviors.

Note. ASD=autism spectrum disorder; OCD=obsessive-compulsive disorder.

jority of collectors do not meet the diagnostic criteria for HD. Distinguishing hoarding from culturally typical (even eccentric) collecting behaviors is generally a straightforward endeavor.

Clinician- and Self-Administered Measures of Hoarding Severity and Associated Features

Once the HD diagnosis is made, a number of clinician- and self-administered measures can be used to assess the nature and severity of symptoms in patients with this diagnosis (see Table 4–2). Measures of this kind permit key hoarding symptoms to be rated on varying, Likert-type scales that correspond to increasing severity of the behavior.

Additional measures that assess problematic acquisition (e.g., Compulsive Acquisition Scale; Frost et al. 2002), self-reported squalor (e.g., Home Environment Index; Rasmussen et al. 2014), and caregiver burden and accommodation (e.g., Family Impact Scale for Hoarding Disorder; Nordsletten et al. 2013b) are available and may prove useful for clarifying the clinical picture.

Etiology and Risk Factors

Research into the causes and risk factors of HD is in its infancy. As in most psychiatric disorders, it would be expected that a complex interplay between genetic and environmental factors confers risk of developing HD.

Although controlled family studies have not yet been carried out, patient self-report suggests that hoarding runs in families (Pertusa et al. 2008). Consistently, a handful of twin studies conducted in large, population-based adult twin samples suggest that this familiality is largely attributable to additive genetic factors (with heritabilities ranging between 36% and 50%), with the remaining variance attributable to nonshared environmental factors and measurement error (Iervolino et al. 2009; Mathews et al. 2014). Of interest, recent work in adolescent Swedish twins has indicated possible sex-based variations regarding the role of genes and environment in hoarding symptoms, suggesting that the etiology of HD may be dynamic across the life span, with the roles of genes and environment varying over time and between the sexes (Ivanov et al. 2013).

Additional research in twins suggests substantial, yet incomplete, genetic overlap between core symptoms of HD (i.e., difficulties discarding) and theoretically linked behaviors (i.e., excessive acquisition), while nonshared environmental influences appear to be more specific to each of these traits (Nordsletten et al. 2013d). This work lends some support to the placement of excessive acquisition as a specifier of HD rather than as a core criterion.

TABLE 4–4. Features differentiating hoarding disorder (HD) from normative collecting

Feature	Normative collecting	Hoarding disorder
Object content	Focused; objects are bound by a cohesive theme and the accumulation is confined to a narrow range of object "types."	Unfocused; objects lack a cohesive theme and the accumulation consists of a broad range of object "types."
Acquisition process	Structured; acquisition of collected items is carried out in structured stages, including planning, hunting, and organizing.	Unstructured; acquisition is frequent and often impulsive, characterized by a lack of advanced planning, focused searching, and/or organization.
Excessive acquisition	Possible; estimates indicate that a minority of collectors (≤40%) endorse the excessive acquisition specifier; when present, acquisition is most often focused on "bought items."	Common; estimates suggest that the vast majority of individuals with HD (≥80%) engage in this behavior; when present, excessive acquisition typically extends to both free and bought items.
Level of organization	High; collectors' rooms are characterized by functionality, with collected items arranged, stored, or displayed in an orderly fashion.	Low; individuals with HD are typified by the disorganization of their living spaces, with the functionality of rooms compromised by pervasive, haphazard clutter.

TABLE 4–4. Features differentiating hoarding disorder (HD) from normative collecting (*continued*)

Feature	Normative collecting	Hoarding disorder
Presence of distress	Rare; the majority of collectors derive pleasure from their activity; for a minority, collecting may result in distress, most often due to factors unrelated to clutter (e.g., financial burden of acquiring desired pieces).	Required for diagnosis; this distress often stems from the presence of excessive clutter and the limitations this clutter imposes on the person's functionality.
Social impairment	Minimal; collectors show typical rates of marriage and often engage in social relationships (e.g., hobby clubs, collector societies) as part of their collecting behavior.	Severe; those individuals who hoard consistently show reduced rates of marriage and increased rates of relationship conflict and social withdrawal. These issues are often attributed directly to their hoarding activities.
Occupational interference	Rare; scores on objective measures, such as the Work and Social Adjustment Scale, indicate that collectors experience little impairment in their work attendance or productivity.	Common; research indicates that as hoarding severity increases, so too does the person's level of occupational impairment and nonparticipation in work activities.

Source. Adapted from Nordsletten et al. 2013c.

The mechanism by which either genetic or environmental features, or their interaction, confer risk for the development of HD remains unknown; as yet, specific genes have not been consistently identified, and although research has suggested some unique environmental risk factors (e.g., traumatic life events), small samples and retrospective self-report methods leave unclear the role of such exposures in the onset or exacerbation of HD (Iervolino et al. 2009; Landau et al. 2011). Anecdotal links between material deprivation and hoarding activity have, meanwhile, received no support in the relevant literature (Landau et al. 2011).

Future work is warranted to understand how specific genetic and environmental risk factors interact to confer risk to individuals carefully diagnosed as having HD. It is likely that these genetic and environmental risk factors will be, at least in part, shared with related conditions such as OCD and other related disorders, as recently suggested in a population-based twin study using self-report measures (Monzani et al. 2014). The etiological links between HD and other neuropsychiatric conditions (e.g., anxiety and DSM-IV-TR mood disorders, attention-deficit/hyperactivity disorder) remain to be explored.

It is difficult to draw firm conclusions from early reports on the neuropsychology and neural substrates of HD (see Mataix-Cols et al. 2011). Many of the initial neuropsychological studies recruited OCD patients with hoarding symptoms (with different degrees of severity), whereas others recruited individuals with severe hoarding but predominantly without OCD. The neuropsychological tests employed have been heterogeneous and have tapped into different domains, and few employed psychiatric control groups. Findings to date suggest possible impairments in spatial planning, visuospatial learning and memory, sustained attention/working memory, organization, response inhibition, set shifting, probabilistic learning, and reversal (Mataix-Cols et al. 2011; Woody et al. 2014).

The neural substrates of hoarding behavior in nonhuman animals are well established, but much less is known about normal and abnormal hoarding behavior in humans. Useful clues come from case studies of brain-damaged patients and of individuals with dementia, particularly of the frontotemporal type. This research suggests that the ventromedial prefrontal/anterior cingulate cortices as well as medial temporal regions may be implicated in hoarding behavior (Mataix-Cols et al. 2011). One theory is that the former cortical regions modulate or suppress subcortically driven predispositions to acquire and collect and adjust these predispositions to environmental context (Anderson et al. 2005). Damage to these cortical regions may result in dysregulated collecting and hoarding behavior. The neuroimaging literature of "non-organic" hoarding has also implicated the ventromedial prefrontal/anterior cingulate cortices and subcortical limbic structures (e.g., amygdala/hippocampus) in hoarding patients. However, the evidence is preliminary, was obtained from small samples, and is confounded in many cases by the presence of comorbid OCD symptoms (Mataix-Cols et al. 2011). Future work in this area should include carefully characterized samples of individuals meeting strict criteria for HD.

Treatment

There are no large-scale, definitive clinical trials to guide treatment of HD. Also, there is a good deal of evidence from studies of patients with OCD that the presence of hoarding symptoms in individuals with OCD is associated with a worse response to both pharmacotherapy and psychotherapy (Bloch et al. 2014). Nevertheless, pharmacological (serotonin reuptake inhibitors) and psychological (cognitive-behavioral therapy [CBT] that incorporates exposure and response prevention) therapies that have demonstrated efficacy for nonhoarding OCD may be helpful for some patients with HD, so they are the first-line interventions for this condition (Pertusa et al. 2010a; Saxena 2011).

Because individuals with HD appear to often have poor insight, use of motivational interviewing strategies may be needed to encourage patients to obtain and stay in treatment. Although there are no systematic trials comparing pharmacotherapy and psychotherapy in HD, the research data suggest that each modality is equally efficacious, and clinical experience suggests that combined pharmacotherapy and psychotherapy may be useful (Saxena 2011). Clinical judgment, relying in part on data from other OCRDs, may also influence treatment decisions; for example, patients with HD and comorbid depression may well require robust intervention with serotonin reuptake inhibitors or venlafaxine.

In an open comparison of consecutive cases, paroxetine was as effective for HD ($n=32$; 28% responders) as for nonhoarding OCD ($n=47$; 32% responders), although the overall outcomes were modest in both groups (Saxena et al. 2007). In another small ($N=24$) open-label trial, venlafaxine monotherapy led to significant decreases in hoarding symptom severity, with 16 of the 23 completers (70%) being classified as responders after 12 weeks of treatment (Saxena and Sumner 2014). The literature on pharmacotherapy of treatment-refractory HD is sparse, but it is noteworthy that there are a few case reports of patients with prominent hoarding symptoms responding to glutamate modulators (Saxena 2011). Randomized placebo-controlled trials of selective serotonin reuptake inhibitors and other medications are now needed in carefully diagnosed patients with primary HD.

Currently, the intervention that has the strongest evidence base is a multicomponent psychological treatment based on a cognitive-behavioral model of hoarding (Frost and Hartl 1996). The treatment incorporates education about hoarding, goal setting and motivational enhancement techniques, organizing and decision-making skills training, practice with sorting and discarding objects, practice with resisting acquiring objects, and cognitive techniques designed to alter dysfunctional beliefs about the importance of possessions (Steketee and Frost 2013).

This intervention was initially tried in small case series and uncontrolled pilot studies and was more recently evaluated in a two-site wait-list controlled trial involving 46 patients (Steketee et al. 2010). After 12 weeks of CBT, 10 of 23 patients (43.5%) were rated as much or very much improved, compared with none of the wait-list patients ($P=0.001$). At this point, wait-list patients were also offered this CBT treatment. After 26 weeks of treatment, 29 of the 41 patients (71%) who had received treatment (both groups combined) were considered improved. However, 27 of the 73 eligible participants (37%) declined to participate in the trial. The therapy gains were maintained up to 1 year later, with 62% of the patients who completed the original treatment phase (23 of 37 patients) rated as much or very much improved. This intervention involves more than 25 weekly, 60-minute individual therapy sessions plus home visits over 9–12 months. A detailed manualized treatment guide that clinicians can use when treating patients with HD is available (Steketee and Frost 2013).

More cost-effective treatments (e.g., group therapy, bibliotherapy self-help, peer-led support groups, or Internet CBT) have recently been developed and tested in small open or wait-list controlled trials, with comparable results to those of individual face-to-face treatment (e.g., Frost et al. 2012; Muroff et al. 2012). However, additional research that uses a more rigorous trial design is needed to further test these treatments' efficacy and whether they really are as effective as treatment provided by clinicians.

Two additional open CBT trials in geriatric patients with HD suggest higher dropout rates (Turner et al. 2010) and lower response rates (Ayers et al. 2011; Turner et al. 2010) compared with studies in younger individuals, indicating that elderly patients may be particularly challenging to engage and treat. A recent pilot open trial in this age group tested a behavioral intervention that includes cognitive rehabilitation techniques targeting memory and executive dysfunction and emphasizing therapist-guided exposure to discarding and not acquiring. The results were more encouraging, with 8 of the 11 participants rated as much improved (Ayers et al. 2014; Saxena et al. 2007).

Much treatment research is greatly needed. Available studies had small samples and were not adequately controlled. Clinical trials are needed to assess the short- and longer-term efficacy of psychological and pharmacological treatments, alone and in combination, in carefully diagnosed individuals with primary HD. Well-controlled studies are needed, using pill placebo in medication studies and a comparison treatment that controls for therapist time and attention in psychotherapy studies. Direct comparisons between different active treatments are also needed. Evaluation of interventions aimed at improving cognitive functioning (e.g., attention, organization) in individuals with HD is warranted, as is the development and evaluation of family-centered interventions, because HD has a negative impact on the entire family (Drury et al. 2014). Studies of interventions adapted for special populations—for example, comorbid HD in individuals with ASDs or intellectual disabilities—are also needed.

Although the current psychological treatments emphasize the importance of motivational interviewing techniques, the patients included in the trials mentioned here had "enough" insight to at least seek help. It is currently unclear how to best approach individuals with absent or delusional insight who may only come to the attention of mental health services against their will. The clinical management of these cases may require a high level of interagency coordination. Several countries have set up local or federal multiagency task forces (often including mental health, fire, pest control, housing, legal, and social services) to tackle the most severe cases of hoarding in which the person does not voluntarily seek or want help (Bratiotis 2013).

Key Points

- Hoarding disorder (HD) is a new mental disorder included in the new "Obsessive-Compulsive and Related Disorders" chapter of DSM-5.

- The main clinical feature of HD is a persistent difficulty in parting with possessions, which results in severely cluttered living spaces and clinically significant distress or impairment in functioning, and which is not attributable to another medical or mental disorder.

- The majority of people diagnosed with HD excessively acquire items that they do not need or for which no space is available. In those cases, the "excessive acquisition" specifier is endorsed.

- A conservative estimate of the disorder's prevalence is 1.5% for both men and women.

- The causes of HD are currently unknown, but the condition runs in families and is moderately heritable.

- HD is easily diagnosed by means of a clinical interview with the affected person, ideally conducted in the person's home to assess the extent of the clutter and impairment. When home visits are not feasible, it is useful to request photographs of the living environments.

- Many persons with HD have limited insight into their difficulties and are reluctant to seek help. Motivation-enhancing techniques may be helpful to increase compliance with treatment and improve outcomes, at least for those patients who decide to seek help.

- Currently, the intervention with the strongest evidence base is cognitive-behavioral therapy that is specifically tailored to hoarding difficulties. A detailed manualized treatment guide that clinicians can use when treating patients with HD is available (Steketee and Frost 2013).

References

American Psychiatric Association: Diagnostic and Statistical Manual of Mental Disorders, 4th Edition. Washington, DC, American Psychiatric Association, 1994

American Psychiatric Association: Diagnostic and Statistical Manual of Mental Disorders, 4th Edition, Text Revision. Arlington, VA, American Psychiatric Association, 2000

American Psychiatric Association: Diagnostic and Statistical Manual of Mental Disorders, 5th Edition. Arlington, VA, American Psychiatric Association, 2013

Anderson SW, Damasio H, Damasio AR: A neural basis for collecting behaviour in humans. Brain 128 (Pt 1):201–212, 2005 15548551

Ayers CR, Saxena S, Golshan S, et al: Age at onset and clinical features of late life compulsive hoarding. Int J Geriatr Psychiatry 25(2):142–149, 2010 19548272

Ayers CR, Wetherell JL, Golshan S, et al: Cognitive-behavioral therapy for geriatric compulsive hoarding. Behav Res Ther 49(10):689–694, 2011 21784412

Ayers CR, Saxena S, Espejo E, et al: Novel treatment for geriatric hoarding disorder: an open trial of cognitive rehabilitation paired with behavior therapy. Am J Geriatr Psychiatry 22(3):248–252, 2014 23831173

Bloch MH, Bartley CA, Zipperer L, et al: Meta-analysis: hoarding symptoms associated with poor treatment outcome in obsessive-compulsive disorder. Mol Psychiatry 19(9):1025–1030, 2014 24912494

Bratiotis C: Community hoarding task forces: a comparative case study of five task forces in the United States. Health Soc Care Community 21(3):245–253, 2013 23199135

Drury H, Ajmi S, Fernández de la Cruz L, et al: Caregiver burden, family accommodation, health, and well-being in relatives of individuals with hoarding disorder. J Affect Disord 159:7–14, 2014 24679383

Fernández de la Cruz L, Nordsletten AE, Billotti D, et al: Photograph-aided assessment of clutter in hoarding disorder: is a picture worth a thousand words? Depress Anxiety 30(1):61–66, 2013 22930673

Frost RO, Hartl TL: A cognitive-behavioral model of compulsive hoarding. Behav Res Ther 34(4):341–350, 1996 8871366

Frost RO, Steketee G, Williams L: Hoarding: a community health problem. Health Soc Care Community 8(4):229–234, 2000

Frost RO, Steketee G, Williams L: Compulsive buying, compulsive hoarding, and obsessive-compulsive disorder. Behav Ther 33:201–214, 2002

Frost RO, Steketee G, Grisham J: Measurement of compulsive hoarding: saving inventory—revised. Behav Res Ther 42(10):1163–1182, 2004 15350856

Frost RO, Steketee G, Tolin D, et al: Development and validation of the Clutter Image Rating. J Psychopathol Behav Assess 30(3):193–203, 2008

Frost RO, Tolin D, Maltby N: Insight-related challenges in the treatment of hoarding. Cogn Behav Pract 17(4):404–413, 2010

Frost RO, Steketee G, Tolin DF: Comorbidity in hoarding disorder. Depress Anxiety 28(10):876–884, 2011 21770000

Frost RO, Ruby D, Shuer LJ: The Buried in Treasures Workshop: waitlist control trial of facilitated support groups for hoarding. Behav Res Ther 50(11):661–667, 2012 22982080

Fullana MA, Vilagut G, Rojas-Farreras S, et al: Obsessive-compulsive symptom dimensions in the general population: results from an epidemiological study in six European countries. J Affect Disord 124(3):291–299, 2010 20022382

Grisham JR, Frost RO, Steketee G, et al: Age of onset of compulsive hoarding. J Anxiety Disord 20(5):675–686, 2006 16112837

Grisham JR, Brown TA, Savage CR, et al: Neuropsychological impairment associated with compulsive hoarding. Behav Res Ther 45(7):1471–1483, 2007 17341416

Iervolino AC, Perroud N, Fullana MA, et al: Prevalence and heritability of compulsive hoarding: a twin study. Am J Psychiatry 166(10):1156–1161, 2009 19687130

Ivanov VZ, Mataix-Cols D, Serlachius E, et al: Prevalence, comorbidity and heritability of hoarding symptoms in adolescence: a population based twin study in 15-year olds. PLoS One 8(7):e69140, 2013 23874893

Landau D, Iervolino AC, Pertusa A, et al: Stressful life events and material deprivation in hoarding disorder. J Anxiety Disord 25(2):192–202, 2011 20934847

Lucini G, Monk I, Szlatenyi C: An Analysis of Fire Incidents Involving Hoarded Households. Worcester, MA, Worcester Polytechnic Institute, 2009

Mataix-Cols D, Pertusa A: Annual research review: hoarding disorder: potential benefits and pitfalls of a new mental disorder. J Child Psychol Psychiatry 53(5):608–618, 2012 21895651

Mataix-Cols D, Frost RO, Pertusa A, et al: Hoarding disorder: a new diagnosis for DSM-V? Depress Anxiety 27(6):556–572, 2010 20336805

Mataix-Cols D, Pertusa A, Snowden J: Neuropsychological and neural correlates of hoarding: a practice-friendly review. J Clin Psychol 67(5):467–476, 2011 21351104

Mataix-Cols D, Billotti D, Fernández de la Cruz L, et al: The London Field Trial for Hoarding Disorder. Psychol Med 43(4):837–847, 2013 22883395

Mathews CA, Delucchi DK, Cath DC, et al: Partitioning the etiology of hoarding and obsessive-compulsive symptoms. Psychol Med 44(13):2867–2876, 2014 25066062

Monzani B, Rijsdijk F, Harris J, et al: The structure of genetic and environmental risk factors for dimensional representations of DSM-5 obsessive-compulsive spectrum disorders. JAMA Psychiatry 71(2):182–189, 2014 24369376

Muroff J, Steketee G, Bratiotis C, et al: Group cognitive and behavioral therapy and bibliotherapy for hoarding: a pilot trial. Depress Anxiety 29(7):597–604, 2012 22447579

Nordsletten AE, Mataix-Cols D: Hoarding versus collecting: where does pathology diverge from play? Clin Psychol Rev 32(3):165–176, 2012 22322013

Nordsletten AE, Reichenberg A, Hatch SL, et al: Epidemiology of hoarding disorder. Br J Psychiatry 203(6):445–452, 2013a 24158881

Nordsletten AE, Fernández de la Cruz L, Drury H, et al: The Family Impact sCcale for Hoarding (FISH): measure development and initial validation. J Obsessive Compuls Relat Disord 3(1):29–34, 2013b

Nordsletten AE, Fernández de la Cruz L, Billotti D, et al: Finders keepers: the features differentiating hoarding disorder from normative collecting. Compr Psychiatry 54(3):229–237, 2013c 22995450

Nordsletten AE, Monzani B, Fernández de la Cruz L, et al: Overlap and specificity of genetic and environmental influences on excessive acquisition and difficulties discarding possessions: implications for hoarding disorder. Am J Med Genet B Neuropsychiatr Genet 162B(4):380–387, 2013d 23533058

Nordsletten AE, Fernández de la Cruz L, Pertusa A, et al: The Structured Interview for Hoarding Disorder (SIHD): development, usage and further validation. J Obsessive Compuls Relat Disord 2:346–350, 2014

Pertusa A, Fullana MA, Singh S, et al: Compulsive hoarding: OCD symptom, distinct clinical syndrome, or both? Am J Psychiatry 165(10):1289–1298, 2008 18483134

Pertusa A, Frost RO, Fullana MA, et al: Refining the diagnostic boundaries of compulsive hoarding: a critical review. Clin Psychol Rev 30(4):371–386, 2010a 20189280

Pertusa A, Frost RO, Mataix-Cols D: When hoarding is a symptom of OCD: a case series and implications for DSM-V. Behav Res Ther 48(10):1012–1020, 2010b 20673573

Phillips KA, Stein DJ, Rauch SL, et al: Should an obsessive-compulsive spectrum grouping of disorders be included in DSM-V? Depress Anxiety 27(6):528–555, 2010 20533367

Rasmussen JL, Steketee G, Frost RO, et al: Assessing squalor in hoarding: the Home Environment Index. Community Ment Health J 50(5):591–596, 2014 24292497

Russio AM, Stein DJ, Chiu WT, et al: The epidemiology of obsessive-compulsive disorder in the National Comorbidity Survey Replication. Mol Psychiatry 15(1):53–63, 2010 18725912

Samuels JF, Bienvenu OJ, Grados MA, et al: Prevalence and correlates of hoarding behavior in a community-based sample. Behav Res Ther 46(7):836–844, 2008 18495084

Saxena S: Pharmacotherapy of compulsive hoarding. J Clin Psychol 67(5):477–484, 2011 21404273

Saxena S, Sumner J: Venlafaxine extended-release treatment of hoarding disorder. Int Clin Psychopharmacol 29(5):266–273, 2014 24722633

Saxena S, Brody AL, Maidment KM, et al: Paroxetine treatment of compulsive hoarding. J Psychiatr Res 41(6):481–487, 2007 16790250

Snowdon J, Pertusa A, Mataix-Cols D: On hoarding and squalor: a few considerations for DSM-5. Depress Anxiety 29(5):417–424, 2012 22553007

Steketee G, Frost RO: Compulsive Hoarding and Acquiring: A Therapist Guide, 2nd Edition. New York, Oxford University Press, 2013

Steketee G, Frost RO, Kyrios M: Cognitive aspects of compulsive hoarding. Cognitive Therapy and Research 27:463–479, 2003

Steketee G, Frost RO, Tolin DF, et al: Waitlist-controlled trial of cognitive behavior therapy for hoarding disorder. Depress Anxiety 27(5):476–484, 2010 20336804

Timpano KR, Exner C, Glaesmer H, et al: The epidemiology of the proposed DSM-5 hoarding disorder: exploration of the acquisition specifier, associated features, and distress. J Clin Psychiatry 72(6):780–786, quiz 878–879, 2011 21733479

Timpano KR, Broman-Fulks JJ, Glaesmer H, et al: A taxometric exploration of the latent structure of hoarding. Psychol Assess 25(1):194–203, 2013 22984803

Tolin DF, Villavicencio A: Inattention, but not OCD, predicts the core features of hoarding disorder. Behav Res Ther 49(2):120–125, 2011 21193171

Tolin DF, Frost RO, Steketee G, et al: The economic and social burden of compulsive hoarding. Psychiatry Res 160(2):200–211, 2008a 18597855

Tolin DF, Frost RO, Steketee G, et al: Family burden of compulsive hoarding: results of an Internet survey. Behav Res Ther 46(3):334–344, 2008b 18275935

Tolin DF, Frost RO, Steketee G: A brief interview for assessing compulsive hoarding: the Hoarding Rating Scale–Interview. Psychiatry Res 178(1):147–152, 2010a 20452042

Tolin DF, Fitch KE, Frost RO, Steketee G: Family informants' perceptions of insight in compulsive hoarding. Cognitive Therapy and Research 34:69–81, 2010b

Turner K, Steketee G, Nauth L: Treating elders with compulsive hoarding: a pilot program. Cogn Behav Pract 17(4):449–457, 2010

Woody SR, Kellman-McFarlane K, Welsted A: Review of cognitive performance in hoarding disorder. Clin Psychol Rev 34(4):324–336, 2014 24794835

World Health Organization: International Statistical Classification of Diseases and Related Health Problems, 10th Revision. Geneva, Switzerland, World Health Organization, 1992

Recommended Readings

Frost RO, Steketee G (eds): The Oxford Handbook of Hoarding and Acquiring. New York, Oxford University Press, 2014

Snowdon J, Halliday G, Banerjee S (eds): Severe Domestic Squalor. Cambridge, United Kingdom, Cambridge University Press, 2012

Steketee G, Frost RO: Compulsive Hoarding and Acquiring: A Therapist Guide, 2nd Edition. New York, Oxford University Press, 2013

CHAPTER 5

Trichotillomania (Hair–Pulling Disorder)

Ivar Snorrason, M.A.
David C. Houghton, M.S.
Douglas W. Woods, Ph.D.

Trichotillomania (hair-pulling disorder)—the persistent habit of pulling out one's hair—has been recognized in the medical literature for more than a century and as a formal diagnostic entity in DSM since 1987 (American Psychiatric Association 1987; Stein et al. 2010). Traditionally, trichotillomania (hair-pulling disorder) has received limited research attention, but since its inclusion in DSM, the empirical literature has increased substantially. This research has shed light on the role of genetic factors, abnormal neural circuitry, and cognitive/affective/behavioral processes in the disorder. At the same time, there have been important advances in the development of effective pharmacological and cognitive-behavioral interventions. In this chapter, we review the current literature on symptom presentation, diagnosis, clinical characteristics, etiology, treatment, and other clinically relevant aspects of trichotillomania (hair-pulling disorder).

Diagnostic Criteria and Symptomatology

The DSM-5 diagnostic criteria for trichotillomania (hair-pulling disorder) (American Psychiatric Association 2013) are presented in Box 5–1. In DSM-III-R and DSM-IV (American Psychiatric Association 1987, 1994), Criterion A specified recurrent hair pulling resulting in "noticeable hair loss." Given that hair loss in hair-pulling patients is not always clearly visible (e.g., sometimes pulling is widely distributed), the word *noticeable* was deleted from the criteria for DSM-5 (Stein et al. 2010). Also, unlike previous DSM criteria for trichotillomania, the DSM-5 criteria do not include requirements of tension or arousal preceding hair pulling or gratification or relief during the act. The decision to delete this criterion was based on data showing that individuals with clinically significant hair-pulling problems do not necessarily endorse these experiences, or they do so inconsistently (Lochner et al. 2012). Some studies have shown a correlation between these symptoms and severity of trichotillomania (hair-pulling disorder); however, these findings have not been consistently replicated (Lochner et al. 2012). Researchers have also failed to find meaningful differences in clinical characteristics between individuals with and without tension/arousal and relief/gratification (Lochner et al. 2012). To differentiate trichotillomania (hair-pulling disorder) from normal or nonpathological hair pulling/plucking, DSM-5 retained the criterion that pulling must cause clinically significant distress or impairment in psychosocial functioning and also included a requirement of repeated failed attempts to decrease or stop the behavior.

BOX 5–1. DSM-5 Diagnostic Criteria for Trichotillomania (Hair-Pulling Disorder)

A. Recurrent pulling out of one's hair, resulting in hair loss.
B. Repeated attempts to decrease or stop hair pulling.
C. The hair pulling causes clinically significant distress or impairment in social, occupational, or other important areas of functioning.
D. The hair pulling or hair loss is not attributable to another medical condition (e.g., a dermatological condition).
E. The hair pulling is not better explained by the symptoms of another mental disorder (e.g., attempts to improve a perceived defect or flaw in appearance in body dysmorphic disorder).

Reprinted from American Psychiatric Association: *Diagnostic and Statistical Manual of Mental Disorders*, 5th Edition. Arlington, VA, American Psychiatric Association. Copyright 2013, American Psychiatric Association. Used with permission.

The majority of trichotillomania (hair-pulling disorder) patients pull hair daily, either in several episodes throughout the day or in fewer isolated episodes. Most use their fingers to pull out hairs one by one, and some also use tweezers or other instruments (Christenson et al. 1991). Studies show that preschool-age children with trichotillomania (hair-pulling disorder) tend to pull only from the scalp (Walther et al. 2014), presumably because of a relative lack of hair elsewhere on the body. Older individuals pull from more diverse regions of the body. Table 5–1 shows the most common pulling sites in children, adolescents, and adults with trichotillomania (hair-pulling disorder). Scalp, eyebrows, and eyelashes are the most common pulling areas, regardless of age group; the number of targeted pulling sites increases with age.

TABLE 5–1.   Common pulling sites by age group

Body area	Children ages 0–10 years,[a] %	Adolescents ages 10–17 years,[b] %	Adults ages 18+ years,[c] %
Scalp	83	86	73
Eyebrows	39	38	56
Eyelashes	52	52	52
Pubic region	–	27	51
Legs	13	19	22
Arms	16	9	12
More than one	40	58	97

Source.   [a]Walther et al. 2014; [b]Franklin et al. 2008; [c]Woods et al. 2006a.

Individuals often engage in (and gain pleasure from) certain habitual behaviors before and after pulling (Christenson et al. 1991). Prepulling activities typically include stroking the hair and/or searching for a "good" hair to pull. Postpulling activities may involve oral or tactile stimulation obtained by rolling the hair between the fingers or stroking it against the lips. A minority of patients consume the hair (trichophagia), often by biting off the hair root and swallowing it. In one study, nearly 30% of individuals with trichotillomania (hair-pulling disorder) reported at least occasionally engaging in one or more of the following: stroking the hair against the lips, biting the hair root, or swallowing the pulled hair or hair root (Grant and Odlaug 2008). Some individuals, particularly children, pull hair from other people, pets, dolls, or other objects.

In some instances, the individual is unaware that she or he is pulling while the behavior occurs (Christenson et al. 1991; Flessner et al. 2007, 2008). Such "automatic" episodes typically take place when the individual is engaged in another activity such as reading, watching television, driving, or talking on the telephone. More commonly, people are fully aware of the behavior, experience an urge or impulse to pull hair, and feel gratification or relief during the act (Lochner et al. 2012). It is also common for boredom, stress, or frustration to trigger hair-pulling episodes, and pulling may temporarily reduce these experiences (Snorrason et al. 2012). Most people with trichotillomania (hair-pulling disorder) report both automatic and focused pulling episodes, although individuals vary in terms of how frequently they engage in each type (Flessner et al. 2007, 2008). Studies show that children (especially preschool-age children) are less likely to experience preceding urge or tension and are more likely to pull automatically, without reflective awareness (Walther et al. 2014).

Case Example: Mary

Mary, a 37-year-old white woman, worked in an office, was married, and had a young daughter. Mary had started pulling out hairs from her eyebrows and scalp in her early teen years. Since then, she had pulled hairs almost every day, with the exception of a 1-month period during her honeymoon while she was in her early 20s. She typically pulled in the evenings, when alone in the bathroom. Mary's pulling episodes often lasted for hours. Even though Mary "hated" the habit, she often experienced an irresistible desire to pull hair and a sense of gratification or relief when the hair was pulled out. She especially enjoyed hair pulling when she pulled out a hair with a root on it. This gave her a thrill, and she often scrutinized the root, bit it off, and consumed it.

Mary was intensely embarrassed about this behavior and distressed by her inability to control it. She had a bald patch the size of an orange on the top of her head, which extended downward on the right side. She also had substantial thinning of the hair on the front of her head, and a significant portion of both eyebrows was missing. Mary attempted to hide her bald spots by combing hair over them or wearing hats or scarves. She also avoided any situations or activities that might expose her bald spots (e.g., she would not go swimming with her children). During stressful periods, when pulling was frequent and bald patches were larger than usual, she avoided all social activities.

Epidemiology

Surveys among college students and adults in the general population have shown that 10%–15% of respondents engage in some noncosmetic hair pulling (e.g., Duke et al. 2009), although the behavior reported in these studies does not necessary meet all required DSM-5 diagnostic criteria. Between 1% and 3% endorse hair pulling that results in distress, impairment, or hair loss, possibly reflecting the trichotillomania (hair-pulling disorder) diagnosis. Similar findings have been reported among adolescents (King et al. 1995).

The prevalence of trichotillomania (hair-pulling disorder) among children in the general population has not been investigated.

Most surveys indicate a preponderance of females among individuals with trichotillomania (hair-pulling disorder), although a few surveys have reported an equal gender ratio among those with symptoms that meet full DSM-IV criteria (e.g., Duke et al. 2009). In general, however, samples of individuals who are seeking treatment or participating in research (Snorrason et al. 2012) consistently contain a large majority of females (around 90%). Findings concerning gender ratio in pediatric samples are more mixed, with some studies showing an equal gender ratio but a majority showing a significant female preponderance, albeit less than in adult samples (57%–87%; Snorrason et al. 2012; Walther et al. 2014). Overall, existing data indicate that trichotillomania (hair-pulling disorder) is more common among females, although this may reflect gender differences in treatment-seeking behaviors (i.e., females may be more likely to seek help or treatment).

Comorbidity

Common Comorbid Psychiatric Disorders

Data from clinical trials and specialty clinics suggest that 40%–50% of individuals with trichotillomania (hair-pulling disorder) have current comorbid psychiatric disorders (Lochner et al. 2012; Odlaug et al. 2010; Tolin et al. 2007). For example, Odlaug et al. (2010) interviewed 70 adults with trichotillomania who had participated in treatment trials. More than half (37/70; 53%) had at least one additional current Axis I diagnosis, most commonly a mood disorder (20/70; 29%), an anxiety disorder (17/70; 25%), or attention-deficit/hyperactivity disorder (5/70; 7%). Tolin et al. (2007) found that 38% of children and adolescents participating in a treatment trial ($N=46$) had at least one comorbid diagnosis. About one-third (30%) had an anxiety disorder (primarily generalized anxiety disorder), and 11% had an externalizing disorder (primarily attention-deficit/hyperactivity disorder). Studies in general outpatient settings have reported somewhat higher comorbidity rates but similar patterns of comorbidities (e.g., Christenson et al. 1991).

Comorbid Obsessive-Compulsive and Related Disorders

Trichotillomania (hair-pulling disorder) and excoriation (skin-picking) disorder are similar with respect to phenomenology and clinical characteristics, and they probably share common genetic underpinnings (Monzani et al. 2014). The lifetime prevalence of excoriation (skin-picking) disorder among outpatients with trichotillomania (hair-pulling disorder) ranges from 10% to 34% (Snorrason et al. 2012). Both trichotillomania (hair-pulling disorder) and excoriation (skin-picking) disorder frequently co-occur with other problematic body-focused repetitive behaviors (Stein et al. 2008). For example, in a large online sample ($N = 990$) of self-identified hair-pulling disorder patients (Stein et al. 2008), 74% endorsed a lifetime history of at least one problematic body-focused repetitive behavior (defined as a recurrent habit resulting in physical damage, such as skin lesions). The most commonly endorsed problems were excessive skin picking (54%), nail biting (32%), lip/cheek biting (26%), and nose picking (13%). Also, clinical impression suggests that habitual thumb sucking is common among young children with trichotillomania (hair-pulling disorder).

The prevalence of current obsessive-compulsive disorder (OCD) in samples of individuals with trichotillomania (hair-pulling disorder) ranges from 8% to 30% (Christenson et al. 1991; Odlaug and Grant 2008), and data suggest the two disorders tend to run in families (Bienvenu et al. 2012). The prevalence of current trichotillomania (hair-pulling disorder) may be higher among individuals with OCD than among individuals with anxiety disorders, although findings have been mixed (Lochner and Stein 2010).

Given that hoarding symptoms tend to be more acceptable to the individual than OCD symptoms (i.e., the symptoms themselves tend not to bother hoarding disorder patients as much as OCD patients), it has been speculated that trichotillomania (hair-pulling disorder) may have greater overlap with hoarding than OCD. Some studies have found that hair pulling is more common in OCD patients with hoarding disorder than in OCD patients without hoarding disorder; however, other studies have failed to find such differences (Torres et al. 2012).

The relationship between body dysmorphic disorder (BDD) and hair-pulling disorder has not received much attention. Further, the association between these disorders is complicated by the fact that hair pulling can negatively affect appearance and also by the fact that hair pulling can be a symptom of BDD and in such cases can be misdiagnosed as trichotillomania (hair-pulling disorder). An early study (Soriano et al. 1996) using a dimensional self-report measure of BDD showed high prevalence of BDD symptoms (22%) among individuals with trichotillomania. However, more recent studies using structured diagnostic interviews indicate low comorbidity between the two disorders. Lochner et al. (2012) interviewed 84 adults with trichotillomania, none of whom met diagnostic criteria for current BDD. Similarly, Grant et al. (2006) found that only 2.3% of a BDD sample ($N = 176$) reported a history of trichotillomania.

Course and Prognosis

Trichotillomania (hair-pulling disorder) most frequently has onset in early adolescence (Snorrason et al. 2012), but early childhood onset is also common (Walther et al. 2014). In adult and adolescent treatment-seeking populations, the course of the disorder tends to be chronic, with no lengthy symptom-free periods (Snorrason et al. 2012). Some evidence (Swedo et al. 1992) indicates that children with early onset (<5 years old) are more likely than those with later onset to have a remitting course and spontaneous recovery within a few years after onset. It has therefore been speculated that early-onset cases may represent a distinct subtype with a more favorable prognosis (Swedo et al. 1992). However, a substantial portion of adults with trichotillomania (hair-pulling disorder) report very early onset and a chronic course (Snorrason et al. 2012). Furthermore, it is possible that parents of young children with hair pulling are more willing to seek professional help than older individuals with a remitting course. In other words, adults may not seek help unless the hair pulling is relatively chronic, whereas parents of toddlers with hair pulling may have a lower threshold for help seeking. This would lead to an overrepresentation of toddler-onset cases with a remitting course in treatment-seeking populations. More research is needed to understand factors that contribute to the chronicity of hair-pulling problems, and longitudinal research is needed to determine if there is in fact a distinct early-onset subtype.

Psychosocial Impairment

Trichotillomania (hair-pulling disorder) can be a severe condition. Affected individuals often spend a significant amount of time daily pulling hairs or dealing with the consequences of hair pulling. Some patients have very noticeable hair loss that is difficult to conceal. A small minority of children and adults who ingest the pulled hairs develop a hair ball (trichobezoar) in the gastrointestinal tract, which can lead to serious and even life-threatening medical complications, such as perforation of the stomach or intestine and gastric ulcer. Surgical removal of the trichobezoar may be required (Grant and Odlaug 2008). Although numerous case reports describing this condition in trichotillomania (hair-pulling disorder) have been published, the prevalence is unknown. An early study among 24 females with trichotillomania showed that 25% had trichobezoars; however, a more recent study of 68 adults (9 of whom currently ingested the pulled hair) did not find physical problems suggestive of trichobezoar in any of the patients (Grant and Odlaug 2008).

Significant emotional distress is frequently reported. Repeated failures to control the behavior can lead to frustration, hopelessness, and despair. Some patients experience deep shame and embarrassment because of their hair pulling, and studies show a relationship between trichotillomania (hair-pulling disorder) and low self-esteem (Soriano et al. 1996). Social interference is common and may include intense fear of being "found out," time-consuming cover-up routines, and avoidance of situations or activities where the hair loss may be exposed. One study (Odlaug et al. 2010) found that adults with trichotillomania reported significantly lower quality of life compared with healthy control subjects, with about one-third reporting "low" or "very low" quality of life. Large online surveys of adults (Woods et al. 2006a) and adolescents (Franklin et al. 2008) with trichotillomania showed that the majority of respondents experienced mild to moderate impairment in occupational, academic, or social functioning.

Developmental Considerations

Even though symptoms of hair-pulling disorder are very similar in children and adults, some differences have been noted, especially among preschool-age children. Young children are less likely to endorse urges or arousal prior to pulling or gratification and relief during pulling and are more likely to pull without awareness. These findings possibly reflect underdeveloped cognitive capacities and limited ability to report such experiences among children (Walther et al. 2014). Also, a comparison (Walther et al. 2014) of samples of children, adolescents, and adults with trichotillomania (hair-pulling disorder) showed that young children, particularly preschool-age children, experience less distress and impairment due to their illness than do adolescents and adults. In contrast, pulling severity was similar across all age groups.

Case Example: Alex

Alex, a 4-year-old white child, was the youngest of four siblings and lived with both parents. He began pulling hairs from his scalp when he was 9 months old. He almost always sucked his thumb while pulling hair. His parents reported that the behavior appeared to soothe him. For the past year, he had pulled primarily in the evenings while alone in bed and occasionally pulled his hair and sucked his thumb while sleeping. He had a very large bald spot on the crown of his head.

The hair-pulling behavior had interfered with his parents' child-rearing practices (e.g., caused them to be frustrated and impatient with him, reduced the frequency of positive interactions). His parents had attempted to control the behavior with different methods, including reprimanding Alex for pulling, distracting him as soon as he started, and having him wear gloves in bed. None of these strategies had been effective. On two occasions, they shaved off all his hair; however, he started pulling as soon as the hair grew back. The onset of the hair-pulling problem coincided with the family's moving to a new city, but the parents reported no significant stressors in Alex's life. A detailed assessment indicated that other than the excessive hair pulling, Alex did not have any developmental, psychiatric, or physical problems.

Gender-Related Issues

Because more than 90% of trichotillomania (hair-pulling disorder) patients and research subjects are female, little is known about gender differences in hair pulling. The few studies that have compared males and females with hair-pulling disorder found more similarities than differences in symptom presentation and clinical characteristics. One study (Lochner et al. 2010) found that in comparison to females with trichotillomania, males with the disorder were less likely to report positive affect as cues for hair pulling and had a later age at onset, more comorbidity with OCD and tics, and less trichotillomania-related disability. Males were also more likely than females to pull hairs from their face, chest, and other areas. Another study (Grant and Christenson 2007) examined a combined sample of individuals with trichotillomania and excoriation (skin-picking) disorder. The results (which were not reported for each disorder separately) showed that males reported greater functional impairment and more comorbid anxiety disorders than females. Additionally, one study showed that trichotillomania patients who endorsed mouthing (putting hairs against the lips), biting, or consuming hairs or hair roots after pulling (trichophagia) were more likely to be male (Grant and Odlaug 2008).

Cultural Aspects of Phenomenology

Very limited data exist on cultural factors in trichotillomania (hair-pulling disorder). In general, symptoms appear to be similar across cultures, although data from non-Western cultures are scarce. Surveys that have compared African American to non–African American college students showed similar prevalence and characteristics of excessive hair pulling (although most did not have symptoms that met full criteria for the disorder); however, some evidence suggests that African American students are less likely to report distress due to their pulling (Mansueto et al. 2007). In addition, an Internet survey of U.S. adults with self-reported trichotillomania found that responders from minority groups were less likely than Caucasian responders to report tension prior to pulling and were less likely to pull from their eyebrows and eyelashes (Neal-Barnett et al. 2010).

Assessment and Differential Diagnosis

Assessment

The diagnosis of trichotillomania (hair-pulling disorder) primarily involves establishing the occurrence of recurrent hair pulling that is not due to normal cosmetic reasons, the use of drugs, other psychiatric disorders (such as BDD), or medical conditions. Table 5–2 gives examples of screening questions for hair-pulling disorder.

TABLE 5–2.   Screening questions for trichotillomania (hair-pulling disorder)

Do you repeatedly pull out your hairs from the scalp, eyebrows, eyelashes, or other areas of the body?

How frequently do you pull hair? On average, how many episodes (per day), and how long are the episodes?

Do you want to stop pulling hair or do it less? Why? Have you ever tried to stop pulling or do it less?

Has hair pulling caused you any emotional distress (e.g., made you really unhappy with yourself; caused significant shame, embarrassment, hopelessness, frustration)?

Has hair pulling interfered with your academic or work functioning (e.g., caused you to show up late or skip work/school, made it difficult to focus on tasks)?

Has hair pulling made you avoid activities, places, or people (e.g., social events, swimming pools) or interfered with your relationships in any way?

Why do you pull hair (e.g., do you pull in order to correct the appearance of the hair)?

Is there any medical condition (e.g., dermatological problem) that causes you to pull hairs? What is the condition called? Would you still pull if you did not have it?

A potential complication in diagnosing trichotillomania (hair-pulling disorder) occurs when the individual denies pulling hair. This can happen for at least two reasons. First, some patients, especially children, are unaware of the behavior. As a result, they may underreport the extent of their pulling or deny it altogether. Second, some individuals may not want to admit that they pull their hair (e.g., because of shame or embarrassment). Again, this is perhaps more common among children and adolescents than adults. In situations when the patient denies pulling hair but there is a strong suspicion that trichotillomania (hair-pulling disorder) may be present, it may be necessary to rely primarily on information from other sources (e.g., parents). Dermatological examination may help rule out other causes of alopecia and establish a trichotillomania (hair-pulling disorder) diagnosis.

In addition to establishing the diagnosis, it is important to assess characteristics of the disorder, including pulling sites, pre- and postpulling activities, trichophagia, and proxy pulling. Assessment of symptom severity is also important, especially during treatment. Table 5–3 lists methods and instruments that can be helpful in determining the diagnosis, characteristics, and severity of trichotillomania (hair-pulling disorder).

Differential Diagnosis

Individuals who pull/pluck hair solely for cultural or cosmetic reasons (e.g., plucking eyebrows) should not be diagnosed with trichotillomania (hair-pulling disorder). DSM-5 also excludes repetitive/habitual hair manipulation that does not involve pulling out the hair (e.g., hair twirling or hair biting without hair removal). When such habits become clinically significant problems, they should be diagnosed as an other specified obsessive-compulsive and related disorder ("other body-focused repetitive behavior disorder").

Trichotillomania (hair-pulling disorder) has some similarities with OCD, in that it is marked by repetitive tension-reducing motor behavior that is difficult to control. However, there are substantial phenomenological differences between the two disorders. Individuals with trichotillomania (hair-pulling disorder) may feel compelled to pull hair, but it is not because of fear or discomfort as commonly drives OCD rituals (e.g., a sense of looming danger/harm or disgust). Rather, trichotillomania (hair-pulling disorder) patients typically experience a longing to pull hair and gratification or pleasure when pulling. If hair pulling is solely due to obsessive intrusions related to OCD, trichotillomania (hair-pulling disorder) should not be diagnosed.

Individuals with BDD may engage in excessive hair pulling aimed at correcting perceived (i.e., nonexistent or slight) flaws in the appearance of their hair (e.g., "excessive," "thick," or "asymmetrical" hair that is considered ugly or unattractive). Similarly, patients with trichotillomania (hair-pulling disorder) may report pulling out hairs to obtain symmetry (e.g., pulling evenly from both eyebrows) or for an appearance-related reason (e.g., preference for pulling out hairs that are gray or wiry). However, in trichotillomania (hair-pulling disorder) these behaviors are not driven by concerns that the hair looks ugly, abnormal, or unattractive. A diagnosis of trichotillomania (hair-pulling disorder) should not be given if hair pulling is *solely* driven by appearance concerns, as in BDD.

Similarly, if hair pulling is done solely in response to hallucinations or delusions or is attributable to the use of substances, trichotillomania (hair-pulling disorder) is not diagnosed. Finally, several medical or dermatological conditions can cause alopecia (e.g., alopecia areata, telogen effluvium, tinea capitis, lichen planopilaris, or alopecia mucinosa). In such cases, if hair pull-

TABLE 5–3. Instruments and methods for the assessment of trichotillomania (hair-pulling disorder)

Instrument/Method	Description	Scores/Diagnoses
Interviews		
Trichotillomania Diagnostic Interview (TDI; Rothbaum and Ninan 1994)	Semistructured diagnostic interview designed to determine the diagnosis of trichotillomania. TDI was originally designed for DSM-III-R criteria and was modified for DSM-IV.	DSM-III-R/DSM-IV diagnosis of trichotillomania
National Institute of Mental Health Trichotillomania Questionnaire (Swedo et al. 1992)	Semistructured interview designed to assess clinical severity of trichotillomania.	Severity score Impairment score Total score
Questionnaires		
Massachusetts General Hospital Hairpulling Scale (Keuthen et al. 2007)	Seven-item self-report questionnaire that measures trichotillomania severity over the past week. The scale assesses urges to pull, time spent pulling, control over pulling, interference due to pulling, etc.	Severity score Resistance/Control score Total score
Trichotillomania Scale for Children (Tolin et al. 2008)	A 12-item self-report questionnaire designed to assess severity of hair-pulling disorder in children and adolescents. The scale has parallel child and parent versions.	Severity score Distress/Impairment score Total score
Milwaukee Inventory for Subtypes of Trichotillomania— Adult Version (Flessner et al. 2008)	A 15-item self-report questionnaire that assesses tendency to engage in two styles of pulling: 1) focused pulling (pulling in response to urges, negative affect, etc.) and 2) automatic pulling (pulling without reflective awareness).	Automatic hair-pulling score Focused hair-pulling score

TABLE 5–3. Instruments and methods for the assessment of trichotillomania (hair-pulling disorder) *(continued)*

Instrument/Method	Description	Scores/Diagnoses
Questionnaires *(continued)*		
Milwaukee Inventory for Styles of Trichotillomania–Child Version (Flessner et al. 2007)	A 17-item self-report questionnaire for the assessment of automatic and focused hair pulling in children and adolescents.	Automatic hair-pulling score Focused hair-pulling score
Obsessive-Compulsive Spectrum Disorder Scales for DSM-5 (LeBeau et al. 2013)	Four five-item self-report scales that assess past-week severity and impairment of trichotillomania (hair-pulling disorder), excoriation (skin-picking) disorder, body dysmorphic disorder, and hoarding disorder.	Hair-pulling severity/impairment score (also yields score for excoriation (skin-picking) disorder, body dysmorphic disorder, and hoarding disorder)
Other measures		
Self-monitoring	During treatment, it is often useful to have patients engage in daily self-monitoring. For example, they can be asked to record minutes spent pulling per day or number of "submits" (how often they pulled) versus "resists" (how often they wanted to pull but did not) each day.	Minutes spent pulling per day (or other outcomes)
Photographs	It may be useful to take photographs of pulled areas to have objective assessment of progress.	Photographs of bald spots
Hair collection	Ask patient to collect (and count) pulled hairs. This can be a helpful and objective way of monitoring progress.	Counts of pulled hairs

ing or hair loss is solely explained by an underlying medical condition, trichotillomania (hair-pulling disorder) should not be diagnosed. The major differential diagnoses for hair-pulling disorder are presented in Table 5–4.

Etiology and Pathophysiology

Genetics/Neurobiology

A large family study found that trichotillomania (hair-pulling disorder) subjects had a significantly higher proportion of family members with the disorder compared with control subjects without trichotillomania (hair-pulling disorder) (Keuthen et al. 2014). Two twin studies, both of which relied on self-report assessment of symptoms, found a significantly higher concordance for trichotillomania among identical twins than fraternal twins, yielding heritability estimates of 32% and 76% (Monzani et al. 2014; Novak et al. 2009).

Trichotillomania (hair-pulling disorder) appears to aggregate in families with OCD and other obsessive-compulsive and related disorders (Bienvenu et al. 2012; Monzani et al. 2014). For example, Monzani et al. (2014) examined self-reported symptom severity of trichotillomania (hair-pulling disorder), BDD-like symptoms, hoarding disorder, and excoriation (skin-picking) disorder among 5,409 female twins from the general U.K. population. The data supported two latent liability factors that were both largely heritable. The first factor represented a general vulnerability underlying all five symptom dimensions (particularly OCD, BDD-like symptoms, and hoarding disorder), and the second factor represented a more specific liability shared only by trichotillomania (hair-pulling disorder) and excoriation (skin-picking) disorder. Trichotillomania (hair-pulling disorder) and excoriation (skin-picking) disorder shared most of their genetic underpinnings. However, Keuthen et al. (2014) failed to find elevated rates of excoriation (skin-picking) disorder in first-degree family members of trichotillomania (hair-pulling disorder) subjects.

Understanding of a specific genetic underpinning of trichotillomania (hair-pulling disorder) is currently limited, and the few studies conducted so far need replication (Stein and Lochner 2012). For instance, studies have found a link between a variant of the gene *SAPAP3* and overgrooming in mice as well as pathological hair pulling, skin picking, and nail biting in humans. Other studies have linked trichotillomania (hair-pulling disorder) with the gene *SLITRK1* and another gene involving serotonin receptors (Stein and Lochner 2012).

Because hair pulling is difficult to control, often provides pleasure or gratification, and may regulate stress reactions or negative affect, it has been sug-

TABLE 5–4. Differential diagnosis for trichotillomania (hair–pulling disorder)

	Trichotillomania (hair-pulling disorder) should NOT be diagnosed:
Nonpathological hair pulling	If hair pulling is solely part of normal grooming practices (plucking eyebrows).
Obsessive-compulsive disorder (OCD)	If hair pulling is solely in response to obsessions in OCD.
Body dysmorphic disorder (BDD)	If hair pulling is solely caused by preoccupation with nonexistent or slight defects or flaws involving the appearance of the hair, with hair pulling an attempt to improve the perceived flaws. BDD should be diagnosed rather than trichotillomania (hair-pulling disorder).
Psychotic disorders	If hair pulling is due to hallucinations or delusions in psychotic disorders.
Medical conditions	If hair pulling is solely due to a medical condition such as a dermatological problem.
Substance use	If hair pulling is solely due to the use of drugs.

gested that trichotillomania (hair-pulling disorder) results from dysfunctions in brain circuitry involving behavioral control, reward processing, and affect or stress regulation (Stein and Lochner 2012). Current brain imaging data are somewhat consistent with this notion, although the literature is small and findings are mixed. In short, some neuroimaging studies (e.g., Chamberlain et al. 2010; White et al. 2013) have reported that individuals with trichotillomania (hair-pulling disorder) show aberrant brain activity in a number of regions when compared with healthy control subjects. These regions include those involved in reward processing (e.g., nucleus accumbens), top-down action regulation (e.g., anterior cingulate, presupplementary motor area), affect regulation (e.g., amygdalo-hippocampal complex), and habit learning (e.g., striatum). In contrast, other studies have failed to find differences in brain activity between trichotillomania (hair-pulling disorder) subjects and control subjects or have found abnormalities only among individuals with greater severity and longer duration of illness (Roos et al. 2013). However, it should be noted that the imaging studies conducted so far have used small samples, and failure to detect group differences may be due to lack of statistical power.

We do not know of any neuropsychological work examining stress/affect regulation or reward processing in trichotillomania (hair-pulling disorder). However, a few studies have found that adults with trichotillomania (hair-pulling disorder) perform poorly on motor inhibition tasks (e.g., the stop-signal task) compared with healthy control subjects, although these findings have not been consistently replicated (Chamberlain et al. 2009). Subjects with trichotillomania (hair-pulling disorder) also perform worse than or differently from healthy control subjects on tasks assessing divided attention, visuospatial learning, spatial working memory (Chamberlain et al. 2009), and attentional processing of hair-related cues (Lee et al. 2012). These findings require replication and clarification regarding how such deficits may play a role in the disorder.

Environmental/Sociocultural

Twin research (Monzani et al. 2014) shows substantial environmental underpinnings of trichotillomania (hair-pulling disorder). However, the specific environmental risk factors have not been identified, and gene-by-environment interactions are poorly understood. Clinical observation and uncontrolled studies have linked the onset and severity of trichotillomania (hair-pulling disorder) with life stress, and some evidence suggests higher levels of childhood trauma in samples with the disorder compared with healthy control subjects (Stein and Lochner 2012). Thus, it is possible that stress or trauma plays a role in onset of the disorder for some individuals, although additional studies are needed.

Treatment

General Approaches to Treatment and Special Considerations

In milder cases, and possibly some early-onset cases, individuals with trichotillomania (hair-pulling disorder) may experience lasting remission, either spontaneously or in response to minimal interventions. In general, however, trichotillomania (hair-pulling disorder) tends to be a chronic problem that is difficult to treat, and the behavior is prone to relapse. A form of cognitive-behavioral therapy (CBT) that emphasizes habit reversal training (HRT) and stimulus control (SC) techniques should be the first line of treatment. Medication may also be beneficial, either as monotherapy or in combination with CBT (Bloch et al. 2007).

Pharmacotherapy

Three medications have been shown to produce greater symptom reduction than pill placebo or comparison treatment in double-blind randomized controlled trials: clomipramine, olanzapine, and N-acetylcysteine. Clomipramine has been investigated in two randomized trials (see Bloch et al. 2007). An early crossover trial compared the efficacy of 5 weeks of clomipramine (average maximal dosage, 180 mg/day) and 5 weeks of desipramine (average maximal dosage, 173 mg/day) in the treatment of 13 females with trichotillomania. Participants showed significantly greater symptom reduction during the clomipramine treatment compared with the desipramine treatment. During the clomipramine phase, nine participants (69%) had at least 50% reduction in symptoms (clinician-rated symptom severity); three of these patients had complete remission of hair pulling.

Another study compared the efficacy of 9 weeks of clomipramine treatment (average dosage, 116 mg/day) with that of pill placebo and of CBT involving HRT/SC interventions (see subsection "Psychotherapy" later in this chapter). Intention-to-treat analyses showed that all five participants in the CBT condition, four of six participants in the clomipramine condition, and none of the five participants in the placebo condition responded (defined as "much or very much improvement" on the clinician-rated Clinical Global Impression–Improvement scale; CGI-I). Clomipramine resulted in greater symptom reduction than placebo, but the difference was not statistically significant, presumably because of lack of power. A meta-analysis of the two clomipramine studies indicated a significant treatment effect (Bloch et al. 2007).

Studies also indicate that olanzapine may be effective in reducing trichotillomania (hair-pulling disorder) symptoms. Van Ameringen et al. (2010)

randomly assigned adults with trichotillomania to receive 12 weeks of placebo treatment or 12 weeks of olanzapine treatment (flexible titrated dosages, starting at 2.5 mg/day and reaching up to 20 mg/day at the end of treatment). Many participants in the treatment group (11/13, 85%) reported adverse side effects (e.g., increased appetite, fatigue, headaches, and dry mouth); however, none withdrew from the study early. At posttreatment, 11 of 13 patients (85%) in the treatment group were classified as treatment responders (i.e., "much or very much improved" on the CGI-I). Only 2 of the 12 patients (17%) in the placebo group were classified as responders. Difference between groups became significant after 6 weeks of treatment.

Evidence suggests that N-acetylcysteine, a glutamate modulator, may benefit adults but not children with trichotillomania (hair-pulling disorder). N-Acetylcysteine is an over-the-counter medication that is well tolerated and has minimal side effects. Grant et al. (2009) randomly assigned 50 adults with trichotillomania to 9 weeks of treatment with placebo or N-acetylcysteine (dosages ranged from 1,200 to 2,400 mg/day). At posttreatment, 56% (14/25) of the participants in the N-acetylcysteine group versus only 16% (4/25) of the placebo group were judged "much improved" or "very much improved" (on the CGI-I). Statistically significant group differences emerged after 9 weeks of treatment. No participants in the N-acetylcysteine group reported adverse side effects.

However, a similar placebo-controlled trial (Bloch et al. 2013) in pediatric trichotillomania (N=39) failed to replicate the results from the adult sample (Grant et al. 2009). In this study, 39 children (8–17 years old) were randomly assigned to receive 12 weeks of placebo or N-acetylcysteine treatment (dosages titrated up to a maximum of 2,400 mg/day). At posttreatment, 25% (5/20) of the N-acetylcysteine group and 21% (4/19) of the placebo group were judged to be treatment responders (i.e., "much or very much improved" on the CGI-I). A full body rash was reported in one girl receiving N-acetylcysteine, although overall rates of reported side effects were not elevated in the treatment group compared with the placebo group.

Even though uncontrolled trials have shown that selective serotonin reuptake inhibitors (SSRIs) may be effective in the treatment of trichotillomania (hair-pulling disorder), the four placebo-controlled trials conducted thus far have all failed to show treatment effect (Bloch et al. 2007). Three of the trials examined fluoxetine and one trial examined sertraline; all included small samples (9–16 patients in the treatment groups) and thus were underpowered to detect treatment differences. Meta-analyses of these four studies showed no treatment effect of SSRIs (Bloch et al. 2007). Some evidence, however, suggests that SSRIs in combination with psychotherapy may be more beneficial than either treatment alone, at least for some individuals; this possibility warrants further empirical attention (Dougherty et al. 2006).

Venlafaxine showed promise in uncontrolled examination but did not show efficacy in a small controlled trial (Ninan 2000). Eight of 12 responders to a 12-week venlafaxine trial (dosages titrated to 150–375 mg/day) were randomly assigned to continued venlafaxine ($n=4$) versus placebo ($n=4$) treatment (24 weeks). All participants in the venlafaxine group had relapsed by week 14. Another study (Grant et al. 2014) examined 8 weeks of naltrexone treatment in a placebo-controlled trial ($n=51$). At posttreatment, there was no significant difference between the groups; 36% of the naltrexone group and 35% of the placebo group were classified as treatment responders ("much or very much improvement" on the CGI-I).

In conclusion, although the current literature is underdeveloped and many studies were insufficiently powered, some preliminary recommendations for pharmacotherapy can be offered. Surveys show that there is a tendency among clinicians to proscribe SSRIs to trichotillomania (hair-pulling disorder) patients; however, as noted earlier, randomized trials suggest these medications (at least fluoxetine and sertraline) may not provide benefits above placebo effects (although studies were very small). On the other hand, both clomipramine and olanzapine appear effective in reducing symptoms, although adverse side effects need to be considered. Given the tolerability of *N*-acetylcysteine, and favorable response in one large trial (Grant et al. 2009), at present this drug may be considered a first-line medication treatment for adult trichotillomania (hair-pulling disorder). To date, no controlled study has demonstrated effective drug treatment for pediatric trichotillomania (hair-pulling disorder).

Psychotherapy

The therapy with the most empirical support is a behavioral intervention consisting of HRT with SC techniques. HRT has three treatment components: 1) awareness training, 2) competing response training, and 3) social support. In awareness training, the patient is taught to become aware of the behavior and "warning signs" preceding it (e.g., urges to pull or movement of hands toward pulling sites). Awareness training often involves having the patient perform daily self-monitoring of pulling behavior and antecedents, describe pulling episodes in great detail, and participate in in-session exercises (e.g., the patient is asked to act out and identify pulling behavior or "warning signs" during conversation with the clinician). In competing response training, the patient is instructed to perform an incompatible action (e.g., gently clenching the fist) when "warning signs" or the pulling behavior occurs. A "social support person" (e.g., a parent or spouse) is sometimes recruited to reinforce the patient's use of the competing response and compliance with the treatment (this may be especially relevant for pediatric patients). Finally, SC techniques involve changing the patient's environment so that engaging in hair pulling becomes more effortful and/or less reinforcing (e.g., wearing gloves or covering mirrors).

Several randomized controlled trials have consistently shown that HRT/SC is effective in reducing hair pulling among children and adults with trichotillomania (hair-pulling disorder). In general, studies show that 40%–60% of patients show clinically significant improvement in symptoms at posttreatment (Bloch et al. 2007; Franklin et al. 2011). Furthermore, a meta-analysis (Bloch et al. 2007) of studies in adults with trichotillomania showed that HRT/SC was superior to clomipramine.

Studies also suggest that Web-based self-help programs involving HRT/SC may benefit some individuals with trichotillomania (hair-pulling disorder). In a recent study, Rogers et al. (2014) investigated a stepped-care program. In step 1, 60 adults with trichotillomania (hair-pulling disorder) were randomly assigned either to a wait-list condition or to immediate self-help HRT/SC (a 10-week self-help Web-based HRT/SC program at StopPulling.com). The results showed moderate but significant treatment effect according to blinded clinician-rated symptom severity. In step 2, 76% (46/60) of the participants from the first step chose to participate in eight-session in-person HRT (patients with greater severity at posttreatment were more likely to enroll in step 2). One half (50%) of the patients gained significant improvement; the proportion of participants with symptoms that met DSM-IV diagnostic criteria dropped from 95% to 54% in step 2. However, at 3-month follow-up, 67% still had symptoms that met the diagnostic criteria.

To enhance long-term outcome and to more effectively treat patients with severe symptoms, researchers have attempted to augment HRT/SC with strategies aimed at helping patients to better manage internal experiences, such as urges, impulses, negative affect, or stress reactions. Such strategies have been chosen because these experiences tend to trigger hair pulling, and the behavior tends to reduce them. Additionally, augmented treatment protocols often include strategies aimed at enhancing motivation and preventing relapse. Motivation is important to address when treating trichotillomania (hair-pulling disorder), because many patients gain pleasure and emotion or stress reduction from pulling episodes, and thus they may be ambivalent about stopping. To enhance motivation, it can be helpful to carefully review with the patient the psychosocial impact of the disorder and evaluate the costs and benefits associated with hair pulling. Relapse prevention typically involves emphasizing the difference between lapse and relapse and creating strategies the patient can use in future situations that may trigger relapse. Finally, because relapse often occurs when patients stop using strategies learned in treatment, booster sessions may be necessary to maintain treatment gains (e.g., offer sessions every few weeks or months in which the patient and clinician can review treatment strategies and problem-solve new challenges).

Randomized controlled trials in adults with trichotillomania (hair-pulling disorder) have demonstrated the efficacy of HRT/SC augmented with dialectical behavior therapy (Keuthen et al. 2012) and with acceptance and commitment therapy (Woods et al. 2006b), with maintenance of gains at 3 and 6 months after treatment (Keuthen et al. 2012; Woods et al. 2006b). Furthermore, in these studies, symptom improvement and long-term outcome were partly mediated by increased ability to effectively manage or accept internal states (i.e., better emotion regulation ability or less experiential avoidance; Keuthen et al. 2012; Woods et al. 2006b). Researchers have also augmented HRT/SC with cognitive therapy. For example, a controlled trial (Franklin et al. 2011) among children with trichotillomania showed that HRT/SC-enhanced cognitive therapy resulted in significantly greater symptom improvement at the end of treatment compared to a minimal attention control condition; these gains were maintained 2 months later.

Overall, the available literature suggests that cognitive-behavioral strategies, in particular HRT/SC, are effective in significantly reducing trichotillomania (hair-pulling disorder) symptoms at posttreatment for both children and adults. Data on long-term follow-up beyond 3–6 months are limited, but clinical experience suggests that relapse is common. It has been suggested that automatic and focused pulling behaviors may respond differentially to different interventions (Flessner et al. 2007, 2008). HRT/SC interventions may be particularly important for individuals who primarily engage in automatic pulling without awareness. Also, given that children often appear to engage in automatic pulling, HRT/SC may be important in the treatment of many pediatric cases. Alternatively, strategies aimed at managing urges, emotions, and other internal events (acceptance and commitment therapy, dialectical behavior therapy, and cognitive therapy) may be more helpful for individuals with focused pulling. However, this matching hypothesis has not been tested empirically. In our clinical experience, most adolescents and adults with trichotillomania (hair-pulling disorder) report both automatic and focused pulling and benefit from a combination of HRT/SC and strategies aimed at internal events.

Key Points

- Diagnosis of trichotillomania (hair-pulling disorder) is relatively straightforward and involves establishing the occurrence of recurrent hair pulling, although denial or poor awareness of hair-pulling behavior may complicate diagnosis and assessment.

- Trichotillomania (hair-pulling disorder) should not be diagnosed if hair pulling is solely due to concerns about imagined or minor appearance flaws in body dysmorphic disorder, obsessive intrusions in obsessive-compulsive disorder, hallucinations or delusions in psychotic disorders, or underlying medical or dermatological conditions.

- Many individuals with hair-pulling disorder are intensely embarrassed about their hair pulling, feel inadequate for not being able to control it, or are ashamed about certain features of the behavior (e.g., pulling from pubic regions, eating the hairs). Thus, acceptance and understanding by the clinician are important for forming a productive therapeutic alliance.

- Because hair pulling tends to produce pleasurable feelings, patients may have some ambivalence about stopping the behavior. It is therefore important to cultivate motivation to break the habit early in treatment, including in pharmacotherapy treatment.

- Relapse after treatment appears common; thus, relapse prevention strategies should be emphasized before terminating treatment.

- One reason trichotillomania (hair-pulling disorder) patients relapse after cognitive-behavioral therapy is that they stop using the strategies taught in treatment. Thus, booster sessions may be necessary.

- Habit reversal training and stimulus control may possibly be better suited to treating automatic hair pulling, whereas acceptance and commitment therapy, dialectical behavior therapy, and cognitive therapy may be better suited for focused pulling, although this hypothesis requires testing.

References

American Psychiatric Association: Diagnostic and Statistical Manual of Mental Disorders, 3rd Edition Revised. Washington, DC, American Psychiatric Association, 1987

American Psychiatric Association: Diagnostic and Statistical Manual of Mental Disorders, 4th Edition. Arlington, VA, American Psychiatric Association, 1994

American Psychiatric Association: Diagnostic and Statistical Manual of Mental Disorders, 5th Edition. Washington, DC, American Psychiatric Association, 2013

Bienvenu OJ, Samuels JF, Wuyek LA, et al: Is obsessive-compulsive disorder an anxiety disorder, and what, if any, are spectrum conditions? A family study perspective. Psychol Med 42(1):1–13, 2012 21733222

Bloch MH, Landeros-Weisenberger A, Dombrowski P, et al: Systematic review: pharmacological and behavioral treatment for trichotillomania. Biol Psychiatry 62(8):839–846, 2007 17727824

Bloch MH, Panza KE, Grant JE, et al: N-Acetylcysteine in the treatment of pediatric trichotillomania: a randomized, double-blind, placebo-controlled add-on trial. J Am Acad Child Adolesc Psychiatry 52(3):231–240, 2013 23452680

Chamberlain SR, Hampshire A, Menzies LA, et al: Reduced brain white matter integrity in trichotillomania: a diffusion tensor imaging study. Arch Gen Psychiatry 67(9):965–971, 2010 20819990

Chamberlain SR, Odlaug BL, Boulougouris V, et al: Trichotillomania: neurobiology and treatment. Neurosci Biobehav Rev 33(6):831–842, 2009 19428495

Christenson GA, Mackenzie TB, Mitchell JE: Characteristics of 60 adult chronic hair pullers. Am J Psychiatry 148(3):365–370, 1991 1992841

Dougherty DD, Loh R, Jenike MA, et al: Single modality versus dual modality treatment for trichotillomania: sertraline, behavioral therapy, or both? J Clin Psychiatry 67(7):1086–1092, 2006 16889452

Duke DC, Bodzin DK, Tavares P, et al: The phenomenology of hairpulling in a community sample. J Anxiety Disord 23(8):1118–1125, 2009 19651487

Flessner CA, Woods DW, Franklin ME, et al: The Milwaukee Inventory for Styles of Trichotillomania–Child Version (MIST-C): initial development and psychometric properties. Behav Modif 31(6):896–918, 2007 17932243

Flessner CA, Woods DW, Franklin ME, et al: The Milwaukee Inventory for Subtypes of Trichotillomania–Adult Version (MIST-A): development of an instrument for the assessment of "focused" and "automatic" hair pulling. J Psychopathol Behav Assess 30:20–30, 2008

Franklin ME, Flessner CA, Woods DW, et al: The Child and Adolescent Trichotillomania Impact Project: descriptive psychopathology, comorbidity, functional impairment, and treatment utilization. J Dev Behav Pediatr 29(6):493–500, 2008 18955898

Franklin ME, Edson AL, Ledley DA, et al: Behavior therapy for pediatric trichotillomania: a randomized controlled trial. J Am Acad Child Adolesc Psychiatry 50(8):763–771, 2011 21784296

Grant JE, Christenson GA: Examination of gender in pathologic grooming behaviors. Psychiatr Q 78(1):259–267, 2007 17712636

Grant JE, Odlaug BL: Clinical characteristics of trichotillomania with trichophagia. Compr Psychiatry 49(6):579–584, 2008 18970906

Grant JE, Menard W, Phillips KA: Pathological skin picking in individuals with body dysmorphic disorder. Gen Hosp Psychiatry 28(6):487–493, 2006 17088164

Grant JE, Odlaug BL, Kim SW: N-Acetylcysteine, a glutamate modulator, in the treatment of trichotillomania: a double-blind, placebo-controlled study. Arch Gen Psychiatry 66(7):756–763, 2009 19581567

Grant JE, Odlaug BL, Schreiber LR, et al: The opiate antagonist, naltrexone, in the treatment of trichotillomania: results of a double-blind, placebo-controlled study. J Clin Psychopharmacol 34(1):134–138, 2014 24145220

Keuthen NJ, Flessner CA, Woods DW, et al: Factor analysis of the Massachusetts General Hospital Hairpulling Scale. J Psychosom Res 62(6):707–709, 2007 17540230

Keuthen NJ, Rothbaum BO, Fama J, et al: DBT-enhanced cognitive-behavioral treatment for trichotillomania: a randomized controlled trial. J Behav Addict 1:106–114, 2012

Keuthen NJ, Altenburger EM, Pauls D: A family study of trichotillomania and chronic skin picking. Am J Med Genet B Neuropsychiatr Genet 165:167–174, 2014

King RA, Zohar AH, Ratzoni G, et al: An epidemiological study of trichotillomania in Israeli adolescents. J Am Acad Child Adolesc Psychiatry 34(9):1212–1215, 1995 7559316

LeBeau RT, Mischel ER, Simpson HB, et al: Preliminary assessment of obsessive-compulsive spectrum disorder scales for DSM-5. J Obsessive Compuls Relat Disord 2:114–118, 2013

Lee H-J, Franklin SA, Turkel JE, et al: Facilitated attentional disengagement from hair-related cues among individuals diagnosed with trichotillomania: an investigation based on the exogenous cueing paradigm. J Obsessive Compuls Relat Disord 1:8–15, 2012

Lochner C, Stein DJ: Obsessive-compulsive spectrum disorders in obsessive-compulsive disorder and other anxiety disorders. Psychopathology 43(6):389–396, 2010 20847586

Lochner C, Seedat S, Stein DJ: Chronic hair-pulling: phenomenology-based subtypes. J Anxiety Disord 24(2):196–202, 2010 19932593

Lochner C, Grant JE, Odlaug BL, et al: DSM-5 field survey: hair-pulling disorder (trichotillomania). Depress Anxiety 29(12):1025–1031, 2012 23124891

Mansueto CS, Thomas AM, Brice AL: Hair pulling and its affective correlates in an African-American university sample. J Anxiety Disord 21(4):590–599, 2007 16997529

Monzani B, Rijsdijk F, Harris J, et al: The structure of genetic and environmental risk factors for dimensional representations of DSM-5 obsessive-compulsive spectrum disorders. JAMA Psychiatry 71(2):182–189, 2014 24369376

Neal-Barnett A, Flessner C, Franklin ME, et al: Ethnic differences in trichotillomania: phenomenology, interference, impairment, and treatment efficacy. J Anxiety Disord 24(6):553–558, 2010 20413254

Ninan PT: Conceptual issues in trichotillomania, a prototypical impulse control disorder. Curr Psychiatry Rep 2(1):72–75, 2000 11122936

Novak CE, Keuthen NJ, Stewart SE, et al: A twin concordance study of trichotillomania. Am J Med Genet B Neuropsychiatr Genet 150B(7):944–949, 2009 19199280

Odlaug BL, Grant JE: Trichotillomania and pathologic skin picking: clinical comparison with an examination of comorbidity. Ann Clin Psychiatry 20(2):57–63, 2008 18568576

Odlaug BL, Kim SW, Grant JE: Quality of life and clinical severity in pathological skin picking and trichotillomania. J Anxiety Disord 24(8):823–829, 2010 20594805

Rogers K, Banis M, Falkenstein MJ, et al: Stepped care in the treatment of trichotillomania. J Consult Clin Psychol 82(2):361–367, 2014 24491078

Roos A, Fouche J-P, Stein DJ, et al: White matter integrity in hair-pulling disorder (trichotillomania). Psychiatry Res 211(3):246–250, 2013 23149033

Rothbaum BO, Ninan PT: The assessment of trichotillomania. Behav Res Ther 32(6):651–662, 1994 8085996

Snorrason I, Belleau EL, Woods DW: How related are hair pulling disorder (trichotillomania) and skin picking disorder? A review of evidence for comorbidity, similarities and shared etiology. Clin Psychol Rev 32(7):618–629, 2012 22917741

Soriano JL, O'Sullivan RL, Baer L, et al: Trichotillomania and self-esteem: a survey of 62 female hair pullers. J Clin Psychiatry 57(2):77–82, 1996 8591973

Stein DJ, Lochner C: Psychobiology of hair pulling disorder (trichotillomania) and skin picking disorder, in Trichotillomania, Skin Picking, and Other Body-Focused Repetitive Behaviors. Edited by Grant JE, Stein DJ, Woods DW, et al. Washington, DC, American Psychiatric Publishing, 2012

Stein DJ, Flessner CA, Franklin M, et al: Is trichotillomania a stereotypic movement disorder? An analysis of body-focused repetitive behaviors in people with hair-pulling. Ann Clin Psychiatry 20(4):194–198, 2008 19034750

Stein DJ, Grant JE, Franklin ME, et al: Trichotillomania (hair pulling disorder), skin picking disorder, and stereotypic movement disorder: toward DSM-V. Depress Anxiety 27(6).611–626, 2010 20533371

Swedo SE, Leonard HL, Lenane MC, et al: Trichotillomania: a profile of the disorder from infancy through adulthood. International Pediatrics 7:144–150, 1992

Tolin DF, Franklin ME, Diefenbach GJ, et al: Pediatric trichotillomania: descriptive psychopathology and an open trial of cognitive behavioral therapy. Cogn Behav Ther 36(3):129–144, 2007 17852170

Tolin DF, Diefenbach GJ, Flessner CA, et al: The Trichotillomania Scale for Children: development and validation. Child Psychiatry Hum Dev 39(3):331–349, 2008 18183484

Torres AR, Fontenelle LF, Ferrão YA, et al: Clinical features of obsessive-compulsive disorder with hoarding symptoms: a multicenter study. J Psychiatr Res 46(6):724–732, 2012 22464941

Van Ameringen M, Mancini C, Patterson B, et al: A randomized, double-blind, placebo-controlled trial of olanzapine in the treatment of trichotillomania. J Clin Psychiatry 71(10):1336–1343, 2010 20441724

Walther MR, Snorrason I, Flessner CA, et al: The Trichotillomania Impact Project in Young Children (TIP-YC): clinical characteristics, comorbidity, functional impairment and treatment utilization. Child Psychiatry Hum Dev 45(1):24–31, 2014 23564261

White MP, Shirer WR, Molfino MJ, et al: Disordered reward processing and functional connectivity in trichotillomania: a pilot study. J Psychiatr Res 47(9):1264–1272, 2013 23777938

Woods DW, Flessner CA, Franklin ME, et al: The Trichotillomania Impact Project (TIP): exploring phenomenology, functional impairment, and treatment utilization. J Clin Psychiatry 67(12):1877–1888, 2006a 17194265

Woods DW, Wetterneck CT, Flessner CA: A controlled evaluation of acceptance and commitment therapy plus habit reversal for trichotillomania. Behav Res Ther 44(5):639–656, 2006b 16039603

Recommended Readings

Franklin ME, Tolin DF: Treating Trichotillomania: Cognitive-Behavioral Therapy for Hairpulling and Related Problems. New York, Springer, 2007

Grant JE, Stein DJ, Woods DW, et al: Trichotillomania, Skin Picking, and Other Body-Focused Repetitive Behaviors. Washington, DC, American Psychiatric Publishing, 2007

Keuthen NJ, Stein DJ, Christenson GA: Help for Hair Pullers: Understanding and Coping With Trichotillomania. Oakland, CA, New Harbinger Publications, 2001

Penzel F: The Hair-Pulling Problem: A Complete Guide to Trichotillomania. New York, Oxford University Press, 2003

StopPulling.com: www.stoppulling.com. This Web site offers an interactive treatment protocol for hair-pulling disorder that is based on cognitive-behavioral strategies.

Trichotillomania Learning Center: www.trich.org. This is the Web site of the Trichotillomania Learning Center, a national advocacy organization for hair-pulling disorder and related disorders. Among other things, the website includes a variety of educational material as well as information on support groups and treatment providers.

CHAPTER 6

Excoriation (Skin-Picking) Disorder

Jon E. Grant, J.D., M.D., M.P.H.
Brian L. Odlaug, M.P.H.

Excoriation (skin-picking) disorder, also referred to as *pathological skin picking, neurotic excoriation, dermatillomania,* or *psychogenic excoriation,* is characterized by the repetitive and compulsive picking of skin, leading to tissue damage (American Psychiatric Association 2013). Although new to DSM-5, excoriation (skin-picking) disorder has been described in the medical and dermatological fields since the late nineteenth century. The French dermatologist M.L. Brocq was the first to describe the disorder in detail, discussing a case series of young women who repetitively picked at their acne and thereby made their skin lesions worse (Brocq 1898). Excoriation disorder then sporadically appeared in case reports in the dermatological literature over the next several decades but with no agreed-on diagnostic criteria (Adamson 1913; Michelson 1945; Pusey and Senear 1920; Seitz 1951). It was not until 1978, however, that the first report of the epidemiology of excoriation disorder was published. Robert Griesemer, who was trained as a dermatologist and a psychiatrist, examined 4,576 dermatology patients and found that 2% (92) had lifetime excoriation disorder (Griesemer 1978). With this limited body of scientific evidence, excoriation disorder was relegated to a brief mention in DSM-IV (American Psychiatric Association 1994) as an "impulse-control disorder not otherwise specified."

The inclusion of excoriation (skin-picking) disorder in DSM-5 was in response to the growing body of data emphasizing its prevalence and potentially disabling nature, as well as influence from patients and patient advocates (Stein and Phillips 2013). Data from multiple researchers around the world consistently have shown that excoriation (skin-picking) disorder is fairly common, with clear phenomenological characteristics, important neurobiological findings, and documented responsiveness to treatment. These data suggested substantial diagnostic validity for excoriation (skin-picking) disorder, sufficient for its recognition and inclusion in DSM-5 (Grant et al. 2012). It was also clear from the clinical data that there are significant clinical similarities between excoriation (skin-picking) disorder and other obsessive-compulsive and related disorders such as trichotillomania (hair-pulling disorder), and the DSM-5 diagnostic criteria for the two disorders are very similar. The new diagnostic criteria for excoriation (skin-picking) disorder were supported by a DSM-5-sponsored field survey (Lochner et al. 2012).

Diagnostic Criteria and Symptomatology

The DSM-5 criteria for excoriation (skin-picking) disorder are presented in Box 6–1. Most individuals at some time pick at their skin, either to smooth out irregularities or to improve blemishes or acne, although excoriation (skin-picking) disorder should not be diagnosed if diagnostic criteria for body dysmorphic disorder (BDD) are met (i.e., if patients have distressing or impairing preoccupations with perceived skin defects that lead to skin picking). Clinicians must also differentiate between *normal* grooming behaviors and more *pathological* forms of grooming as seen in excoriation (skin-picking) disorder.

BOX 6–1. DSM-5 Diagnostic Criteria Excoriation (Skin-Picking) Disorder

---

A. Recurrent skin picking resulting in skin lesions.
B. Repeated attempts to decrease or stop skin picking.
C. The skin picking causes clinically significant distress or impairment in social, occupational, or other important areas of functioning.
D. The skin picking is not attributable to the physiological effects of a substance (e.g., cocaine) or another medical condition (e.g., scabies).
E. The skin picking is not better explained by symptoms of another mental disorder (e.g., delusions or tactile hallucinations in a psychotic disorder, at-

tempts to improve a perceived defect or flaw in appearance in body dysmorphic disorder, stereotypies in stereotypic movement disorder, or intention to harm oneself in nonsuicidal self-injury).

Criterion A requires that picking be recurrent and result in skin lesions, thereby reflecting the frequency and intensity of the picking. Many individuals with excoriation (skin-picking) disorder report that the behavior began with the onset of a dermatological condition such as acne (Wilhelm et al. 1999) but that the picking continued even after the dermatological condition cleared. For many, the preoccupation with blemishes is disproportional to the dermatological issues faced by the patient (Zaidens 1951), and consequently, picking behaviors have been reported to worsen preexisting conditions (such as scarring from acne; Fruensgaard et al. 1978).

Although the face is the most common site of picking, other areas, such as the hands, fingers, arms, and legs, are also common targets. Most individuals with this disorder pick from more than one body area (Odlaug and Grant 2012). In fact, a study of 60 patients with excoriation (skin-picking) disorder found that subjects picked from an average of 4.5 sites (Tucker et al. 2011). Many individuals report having a primary body area for picking but may pick at other areas of the body in order to allow the most significantly excoriated areas to heal (Bohne et al. 2002; Odlaug and Grant 2008). For many people with excoriation (skin-picking) disorder, a variety of picking lesions are exhibited, ranging from a few to a few hundred (Gupta et al. 1987; Pusey and Senear 1920).

Although most individuals pick at areas they can physically reach with their fingernails, some also report using knives, scissors, tweezers, pins, needles, letter openers, and other objects to pick (Grant et al. 2007). DSM-5 further requires that the person have tried to decrease or stop the picking. This criterion reflects the intense drive underlying the behavior that is endorsed by those with excoriation (skin-picking) disorder. The repetitive picking behavior suggests underlying dysfunction of motor inhibitory control processes, and neurocognitive data support the idea that individuals with this disorder have difficulty inhibiting motor behaviors once they have been initiated (Grant et al. 2011).

Individuals with excoriation (skin-picking) disorder spend a significant amount of time picking their skin, with a mean of 2.8 hours each day spent resisting the urge to pick or actually picking (Flessner and Woods 2006). A smaller percentage (15%) may pick for more than 8 hours each day (Arnold et al. 1998). Becaue of the amount of time spent picking, many individuals (20.7%–40.2%) report missing or being late for important work or social activities (Flessner and Woods 2006). Medical complications are common and include infections, scarring, septicemia, and ulcerations (Odlaug and Grant

2008). The picking often also leads to problems with self-esteem and in personal relationships (Odlaug and Grant 2012).

Skin picking may be accompanied by a range of behaviors or rituals involving the skin or scabs. Individuals may search for a particular kind of scab to pull or an irregularity of the skin to pick. Skin picking may be preceded by anxiety or boredom and may lead to a feeling of accomplishment or pleasure when the skin has been picked (52%–87% report pleasurable feelings resulting from picking; Flessner and Woods 2006; Odlaug and Grant 2012). Some individuals engage in skin picking that is more focused (i.e., with preceding urges to pick), others pick automatically (i.e., are not fully aware that they are doing it), and some have a mix of both styles of picking (American Psychiatric Association 2013; Grant et al. 2011; Odlaug and Grant 2012; Walther et al. 2009).

Because stimulant drugs such as cocaine and amphetamines can lead to skin picking, the diagnosis of excoriation (skin-picking) disorder should not be made if the picking is only a consequence of drug use. In addition, the diagnosis should not be made when the excoriation behavior is secondary to a dermatological condition such as scabies, atopic dermatitis, or psoriasis. Skin picking may also be a symptom of certain other psychiatric disorders— in particular, BDD, in which patients pick their skin in an attempt to improve the appearance of perceived skin flaws, such as acne. Another is parasitosis, in which individuals excoriate their skin in response to a delusion that their skin is infected with parasites or other vermin. Excoriation (skin-picking) disorder should not be diagnosed in such cases (also see "Differential Diagnosis" section).

Case Example: Ginny

Ginny is a 19-year-old single, white student at a university who picks at her face daily. She began picking at approximately age 14 and has not been able to stop the behavior for more than a few days at a time. She tends to pick more while studying, when stressed, and when her hands are free, and she is not fully aware of the behavior most of the time. She often stops when she is aware of the blood and feels ashamed immediately afterward. The picking has led to social isolation, because she does not want to date or be around other students due to the scarring and scabs created by the picking behavior.

Case Example: Richard

Richard is a 30-year-old African American man who lives alone and is unable to work due to picking. Richard picks only at his face, but the time (3–5 hours each day) and the intensity of the picking have left him covered with scars and scabs. Although he reports urges to pick, most of the time he is completely unaware of his behavior while picking. He reports that while sitting and watching television, he frequently may notice that his fingers are covered with blood, yet he was unaware that he was picking at his skin. The picking behavior has been present for more than 10 years without any relief. He covers his face in public and cannot socialize due to the embarrassment caused by the disfiguring scars. Last year he was admitted to the hospital for intravenous antibiotics due to an infection from picking at his face.

Epidemiology

Although no national epidemiology studies have included excoriation (skin-picking) disorder, two community-based prevalence studies found that the disorder is common. In one study (N=354), 5.4% of participants (19) reported significant picking with associated distress and functional impairment, thereby mirroring the DSM-5 criteria (Hayes et al. 2009). A different study, which used a random digit dialing telephone survey (N=2,513), found that although 10% (251) picked to the point of having noticeable skin damage that was not attributable to a medical condition, when distress or impairment was required in order to meet the criteria, 1.4% (35) had symptoms that met the criteria for excoriation (skin-picking) disorder (Keuthen et al. 2010). In addition, a community-based twin study (N=2,481) found that 1.4% (35) had behavior consistent with the diagnosis of excoriation (skin-picking) disorder (Monzani et al. 2012). Rates of excoriation (skin-picking) disorder in college students have been generally within the range found in the community (4.2%–4.6%) (Bohne et al. 2002; Odlaug et al. 2013).

Comorbidity

Excoriation (skin-picking) disorder is often accompanied by other mental disorders. Commonly co-occurring disorders include obsessive-compulsive disorder (OCD), BDD, trichotillomania (hair-pulling disorder), and major depressive disorder. Rates of current co-occurring OCD are significantly higher in individuals with excoriation (skin-picking) disorder (6%–52%) compared with rates in the community (1%–3%) (Arnold et al. 1998; Calikuşu et al. 2003). One study found that 11 (32%) of the 34 subjects with excoriation disorder also had BDD (Arnold et al. 1998).

Other disorders that are characterized by excessive grooming behavior (i.e., body-focused repetitive behaviors such as trichotillomania [hair-pulling disorder] and nail biting) are also common in individuals with excoriation (skin-picking) disorder (Arnold et al. 1998; Lochner et al. 2002). One study (N=60) found that 36.7% of individuals with excoriation disorder (22) had a lifetime diagnosis of trichotillomania (Odlaug and Grant 2008). This rate is substantially higher than the rate of trichotillomania (hair-pulling disorder) in the general population (0.6%–3.9%; Mansueto and Rogers 2012). A study of 80 subjects with excoriation disorder found a lifetime rate of co-oc-curring major depressive disorder of 26.3% ($n = 21$; Odlaug et al. 2013).

Course and Prognosis

The age at onset for excoriation (skin-picking) disorder varies substantially. Although the mean age at onset seems to be about 12 years (Odlaug and Grant 2008), the disorder may have its onset during childhood (<10 years old), adolescence (mean age approximately 13–15 years), or at a later age (between the ages of 30 and 45) (Bohne et al. 2002; Flessner and Woods 2006; Simeon et al. 1997; Tucker et al. 2011). The disorder frequently begins with a dermatological condition, such as acne.

Although the course of illness varies, when untreated, excoriation (skin-picking) disorder is most often considered a chronic disorder with fluctuations in intensity over time (Odlaug and Grant 2012). Two studies have found a mean duration of illness of 19–20 years (Grant et al. 2007; Keuthen et al. 2000). Many individuals report that the symptoms of their picking, although waxing and waning in intensity over many years, are essentially unchanged with time. Seeking medical help from a physician is uncommon among individuals who pick their skin (Grant et al. 2007). Research indicates that less than 20% of subjects seek treatment for their picking (Flessner and Woods 2006; Grant et al. 2007). Individuals with this disorder often report that they are unaware that viable treatments are available, too embarrassed to mention it, and feel as if they should be able to stop the behavior on their own (Grant et al. 2007).

Psychosocial Impairment

Excoriation (skin-picking) disorder can take an enormous toll. A study of 92 individuals with the disorder found that 17.4% (16) used illegal drugs, 22.8% (21) used tobacco products, and 25.0% (23) used alcohol to relieve feelings (e.g., anxiety, depression, guilt, and shame) associated with excoriation and its physical consequences (Flessner and Woods 2006). In addition, 85.9% of subjects (79) reported anxiety and 66.3% (61) reported depressed mood due to picking (Flessner and Woods 2006). Picking often impacts an individual's social life (40.2% miss social events and 54.3% refrain from intimacy) and career path (12.0% reported not pursuing advancement at work due to picking) (Flessner and Woods 2006).

In addition to the emotional impact of picking, the behavior may result in significant tissue damage and often leads to medical complications such as localized infections and even septicemia (38% report needing some medical intervention because of the picking; Keuthen et al. 2000; Odlaug and

Grant 2008, 2012). Patients are often too ashamed to reveal areas that have become infected or where picking is particularly severe, for fear of being negatively judged by others. A thorough physical examination is often needed to accurately assess the extent and severity of picking. Topical or oral antibiotics may be needed.

The repetitive, excoriative nature of picking in severe cases may even warrant skin grafting (Arnold et al. 1998; Odlaug and Grant 2008). In rare cases, the behavior can be life threatening, as demonstrated by the case report of a 55-year-old man whose picking on his back required multiple blood transfusions due to excessive blood loss (Kondziolka and Hudak 2008).

Developmental Considerations

A study that assessed childhood-onset excoriation (skin-picking) disorder found that its clinical presentation generally did not differ significantly from the clinical presentation of later-onset cases (Odlaug and Grant 2007a). The only differences were that those who started picking in childhood were less likely to pick with full conscious awareness of their behavior, were more likely to wait a considerable time before seeking treatment, and were less likely to seek medication treatment (Odlaug and Grant 2007a).

Gender-Related Issues

Multiple studies that have examined gender have consistently found that women are approximately two to three times more likely to have excoriation (skin-picking) disorder than men (Lovato et al. 2012; Odlaug et al. 2013; Torresan et al. 2013). One study that examined gender differences in the disorder found that men had a significantly later age at onset (approximately 15 years vs. 10 years in women), spent more than twice the amount of time picking compared with women (approximately 3 hours each day vs. 1 hour each day), and reported significantly greater functional impairment due to picking. In addition, men were more likely to report a co-occurring anxiety disorder (Grant and Christenson 2007).

Cultural Aspects of Phenomenology

Little is known about the cultural aspects of excoriation (skin-picking) disorder. From the limited data, however, it appears that the clinical characteristics are the same across age cohorts and across countries and cultures, including Europe (Bohne et al. 2002), Africa (Lochner et al. 2002), North America (Tucker et al. 2011), South America (Arzeno Ferrão et al. 2006), and the Middle East (Calikuşu et al. 2012).

Assessment and Differential Diagnosis

Clinical Evaluation

The clinical evaluation of an individual with excoriation (skin-picking) disorder entails a comprehensive physical and psychiatric examination. The physical examination serves two purposes: first, to assess the extent of the picking and to develop appropriate interventions based on the damage to the skin; and second, to assess for possible dermatological or infectious etiologies of the skin picking. In terms of possible etiologies, there are many dermatological conditions that may result in scratching or picking—for example, scabies, atopic dermatitis, psoriasis, or blistering skin disorders (Mostaghimi 2012). Where there is diagnostic uncertainty, patients may be referred for a thorough dermatological consultation, which may include microscopic examination of lesions for scabies, Wood's lamp examination for fungal infections, patch testing for allergies, skin biopsies, and laboratory investigations of thyroid (e.g., hypothyroidism), parathyroid (e.g., hypoparathyroidism), liver (e.g., bile duct disease), and kidney (e.g., end-stage renal disease) problems, because these may all cause pruritus, scratching or rubbing of the skin, and resultant excoriations (Mostaghimi 2012).

A thorough psychiatric evaluation is also required in order to differentiate excoriation (skin-picking) disorder from other psychiatric conditions, including personality disorders (e.g., borderline personality disorder when the excoriation is part of a broader presentation of self-injurious behavior) and substance use disorders (e.g., cocaine or amphetamine use disorder). In these cases, the picking should not be diagnosed as excoriation (skin-picking) disorder. Skin picking that occurs as a symptom of BDD or parasitosis (a type of delusional disorder, somatic type) should not be diagnosed as excoriation (skin-picking) disorder (see subsection "Differential Diagnosis" later in this section).

In children, examination should also focus on the possibility that skin picking is associated with a pervasive developmental disorder or Prader-Willi syndrome, a rare chromosomal disorder that is often associated with hyperphagia, hypogonadism, and frequent skin picking (Morgan et al. 2010). Up to 95% of individuals with this syndrome may pick at their skin (Morgan et al. 2010); in these cases, Prader-Willi syndrome, not excoriation (skin-picking) disorder, is the appropriate diagnosis.

Measures

Sample screening questions for excoriation (skin-picking) disorder are presented in Table 6–1. Several reliable and valid measures can be used to monitor symptom severity and change in symptoms during treatment. These scales can be used to track the severity of the skin-picking problem along with other aspects of the picking, such as the time spent experiencing urges and thoughts to pick as well as time expended on the picking behavior itself. Two of several available scales are discussed in the following paragraphs.

TABLE 6–1. Screening questions for excoriation (skin-picking) disorder

---

Can you tell me why you pick?

Can you control your picking?

Do you have urges to pick that are difficult for you to control?

Are there activities or other things in your life that you avoid due to your picking?

At what time(s) in the day do you pick? For example, are you around other people or by yourself? Do you pick most while driving or at home watching TV, etc.?

Do you have any triggers to your picking? For example, do you pick when you are tired, stressed, angry, sad, etc.?

Source. Adapted from Grant et al. 2014a.

The Yale-Brown Obsessive Compulsive Scale Modified for Neurotic Excoriation (NE-YBOCS) is a 10-item clinician-administered scale that assesses picking symptoms during the past 7 days (Grant et al. 2010a). The first five items compose the picking urge/thought subscale (time occupied with urges/thoughts; interference and distress due to urges/thoughts; resistance against and control over urges/thoughts). In general, individuals with excoriation (skin-picking) disorder do not have obsessive thoughts about picking, but they often have intense urges, and these first five items may reflect those urges. Items 6 through 10 compose the picking behavior subscale (time spent picking; interference and distress due to picking; ability to resist and control picking behavior). Higher total scores on the NE-YBOCS indicate greater levels of severity.

The Skin Picking Impact Scale (Keuthen et al. 2001) is a 10-item self-report measure that assesses skin picking (e.g., the scale examines the effects of picking on social life, time spent picking, embarrassment due to picking, and relationship problems). The measure has an even shorter four-item version, which has retained the validity and reliability of the longer measure (Snorrason et al. 2013).

A scale has been developed to examine the degree to which those with excoriation (skin-picking) disorder exhibit focused versus automatic picking behavior (Walther et al. 2009).

Differential Diagnosis

Excoriation (skin-picking) disorder is often misdiagnosed as OCD. Conversely, OCD, BDD, and delusional disorder can be misdiagnosed as excoriation (skin-picking) disorder. Proper diagnosis is important because treatments of these various disorders differ (see Table 6–2).

TABLE 6–2.　Major differential diagnosis for excoriation (skin-picking) disorder

Body dysmorphic disorder	If picking is solely performed to improve a perceived defect in appearance of the skin (e.g., perceived acne, bumps, or scars), then body dysmorphic disorder should be diagnosed.
Stimulant use	If picking is performed only when a person is using or withdrawing from illicit or prescription stimulants, then a primary substance use disorder may be more appropriate.
Delusions of parasitosis	When picking is performed because the person is falsely convinced that he or she is infested with parasites, then delusional disorder is the appropriate diagnosis.
Obsessive-compulsive disorder	When excessive washing in response to contamination obsessions is the cause of skin lesions or when a person picks only to remove particles of dirt or other perceived contaminants from the skin, obsessive-compulsive disorder should be diagnosed.

　　BDD is often the most difficult differential diagnosis to make. BDD is characterized by distressing or impairing preoccupation with perceived defects in physical features (see Chapter 3, "Body Dysmorphic Disorder"). Perceived flaws of the skin (e.g., acne, marks, scars) are the most common focus of BDD concerns. Problematic skin-picking behavior occurs in 26%–45% of patients with BDD (Grant et al. 2006). Individuals with BDD pick at their skin to try to improve its appearance, although, as in excoriation (skin-picking) disorder, because skin picking can be so time consuming and involve use of sharp implements, it often creates visible skin lesions or scarring. Individuals who pick their skin as a symptom of BDD should not be diagnosed with excoriation (skin-picking) disorder; those with excoriation (skin-picking) disorder do not pick their skin because of their appearance, and their symptoms do not meet the diagnostic criteria for BDD. A good way to differentiate these disorders is to ask patients why they pick at their skin. If the picking is intended to improve the appearance of perceived skin flaws, BDD is the more appropriate diagnosis (assuming all diagnostic criteria are met). In contrast, those with excoriation (skin-picking) disorder do not pick in response to a particular cognition.

It is also possible that a person may have co-occurring excoriation (skin-picking) disorder and BDD. For example, a person may pick at his or her face to improve its appearance (a clear symptom of BDD) and yet also pick at the legs in an automatic fashion with no obsessive thinking about the appearance of the legs. Both disorders may therefore be diagnosed concurrently. Treatments for these two disorders typically differ (i.e., selective serotonin reuptake inhibitors for BDD and *N*-acetylcysteine for excoriation (skin-picking) disorder, as well as different cognitive-behavioral approaches), so the appropriate diagnosis of these two disorders is crucial.

Use or abuse of stimulants (e.g., cocaine, methamphetamine, and prescription stimulants) may cause skin excoriation due to unpleasant skin sensations (e.g., crawling, itching sensations) or a type of motor tic (i.e., the uncontrollable need to move one's arms or hands) resulting from the uncomfortable agitation caused by the drugs. Therefore, clinicians should rule out stimulant use. It is also possible that a patient may have excoriation (skin-picking) disorder that is worsened by stimulant use. In those cases, the picking may improve after the stimulant is stopped but will most likely still remain in a less severe form and therefore may need to be treated.

Some individuals with OCD may excessively wash their hands in response to contamination obsessions, and the washing may in turn lead to skin lesions. In addition, other individuals with OCD-related contamination obsessions may pick at or scrub their skin to remove contaminants. In either case, OCD would be the more appropriate diagnosis.

Finally, some individuals with delusions or tactile hallucinations are convinced that they are infested with a parasite, which is a form of delusional disorder known as *parasitosis*. Such individuals typically pick at and scratch their skin to uncover and remove the parasites they believe are present. Although a rare disorder, the first-line treatment for this form of delusional disorder consists of an antipsychotic rather than treatment typically used for excoriation (skin-picking) disorder (see section "Treatment" later in this chapter). Thus, accurate differential diagnosis is important.

Etiology and Pathophysiology

Although data are limited, family history data suggest that excoriation (skin-picking) disorder is familial. In a study of 60 patients with the disorder, 28.3% (17/60) of their first-degree family members had it as well (Odlaug and Grant 2012). Direct comparison of subjects with excoriation (skin-picking) disorder and probands with OCD revealed that subjects with excoriation (skin-picking) disorder had higher rates of co-occurring compulsive nail biting and were more likely to have a first-degree relative with a disorder involving excessive grooming (trichotillomania [hair-pulling disorder] and nail biting; Grant et al. 2010b).

One study that examined the prevalence and heritability of skin picking in a sample of 2,518 twins from the Twins U.K. Adult Twin Registry found that clinically significant skin picking was endorsed by 1.2% of twins (30 subjects) (Monzani et al. 2012). In addition, significantly higher correlations between a measure of skin-picking severity (the Skin Picking Scale) for the monozygotic ($r=0.42$) than for the dizygotic ($r=0.09$) twin pairs indicated a strong genetic influence on skin picking. Additive and nonadditive genetic factors accounted for slightly more than 40% of the variance in skin picking, with the remaining variance attributable to nonshared environmental factors (Monzani et al. 2012).

Animal research on several genes has shown promise in developing our understanding of repetitive behaviors such as that seen in excoriation (skin-picking) disorder. The gene encoding SAPAP3, a scaffolding protein found in excitatory glutamate-responsive synapses largely in the striatum (Welch et al. 2007), has been implicated in human disorders that involve excessive grooming, such as excoriation (skin-picking) disorder and trichotillomania (hair-pulling disorder) (Bienvenu et al. 2009). Another candidate model is the gene *Hoxb8*. Mice with mutations of this gene, compared with their control counterparts, groom excessively to the point of skin lesions. Finally, the Slitrk family of proteins (Slitrk1–6) is a family of integral membrane proteins that are thought to control neurite outgrowth during development. Research suggests that starting at the age of 3 months, loss of the neuron-specific transmembrane protein SLIT and NTRK-like protein-5 (Slitrk5) leads to excessive self-grooming in mice (Shmelkov et al. 2010). The genetic research in animals, while perhaps not directly clinically useful at the current time, is important in highlighting pathological mechanisms that may be relevant to a subset of human patients.

In recent years, neurocognitive research has also attempted to elucidate underpinnings of excoriation (skin-picking) disorder. The repetitive physical symptoms suggest underlying dysfunction of motor inhibitory control processes. Motor impulsivity is classically assessed using tasks that require individuals to make simple motor responses on some computer trials but not others. Stop-signal tasks use an individually tailored tracking algorithm to estimate the time the brain takes to suppress an already initiated response. Response inhibition as a cognitive function is dependent on neural circuitry that includes the right inferior frontal gyrus. One study that used a stop-signal task indicated impaired stop-signal inhibitory control in patients with excoriation (skin-picking) disorder compared with healthy volunteers (Odlaug et al. 2010).

In the only neuroimaging study, subjects with excoriation (skin-picking) disorder exhibited disorganization of white matter tracts involved in motor generation and suppression (i.e., bilateral anterior cingulate and right orbitofrontal and inferior frontal cortices). These findings are remarkably similar to those previously reported for trichotillomania (hair-pulling disorder) (Grant et al. 2013).

Treatment

General Approaches to Treatment

If untreated, excoriation (skin-picking) disorder tends to be a chronic illness that often results in substantial psychosocial dysfunction and may lead to life-threatening medical problems. Control of the skin picking is therefore critical for maintaining long-term health and quality of life. The clinician should begin with a thorough psychiatric assessment to establish an accurate diagnosis of excoriation (skin-picking) disorder. Next, the clinician should have the patient undergo a thorough evaluation from a dermatologist with knowledge about excoriation (skin-picking) disorder to assess for underlying dermatological conditions that may cause or worsen skin picking. Additionally, the clinician should maintain collaboration between internal medicine and psychiatric management teams for monitoring and rapid intervention if serious medical sequelae result from the picking.

Somatic Treatments

The treatment data on excoriation (skin-picking) disorder are quite limited. In terms of pharmacotherapy, there are only four double-blind, placebo-controlled clinical trials (Gelinas and Gagnon 2013). All studies were small and thus had limited power to detect differences between treatment groups.

Data regarding the efficacy of serotonin reuptake inhibitors have been mixed, with some studies demonstrating improvement on certain measures of picking behavior. One small 10-week study of fluoxetine in 21 subjects with excoriation disorder found that among the 17 completers (6 fluoxetine, 11 placebo), the fluoxetine group, at a mean dosage of 55 mg/day, improved significantly more than the placebo group after 6 weeks of treatment. However, the intention-to-treat subjects responded on only one of the three outcome measures of skin picking, and full remission was not observed in any patients (Simeon et al. 1997).

In a second fluoxetine study, 15 subjects were given 6 weeks of open-label fluoxetine (dosages varied between 20 and 60 mg/day), followed by 6 weeks of a double-blind discontinuation phase for responders (measured by a 30% reduction in symptoms assessed with the Yale-Brown Obsessive Compulsive Scale). At the end of the 6-week open-label treatment phase, eight subjects (53.3%) were considered responders. The four subjects who were randomly assigned to receive fluoxetine maintained their improvement during the double-blind discontinuation phase, whereas the placebo group returned to baseline levels of picking severity (Bloch et al. 2001).

In a double-blind study of 45 subjects (23 assigned to receive citalopram and 22 assigned to receive placebo) with excoriation disorder who were treated with citalopram (20 mg/day) or placebo for 4 weeks, there was no significant difference between citalopram and placebo on the primary outcome measure, a visual analog scale of picking behavior (Arbabi et al. 2008). However, this study was not adequately powered, and it is likely that both the dosage and the duration of treatment were suboptimal.

In the only other double-blind, placebo-controlled study in excoriation disorder, the efficacy of the anticonvulsant lamotrigine was examined (Grant et al. 2010a). Although a 12-week open-label study in 24 subjects demonstrated benefit in reducing picking symptoms and improving functioning at a mean dosage of 200 mg/day (Grant et al. 2007), the subsequent 12-week double-blind, placebo-controlled study of 32 patients (with the dosage titrated up to 300 mg/day) failed to demonstrate greater benefit than placebo (Grant et al. 2010a). However, this study, too, was powered to detect only very large effects.

Glutamatergic agents, which have shown some promise in trichotillomania (hair-pulling disorder) (Grant et al. 2009), may have a useful role in the treatment of excoriation (skin-picking) disorder. One example is N-acetylcysteine, which has demonstrated benefit in case reports (Odlaug and Grant 2007b). On the basis of data on trichotillomania (hair-pulling disorder), N-acetylcysteine may be useful for reducing the urge to pick. Previous research has used up to 1,200 mg twice a day as a target dosage, with expected clinical benefit emerging after approximately 9 weeks (Grant et al. 2009). Side effects are generally mild and usually only involve feeling bloated and experiencing mild flatulence.

Opioid antagonists (e.g., naltrexone), which reduce self-licking in dogs with acral lick dermatitis, could also represent a viable option for excoriation (skin-picking) disorder (Banga and Connor 2012), although evidence of such benefit has been limited to small samples (case reports of single patients, often with Prader-Willi syndrome) and should therefore be considered very preliminary (Banga and Connor 2012). On the basis of results from an 8-week double-blind, placebo-controlled study of naltrexone (dosing of 50 mg/day up to 150 mg/day) in the treatment of 52 subjects with trichotillomania (hair-pulling disorder), however, naltrexone may potentially be useful for those with excoriation (skin-picking) disorder who have a family history positive for alcohol use disorders (Grant et al. 2014b).

Psychotherapy

As with pharmacotherapy, the research on psychotherapy for excoriation (skin-picking) disorder is very limited (Gelinas and Gagnon 2013). Psychosocial treatment has largely focused on cognitive-behavioral interventions. Early psychosocial treatment studies provided preliminary evidence for skin-picking reduction with habit reversal or acceptance-enhanced behavior therapy (Siev et al. 2012). There are, however, only two controlled psychosocial treatment studies for excoriation (skin-picking) disorder.

Teng et al. (2006) conducted a wait-list controlled study of habit reversal therapy in 25 subjects. The therapy consisted of habit reversal techniques. Subjects first did self-monitoring, recording the number of skin-picking occurrences each day, and those in the habit reversal group then had a 1-hour treatment session followed by two separate 30-minute booster sessions over the next 3 weeks (one session per week). Subjects were made more aware of their skin picking, including its antecedents, and a competing response was then taught, which consisted of clenching their fists for 1 minute. The final component of habit reversal training involved having participants identify a social support person who could provide praise when the competing response was used correctly and provide prompts when the competing response was used incorrectly or not at all. These treatment approaches are very similar to those used in habit reversal training for trichotillomania (hair-pulling disorder) (see Chapter 5, "Trichotillomania [Hair-Pulling Disorder]"). Those assigned to habit reversal had significantly greater reductions in self-reported picking frequency and skin damage at posttreatment and at 3-month follow-up compared with the wait-list group.

Similarly, Schuck et al. (2011) demonstrated the efficacy of a brief, four-session cognitive-behavioral therapy protocol for excoriation (skin-picking) disorder in comparison with a wait-list control in 34 patients with excoriation (skin-picking) disorder. The treatment consisted of four 45-minute sessions of manualized cognitive-behavioral therapy administered across 5 weeks. Treatment components included an initial discussion of the development, course, circumstances, and impact of skin picking followed by psychoeducation regarding skin picking. The second session focused on cognitive interventions; automatic cognitions with regard to skin picking were identified, critically questioned, and eventually replaced by more functional cognitions. In the third session, behavioral interventions focused on enhancing self-control. The fourth, and final, session focused on relapse prevention. Homework was given as part of each session. Assignments included documenting time spent picking and the strength of picking-related dysfunctional cognitions. Subjects in the treatment condition showed a significantly larger reduction on all measured variables in comparison to the wait-list condition, with large effect sizes (0.90–1.89) that were maintained at the 2-month follow-up.

Key Points

- If untreated, excoriation (skin-picking) disorder is an often chronic illness and in many cases results in substantial psychosocial dysfunction and may lead to life-threatening medical problems.

- The evaluation for excoriation (skin-picking) disorder must begin with a thorough psychiatric assessment to establish an accurate diagnosis, assess for co-occurring psychiatric disorders, and rule out other disorders in the differential.

- A thorough evaluation from a dermatologist with knowledge about excoriation (skin-picking) disorder may be necessary to assess for underlying dermatological conditions that may cause or worsen skin picking.

- A thorough physical examination may be needed to accurately assess the extent and severity of picking.

- Cognitive-behavioral therapy focusing on the dysfunctional thought processes underlying the behavior and including behaviors that are incompatible with picking (a competing response) has demonstrated benefit in only a few weeks of therapy. Receiving treatment from someone trained in habit reversal therapy for skin picking is essential to attain good treatment outcomes.

- In terms of pharmacotherapy, there is little evidence that selective serotonin reuptake inhibitors are beneficial, although studies had limited power. On the basis of our clinical experience, however, we find that N-acetylcysteine at dosages of 1,200 mg twice a day has been quite helpful in reducing urges to pick and probably should be considered the first-line pharmacotherapy treatment for excoriation (skin-picking) disorder.

- Coordinating care with a dermatologist is often necessary. Topical or oral antibiotics may be needed to treat localized infections that result from skin picking.

References

Adamson HG: Acne urticata and other forms of neurotic excoriation. Br J Dermatol 27:1–12, 1913

American Psychiatric Association: Diagnostic and Statistical Manual of Mental Disorders, 4th Edition. Arlington, VA, American Psychiatric Association, 1994

American Psychiatric Association: Diagnostic and Statistical Manual of Mental Disorders, 5th Edition. Arlington, VA, American Psychiatric Publishing, 2013

Arbabi M, Farina V, Balighi K, et al: Efficacy of citalopram in treatment of pathological skin picking: a randomized double blind placebo controlled trial. Acta Med Iran 46:367–372, 2008

Arnold LM, McElroy SL, Mutasim DF, et al: Characteristics of 34 adults with psychogenic excoriation. J Clin Psychiatry 59(10):509–514, 1998 9818631

Arzeno Ferrão Y, Almeida VP, Bedin NR, et al: Impulsivity and compulsivity in patients with trichotillomania or skin picking compared with patients with obsessive-compulsive disorder. Compr Psychiatry 47(4):282–288, 2006 16769303

Banga A, Connor DF: Effectiveness of naltrexone for treating pathologic skin picking behavior in an adolescent with Prader-Willi syndrome. J Child Adolesc Psychopharmacol 22(5):396–398, 2012 23083028

Bienvenu OJ, Wang Y, Shugart YY, et al: Sapap3 and pathological grooming in humans: results from the OCD collaborative genetics study. Am J Med Genet B Neuropsychiatr Genet 150B(5):710–720, 2009 19051237

Bloch MR, Elliott M, Thompson H, et al: Fluoxetine in pathologic skin-picking: open-label and double-blind results. Psychosomatics 42(4):314–319, 2001 11496020

Bohne A, Wilhelm S, Keuthen NJ, et al: Skin picking in German students: prevalence, phenomenology, and associated characteristics. Behav Modif 26(3):320–339, 2002 12080904

Brocq ML: Acne excoriée of young women and their treatment [in French]. J Prat Rev Gen Clin Ther 12:193–197, 1898

Calikuşu C, Yücel B, Polat A, et al: The relation of psychogenic excoriation with psychiatric disorders: a comparative study. Compr Psychiatry 44(3):256–261, 2003 12764714

Calikuşu C, Kucukgoncu S, Tecer Ö, et al: Skin picking in Turkish students: prevalence, characteristics, and gender differences. Behav Modif 36(1):49–66, 2012 21937566

Flessner CA, Woods DW: Phenomenological characteristics, social problems, and the economic impact associated with chronic skin picking. Behav Modif 30(6):944–963, 2006 17050772

Fruensgaard K, Hjortshøj A, Nielsen H: Neurotic excoriations. Int J Dermatol 17(10):761–767, 1978 730429

Gelinas BL, Gagnon MM: Pharmacological and psychological treatments of pathological skin-picking: a preliminary meta-analysis. J Obsessive Compuls Relat Disord 2(2):167–175, 2013

Grant JE, Christenson GA: Examination of gender in pathologic grooming behaviors. Psychiatr Q 78(4):259–267, 2007 17712636

Grant JE, Menard W, Phillips KA: Pathological skin picking in individuals with body dysmorphic disorder. Gen Hosp Psychiatry 28(6):487–493, 2006 17088164

Grant JE, Odlaug BL, Kim SW: Lamotrigine treatment of pathologic skin picking: an open-label study. J Clin Psychiatry 68(9):1384–1391, 2007 17915977

Grant JE, Odlaug BL, Kim SW: N-Acetylcysteine, a glutamate modulator, in the treatment of trichotillomania: a double-blind, placebo-controlled study. Arch Gen Psychiatry 66(7):756–763, 2009 19581567

Grant JE, Odlaug BL, Chamberlain SR, et al: A double-blind, placebo-controlled trial of lamotrigine for pathological skin picking: treatment efficacy and neurocognitive predictors of response. J Clin Psychopharmacol 30(4):396–403, 2010a 20531220

Grant JE, Odlaug BL, Kim SW: A clinical comparison of pathologic skin picking and obsessive-compulsive disorder. Compr Psychiatry 51(4):347–352, 2010b 20579505

Grant JE, Odlaug BL, Chamberlain SR: A cognitive comparison of pathological skin picking and trichotillomania. J Psychiatr Res 45(12):1634–1638, 2011 21824627

Grant JE, Odlaug BL, Chamberlain SR, et al: Skin picking disorder. Am J Psychiatry 169(11):1143–1149, 2012 23128921

Grant JE, Odlaug BL, Hampshire A, et al: White matter abnormalities in skin picking disorder: a diffusion tensor imaging study. Neuropsychopharmacology 38(5):763–769, 2013 23303052

Grant JE, Chamberlain SR, Odlaug BL: Clinical Guide to Obsessive Compulsive and Related Disorders. New York, Oxford University Press, 2014a

Grant JE, Odlaug BL, Schreiber LR, et al: The opiate antagonist, naltrexone, in the treatment of trichotillomania: results of a double-blind, placebo-controlled study. J Clin Psychopharmacol 34(1):134–138, 2014b 24145220

Griesemer RD: Emotionally triggered disease in a dermatologic practice. Psychiatr Ann 8:407–412, 1978

Gupta MA, Gupta AK, Haberman HF: The self-inflicted dermatoses: a critical review. Gen Hosp Psychiatry 9(1):45–52, 1987 3817460

Hayes SL, Storch EA, Berlanga L: Skin picking behaviors: an examination of the prevalence and severity in a community sample. J Anxiety Disord 23(3):314–319, 2009 19223150

Keuthen NJ, Deckersbach T, Wilhelm S, et al: Repetitive skin-picking in a student population and comparison with a sample of self-injurious skin-pickers. Psychosomatics 41(3):210–215, 2000 10849452

Keuthen NJ, Deckersbach T, Wilhelm S, et al: The Skin Picking Impact Scale (SPIS): scale development and psychometric analyses. Psychosomatics 42(5):397–403, 2001 11739906

Keuthen NJ, Koran LM, Aboujaoude E, et al: The prevalence of pathologic skin picking in US adults. Compr Psychiatry 51(2):183–186, 2010 20152300

Kondziolka D, Hudak R: Management of obsessive-compulsive disorder–related skin picking with gamma knife radiosurgical anterior capsulotomies: a case report. J Clin Psychiatry 69(8):1337–1340, 2008 18816157

Lochner C, Simeon D, Niehaus DJ, et al: Trichotillomania and skin-picking: a phenomenological comparison. Depress Anxiety 15(2):83–86, 2002 11891999

Lochner C, Grant JE, Odlaug BL, et al: DSM-5 field survey: skin picking disorder. Ann Clin Psychiatry 24(4):300–304, 2012 23145387

Lovato L, Ferrão YA, Stein DJ, et al: Skin picking and trichotillomania in adults with obsessive-compulsive disorder. Compr Psychiatry 53(5):562–568, 2012 22014580

Mansueto CS, Rogers KE: Trichotillomania: epidemiology and clinical characteristics, in Trichotillomania, Skin Picking, and Other Body-Focused Repetitive Behaviors. Edited by Grant JE, Stein DJ, Woods DW, et al. Washington, DC, American Psychiatric Publishing, 2012, pp 3–20

Michelson HE: Psychosomatic studies in dermatology: the motivation of self-induced eruptions. Arch Derm Syphilol 51:245–250, 1945

Monzani B, Rijsdijk F, Cherkas L, et al: Prevalence and heritability of skin picking in an adult community sample: a twin study. Am J Med Genet B Neuropsychiatr Genet 159B(5):605–610, 2012 22619132

Morgan JR, Storch EA, Woods DW, et al: A preliminary analysis of the phenomenology of skin-picking in Prader-Willi syndrome. Child Psychiatry Hum Dev 41(4):448–463, 2010 20405203

Mostaghimi L: Dermatological assessment of hair pulling, skin picking, and nail biting, in Trichotillomania, Skin Picking, and Other Body-Focused Repetitive Behaviors. Edited by Grant JE, Stein DJ, Woods DW, et al. Washington, DC, American Psychiatric Publishing, 2012, pp 97–112

Odlaug BL, Grant JE: Childhood-onset pathologic skin picking: clinical characteristics and psychiatric comorbidity. Compr Psychiatry 48(4):388–393, 2007a 17560962

Odlaug BL, Grant JE: N-Acetyl cysteine in the treatment of grooming disorders. J Clin Psychopharmacol 27(2):227–229, 2007b 17414258

Odlaug BL, Grant JE: Clinical characteristics and medical complications of pathologic skin picking. Gen Hosp Psychiatry 30(1):61–66, 2008 18164942

Odlaug BL, Grant JE: Pathologic skin picking, in Trichotillomania, Skin Picking, and Other Body-Focused Repetitive Behaviors. Edited by Grant JE, Stein DJ, Woods DW, et al. Washington, DC, American Psychiatric Publishing, 2012, pp 21–41

Odlaug BL, Chamberlain SR, Grant JE: Motor inhibition and cognitive flexibility in pathologic skin picking. Prog Neuropsychopharmacol Biol Psychiatry 34(1):208–211, 2010 19913592

Odlaug BL, Lust K, Schreiber LR, et al: Skin picking disorder in university students: health correlates and gender differences. Gen Hosp Psychiatry 35(2):168–173, 2013 23123103

Pusey WA, Senear FE: Neurotic excoriations with report of cases. Arch Derm Syphilol 1:270–278, 1920

Schuck K, Keijsers GP, Rinck M: The effects of brief cognitive-behaviour therapy for pathological skin picking: a randomized comparison to wait-list control. Behav Res Ther 49(1):11–17, 2011 20934685

Seitz PFD: Psychocutaneous aspects of persistent pruritus and excessive excoriation. AMA Arch Derm Syphilol 64(2):136–141, 1951 14856402

Shmelkov SV, Hormigo A, Jing D, et al: Slitrk5 deficiency impairs corticostriatal circuitry and leads to obsessive-compulsive-like behaviors in mice. Nat Med 16(5):598–602, 1p following 602, 2010 20418887

Siev J, Reese HE, Timpano K, et al: Assessment and treatment of pathological skin picking, in The Oxford Handbook of Impulse Control Disorders. Edited by Grant JE, Potenza MN. New York, Oxford University Press, 2012, pp 360–374

Simeon D, Stein DJ, Gross S, et al: A double-blind trial of fluoxetine in pathologic skin picking. J Clin Psychiatry 58(8):341–347, 1997 9515971

Snorrason I, Olafsson RP, Flessner CA, et al: The Skin Picking Impact Scale: factor structure, validity and development of a short version. Scand J Psychol 54(4):344–348, 2013 23682651

Stein DJ, Phillips KA: Patient advocacy and DSM-5. BMC Med 11:133, 2013 23683696

Teng EJ, Woods DW, Twohig MP: Habit reversal as a treatment for chronic skin picking: a pilot investigation. Behav Modif 30(4):411–422, 2006 16723422

Torresan RC, Ramos-Cerqueira AT, Shavitt RG, et al: Symptom dimensions, clinical course and comorbidity in men and women with obsessive-compulsive disorder. Psychiatry Res 209(2):186–195, 2013 23298952

Tucker BT, Woods DW, Flessner CA, et al: The Skin Picking Impact Project: phenomenology, interference, and treatment utilization of pathological skin picking in a population-based sample. J Anxiety Disord 25(1):88–95, 2011 20810239

Walther MR, Flessner CA, Conelea CA, et al: The Milwaukee Inventory for the Dimensions of Adult Skin Picking (MIDAS): initial development and psychometric properties. J Behav Ther Exp Psychiatry 40(1):127–135, 2009 18725154

Welch JM, Lu J, Rodriguiz RM, et al: Cortico-striatal synaptic defects and OCD-like behaviours in Sapap3-mutant mice. Nature 448(7156):894–900, 2007 17713528

Wilhelm S, Keuthen NJ, Deckersbach T, et al: Self-injurious skin picking: clinical characteristics and comorbidity. J Clin Psychiatry 60(7):454–459, 1999 10453800

Zaidens SH: Self-inflicted dermatoses and their psychodynamics. J Nerv Ment Dis 113(5):395–404, 1951 14832646

Recommended Readings

Franklin ME, Tolin DF: Treating Trichotillomania: Cognitive-Behavioral Therapy for Hairpulling and Related Problems. New York, Springer, 2007

Grant JE, Stein DJ, Woods DW, et al (eds): Trichotillomania, Skin Picking, and Other Body-Focused Repetitive Behaviors. Washington, DC, American Psychiatric Publishing, 2012

Grant JE, Chamberlain SR, Odlaug BL: Clinical Guide to Obsessive Compulsive and Related Disorders. New York, Oxford University Press, 2014

CHAPTER 7

Other Obsessive-Compulsive and Related Disorders in DSM-5

Katharine A. Phillips, M.D.
Dan J. Stein, M.D., Ph.D.

This chapter addresses four diagnostic categories in the DSM-5 chapter on obsessive-compulsive and related disorders (OCRDs): substance/medication-induced OCRD, OCRD due to another medical condition, other specified OCRD, and unspecified OCRD (American Psychiatric Association 2013).

Both the "substance/medication-induced" category and the "due to another medical condition" category are used in the disorder chapters throughout DSM-5. To ensure accurate diagnosis and treatment, it is critically important to consider whether a substance, a medication, or a nonpsychiatric medical condition is responsible for presenting symptoms—for example, whether cocaine use or scabies is the cause of compulsive skin picking.

Furthermore, many presenting conditions have similarities to an OCRD but do not quite meet the diagnostic criteria for the disorders discussed in earlier chapters in this book. Presentations such as these that cause clinically significant distress or impairment in functioning are diagnosed as "other specified OCRD" (when the clinician briefly describes the presenting symptoms) or as "unspecified OCRD" (when the clinician does not describe the presenting symptoms). These two categories are equivalent to the "not otherwise specified" category in previous editions of DSM. The "other specified" and "unspecified" categories are also used across DSM-5, for other diagnostic classes of disorders.

One example of an "other specified OCRD" is *body-focused repetitive behavior disorder,* which is characterized by repetitive behaviors, such as lip biting, that are not covered by other DSM-5 categories of body-focused repetitive behaviors (i.e., trichotillomania [hair-pulling disorder] or excoriation [skin-picking] disorder). Another example of an "other specified OCRD" is *olfactory reference syndrome (jikoshu-kyofu),* which involves distressing or impairing preoccupation with emitting an offensive or foul-smelling body odor, which other people cannot perceive. As these and other specified OCRDs are better studied and better understood, they may be included in future editions of DSM as separate diagnostic entities.

Because the OCRD chapter is new to DSM-5, these four diagnoses are new to the nomenclature, although they are analogous to conditions in DSM-IV (American Psychiatric Association 1994). In this chapter we discuss diagnostic criteria for these categories and examples of these presentations. We also consider key aspects of assessment and management.

Substance/Medication–Induced OCRD

Diagnostic Features

Substance/medication-induced OCRD is diagnosed when OCRD symptoms are clinically assessed as having a causal relationship to substance use, withdrawal from a substance, or use of a medication. It may be difficult to determine with certainty that the symptoms are due to a substance or medication; the diagnostic criteria focus largely on a temporal relationship between use of the substance or medication and development of OCRD-like symptoms as well as whether the substance or medication is known to be capable of producing the OCRD symptoms.

Diagnostic criteria for substance/medication-induced OCRD are shown in Box 7–1. The wording of the criteria is very similar to that used for substance/medication-induced diagnoses in other chapters of DSM-5 (e.g., substance/medication-induced anxiety disorder). However, the criteria include some features that are specific to OCRDs; most notably, Criterion A focuses on obsessions, compulsions, skin picking, hair pulling, other body-focused repetitive behaviors, or other symptoms characteristic of the OCRDs, which must predominate in the clinical picture. Criterion B states that there is evidence from the history, physical examination, or laboratory findings that these symptoms developed during or soon after substance intoxication or withdrawal or after exposure to a medication, and that the involved substance/medication is capable of producing the OCRD-like symptoms.

BOX 7–1. DSM-5 Diagnostic Criteria for Substance/Medication-Induced Obsessive-Compulsive and Related Disorder

---

A. Obsessions, compulsions, skin picking, hair pulling, other body-focused repetitive behaviors, or other symptoms characteristic of the obsessive-compulsive and related disorders predominate in the clinical picture.

B. There is evidence from the history, physical examination, or laboratory findings of both (1) and (2):

1. The symptoms in Criterion A developed during or soon after substance intoxication or withdrawal or after exposure to a medication.

2. The involved substance/medication is capable of producing the symptoms in Criterion A.

C. The disturbance is not better explained by an obsessive-compulsive and related disorder that is not substance/medication-induced. Such evidence of an independent obsessive-compulsive and related disorder could include the following:

The symptoms precede the onset of the substance/medication use; the symptoms persist for a substantial period of time (e.g., about 1 month) after the cessation of acute withdrawal or severe intoxication; or there is other evidence suggesting the existence of an independent non-substance/medication-induced obsessive-compulsive and related disorder (e.g., a history of recurrent non-substance/medication-related episodes).

D. The disturbance does not occur exclusively during the course of a delirium.

E. The disturbance causes clinically significant distress or impairment in social, occupational, or other important areas of functioning.

Note: This diagnosis should be made in addition to a diagnosis of substance intoxication or substance withdrawal only when the symptoms in Criterion A predominate in the clinical picture and are sufficiently severe to warrant clinical attention.

Coding note: The ICD-9-CM and ICD-10-CM codes for the [specific substance/medication]-induced obsessive-compulsive and related disorders are indicated in the table below. Note that the ICD-10-CM code depends on whether or not there is a comorbid substance use disorder present for the same class of substance. If a mild substance use disorder is comorbid with the substance-induced obsessive-compulsive and related disorder, the 4th position character is "1," and the clinician should record "mild [substance] use disorder" before the substance-induced obsessive-compulsive and related disorder (e.g., "mild cocaine use disorder with cocaine-induced obsessive-compulsive and related disorder"). If a moderate or severe substance use disorder is comorbid with the substance-induced obsessive-compulsive and related disorder, the 4th position character is "2," and the clinician should record "moderate [substance] use disorder" or "severe [substance] use disorder," depending on the severity of the comorbid substance use disorder. If there is no comorbid substance use disorder (e.g., after a one-time heavy use of the substance), then the 4th position character is "9," and the clinician should record only the substance-induced obsessive-compulsive and related disorder.

		ICD-10-CM		
	ICD-9-CM	With use disorder, mild	With use disorder, moderate or severe	Without use disorder
Amphetamine (or other stimulant)	292.89	F15.188	F15.288	F15.988
Cocaine	292.89	F14.188	F14.288	F14.988
Other (or unknown) substance	292.89	F19.188	F19.288	F19.988

Specify if (see Table 1 in the [DSM-5] chapter "Substance-Related and Addictive Disorders" for diagnoses associated with substance class):
   With onset during intoxication: If the criteria are met for intoxication with the substance and the symptoms develop during intoxication.
   With onset during withdrawal: If criteria are met for withdrawal from the substance and the symptoms develop during, or shortly after, withdrawal.
   With onset after medication use: Symptoms may appear either at initiation of medication or after a modification or change in use.

Criterion C indicates that the disturbance is not better explained by an OCRD that is not substance/medication-induced; this criterion provides guidelines to determine this, again with a focus on a temporal association between the clinical symptoms and use of a medication or substance. These guidelines are not meant to be exhaustive, however. It is useful to consider temporal relationships; for example, if symptoms preceded use of a medication or substance, it is very unlikely that the medication or substance is causing the symptoms. However, clinicians should consider all other available evidence as well.

Criterion D notes that the disturbance does not occur exclusively during the course of a delirium, and Criterion E indicates that the disturbance must cause clinically significant distress or impairment in social, occupational, or other important areas of functioning.

A DSM-5 "note" emphasizes that this diagnosis should be made in addition to a diagnosis of substance intoxication or substance withdrawal only when the symptoms in Criterion A predominate in the clinical picture and are sufficiently severe to warrant clinical attention. The manual also provides three specifiers: with onset during intoxication, with onset during withdrawal, and with onset after medication use.

Assessment and Treatment

The literature on the prevalence, psychobiology, and management of substance/medication-induced OCRD is sparse. Nevertheless, case reports indicate that obsessions, compulsions, hair pulling, skin picking, and other body-focused repetitive behaviors can occur in association with intoxication with stimulants (including cocaine) and other substances, as well as various toxins (Fried 1994; Laplane et al. 1989; Martin et al. 1998). The association between stimulant abuse and stereotypic behaviors (also known as "punding") has long been described, and such behaviors may include skin picking. Toxins that have been associated with obsessive-compulsive-like behavior include carbon monoxide.

These observations are consistent with the known pathophysiology of OCRDs. Stimulants act to increase dopaminergic neurotransmission, and in animal models they induce stereotypic behavior such as abnormal grooming and picking (Ridley 1994), which has similarities to certain repetitive behaviors in humans, including body-focused repetitive behaviors such as skin picking. Carbon monoxide may lead to basal ganglia lesions, and corticostriatal circuitry is thought to mediate obsessive-compulsive symptoms (Laplane et al. 1989).

Thus, it is appropriate for clinicians to consider routinely whether substances or medications are causing OCRD symptoms. In our clinical experience, it is more common to conclude that the relevant substance/medication plays an exacerbating role rather than a causal one; for example, patients with obsessive-compulsive disorder (OCD) may note that their symptoms worsen when they use cocaine.

When a substance/medication-induced OCRD is diagnosed, assessment and treatment should target the relevant substance/medication. For example, severity of cocaine use can be ascertained using standardized substance use scales. Laboratory assessment, such as a urine toxicology screening, may be useful. Substance use–focused psychotherapy or medication can be initiated. When a substance/medication is thought to be primarily responsible for presenting symptoms, it is more appropriate to directly target the substance or medication use rather than instituting a serotonin reuptake inhibitor (SRI), cognitive-behavioral therapy (CBT), or other treatment for an OCRD. However, when a substance/medication is thought to play an exacerbating role in precipitating or perpetuating an OCRD, clinicians may need to focus treatment on both the substance use and the OCRD itself.

A key debate in the literature regards the relationship between prescription psychostimulants, such as methylphenidate, and subsequent onset of tics. One early view was that because psychostimulants have dopaminergic effects, and because tics are mediated by this neurotransmitter system, tics may be an adverse effect of psychostimulants. A contrasting later view is that the emergence of tics in patients with attention-deficit/hyperactivity disorder (ADHD) after appropriate treatment with medications such as methylphenidate merely reflects the high comorbidity of ADHD with tic disorder. Reviews of the literature support this contemporary view (Madruga-Garrido and Mir 2013); the current consensus is that methylphenidate and other prescription stimulants not only do not exacerbate or reactivate tics but may actually improve tics in patients with comorbid ADHD and tic disorder.

OCRD Due to Another Medical Condition

Diagnostic Features

OCRD due to another medical condition is diagnosed when a nonpsychiatric medical disorder is thought to be the cause of OCRD symptoms. It is worth noting a difference in nomenclature between DSM-IV and DSM-5: DSM-IV referred to nonpsychiatric medical conditions as "general medical conditions," whereas DSM-5 refers to them as "*other* medical conditions," based on the fact that psychiatric disorders are themselves medical conditions.

The diagnostic criteria for OCRD due to another medical condition are presented in Box 7–2. The wording of these criteria is very similar to wording used in analogous "due to another medical condition" diagnoses in other DSM-5 chapters. The criteria also have some similarities to those for substance/medication-induced OCRD. Criterion A emphasizes that obsessions, compulsions, preoccupations with appearance, hoarding, hair pulling, skin picking, other body-focused repetitive behaviors, or other symptoms characteristic of the OCRDs predominate in the clinical picture. Criterion B emphasizes the need for evidence that the presenting symptoms are a direct pathophysiological consequence of a medical condition, based on the history, physical examination, or laboratory findings. Criteria C, D, and E indicate that the disturbance is not better explained by another mental disorder, does not occur exclusively during the course of a delirium, and causes clinically significant distress or impairment in social, occupational, or other important areas of functioning. DSM-5 provides several specifiers: with obsessive-compulsive disorder–like symptoms, with appearance preoccupations, with hoarding symptoms, with hair-pulling symptoms, and with skin-picking symptoms.

BOX 7–2. DSM-5 Diagnostic Criteria for Obsessive-Compulsive and Related Disorder Due to Another Medical Condition

---

A. Obsessions, compulsions, preoccupations with appearance, hoarding, skin picking, hair pulling, other body-focused repetitive behaviors, or other symptoms characteristic of obsessive-compulsive and related disorder predominate in the clinical picture.
B. There is evidence from the history, physical examination, or laboratory findings that the disturbance is the direct pathophysiological consequence of another medical condition.
C. The disturbance is not better explained by another mental disorder.
D. The disturbance does not occur exclusively during the course of a delirium.
E. The disturbance causes clinically significant distress or impairment in social, occupational, or other important areas of functioning.

Specify if:
   With obsessive-compulsive disorder–like symptoms: If obsessive-compulsive disorder–like symptoms predominate in the clinical presentation.
   With appearance preoccupations: If preoccupation with perceived appearance defects or flaws predominates in the clinical presentation.
   With hoarding symptoms: If hoarding predominates in the clinical presentation.
   With hair-pulling symptoms: If hair pulling predominates in the clinical presentation.
   With skin-picking symptoms: If skin picking predominates in the clinical presentation.
Coding note: Include the name of the other medical condition in the name of the mental disorder (e.g., 294.8 [F06.8] obsessive-compulsive and related disorder due to cerebral infarction). The other medical condition should be coded and listed separately immediately before the obsessive-compulsive and related disorder due to the medical condition (e.g., 438.89 [I69.398] cerebral infarction; 294.8 [F06.8] obsessive-compulsive and related disorder due to cerebral infarction).

Reprinted from American Psychiatric Association: *Diagnostic and Statistical Manual of Mental Disorders,* 5th Edition. Arlington, VA, American Psychiatric Association. Copyright 2013, American Psychiatric Association. Used with permission.

In some cases, the cause of the OCRD-like symptoms can be determined with reasonable certainty—for example, when excoriation occurs in response to pruritus caused by eczema. In other cases, however, it may be difficult to determine with certainty whether a medical illness is the cause of OCRD-like symptoms. Guidelines that may assist in determining such an etiological relationship include the presence of a clear temporal association between the onset, exacerbation, or remission of the medical condition and the OCRD symptoms; the presence of features that are atypical of a primary OCRD (e.g., atypical age at onset or course); and evidence in the literature that a known physiological mechanism (e.g., striatal damage) causes OCRD symptoms.

Assessment and Treatment

The literature on the prevalence, psychobiology, and treatment of OCRD due to another medical condition is once again fairly sparse. Nevertheless, case reports indicate that obsessions, compulsions, preoccupations with appearance, hoarding, hair pulling, skin picking, or other body-focused repetitive behaviors can occur as a result of a range of medical disorders (Laplane et al. 1989; Mataix-Cols et al. 2010; Stein et al. 2010). These observations are consistent with the known pathophysiology of some OCRDs; for example, a range of neurological conditions may lead to lesions in corticostriatal circuitry and so precipitate obsessive-compulsive symptoms. There are reports of OCD precipitated by cerebral anoxia, with subsequent basal ganglia damage (Laplane et al. 1989). One published report describes a case of body dysmorphic disorder (BDD)–like symptoms associated with onset of subacute sclerosing panencephalitis (Salib 1988). A degenerative disorder, such as neurocognitive disorder associated with frontotemporal lobar degeneration of Alzheimer's disease, can cause hoarding behavior; in such cases, hoarding disorder should not be diagnosed. Skin excoriation or skin picking may be caused by a dermatological condition, such as scabies, or any medical condition that causes pruritus, and thus excoriation (skin-picking) disorder should not be diagnosed in such instances. Similarly, trichotillomania (hair-pulling disorder) should not be diagnosed if the hair pulling is attributable to a medical condition involving inflammation of the skin, such as seborrheic dermatitis or tinea capitis.

Thus, it is appropriate for clinicians to consider routinely whether a nonpsychiatric medical condition is the cause of OCRD symptoms. When OCRD due to another medical condition is diagnosed, assessment and treatment should target the relevant medical condition. For example, if stroke is thought to be the cause of hoarding symptoms, the standard medical evaluation and management of stroke should follow, including appropriate behavioral interventions to address hoarding symptoms.

A key debate in this literature concerns the question of whether OCRDs can be attributed to group A streptococcal infection. It is well established that Sydenham's chorea is a neurological manifestation of rheumatic fever, results from infection with group A *Streptococcus,* and is often accompanied by motor features (e.g., choreas) and psychiatric symptoms (e.g., obsessions, compulsions, tics). Individuals with Sydenham's chorea who present with such symptoms should be diagnosed with an OCRD due to another medical condition (assuming all diagnostic criteria are met). Assessment and treatment should be targeted at the underlying group A streptococcal infection.

Pediatric autoimmune neuropsychiatric disorders associated with streptococcal infections (PANDAS) has been proposed as another postinfection autoimmune disorder characterized by the sudden onset of obsessions, compulsions, or tics, in the absence of chorea, carditis, or arthritis, following infection with group A *Streptococcus* (Swedo et al. 1998). A range of evidence supports the existence of such an entity, and from a clinical perspective it may be useful to ask patients about the relationship of throat infections to onset of OCD and perhaps also to other OCRD symptoms and to manage relevant group A streptococcal infections when they appear to play a substantial clinical role (Swedo and Grant 2005). Although not all published data are entirely consistent, in selected individuals, and in consultation with infectious disease specialists, such management may include the use of prophylactic antibiotic treatments.

Indeed, there is ongoing controversy as to whether neuropsychiatric symptoms are limited specifically to either OCRD symptoms or group A *Streptococcus*. Recent work has proposed an expanded clinical entity, *pediatric acute-onset neuropsychiatric syndrome* (PANS), or *idiopathic childhood acute neuropsychiatric symptoms* (CANS), with a broad range of neuropsychiatric symptoms (e.g., obsessive-compulsive behaviors, aggressiveness, anxiety, anorexia) that have been suggested to be precipitated by a number of infectious agents and other factors (Singer et al. 2012). The pathogenesis of acute onset of OCD and possibly other OCRDs in children requires additional research; it may involve both constitutional and environmental factors. Although there is an absence of consensus on diagnostic criteria and treatment interventions for PANDAS, PANS, and CANS, clinicians should remain aware of these entities so that appropriate cases may be referred to specialized centers for comprehensive medical assessment and treatment.

Other Specified OCRD

Diagnostic Features

The "other specified OCRD" category is used when symptoms characteristic of an OCRD predominate in the clinical picture and cause clinically significant distress or impairment in social, occupational, or other important areas of functioning but full diagnostic criteria for disorders in the OCRD chapter of DSM-5 are not met (see Box 7–3).

BOX 7–3. DSM-5 Diagnostic Criteria for Other Specified Obsessive-Compulsive and Related Disorder

This category applies to presentations in which symptoms characteristic of an obsessive-compulsive and related disorder that cause clinically significant distress or impairment in social, occupational, or other important areas of functioning predominate but do not meet the full criteria for any of the disorders in the obsessive-compulsive and related disorders diagnostic class. The other specified obsessive-compulsive and related disorder category is used in situations in which the clinician chooses to communicate the specific reason that the presentation does not meet the criteria for any specific obsessive-compulsive and related disorder. This is done by recording "other specified obsessive-compulsive and related disorder" followed by the specific reason (e.g., "body-focused repetitive behavior disorder").

Examples of presentations that can be specified using the "other specified" designation include the following:

1. **Body dysmorphic–like disorder with actual flaws:** This is similar to body dysmorphic disorder except that the defects or flaws in physical appearance are clearly observable by others (i.e., they are more noticeable than "slight"). In such cases, the preoccupation with these flaws is clearly excessive and causes significant impairment or distress.

2. **Body dysmorphic–like disorder without repetitive behaviors:** Presentations that meet body dysmorphic disorder except that the individual has not performed repetitive behaviors or mental acts in response to the appearance concerns.

3. **Body-focused repetitive behavior disorder:** This is characterized by recurrent body-focused repetitive behaviors (e.g., nail biting, lip biting, cheek chewing) and repeated attempts to decrease or stop the behaviors. These symptoms cause clinically significant distress or impairment in social, occupational, or other important areas of functioning and are not better explained by trichotillomania (hair-pulling disorder), excoriation (skin-picking) disorder, stereotypic movement disorder, or nonsuicidal self-injury.

4. **Obsessional jealousy:** This is characterized by nondelusional preoccupation with a partner's perceived infidelity. The preoccupations may lead to repetitive behaviors or mental acts in response to the infidelity concerns; they cause clinically significant distress or impairment in social, occupational, or other important areas of functioning; and they are not better explained by another mental disorder such as delusional disorder, jealous type, or paranoid personality disorder.

5. ***Shubo-kyofu:*** A variant of *taijin kyofusho* (see "Glossary of Cultural Concepts of Distress" in the [DSM-5] Appendix) that is similar to body dysmorphic disorder and is characterized by excessive fear of having a bodily deformity.

6. ***Koro:*** Related to *dhat syndrome* (see "Glossary of Cultural Concepts of Distress" in the [DSM-5] Appendix), an episode of sudden and intense anxiety that the penis (or the vulva and nipples in females) will recede into the body, possibly leading to death.

7. *Jikoshu-kyofu:* A variant of *taijin kyofusho* (see "Glossary of Cultural Concepts of Distress" in the [DSM-5] Appendix) characterized by fear of having an offensive body odor (also termed *olfactory reference syndrome*).

Reprinted from American Psychiatric Association: *Diagnostic and Statistical Manual of Mental Disorders*, 5th Edition. Arlington, VA, American Psychiatric Association. Copyright 2013, American Psychiatric Association. Used with permission.

This category allows clinicians to indicate that a clinically significant entity is present and to communicate the specific reason that the presentation does not meet the criteria for any specific DSM-5 OCRD. This is done by recording "other specified OCRD," followed by the specific reason (e.g., "body dysmorphic–like disorder without repetitive behaviors").

DSM-5 provides a number of examples of other specified OCRD. However, these examples are not meant to be exhaustive; any clinical presentation that fulfills the guidelines may be diagnosed as other specified OCRD.

Body Dysmorphic–Like Disorder With Actual Flaws

Body dysmorphic–like disorder with actual flaws is similar to BDD except that the defects or flaws in physical appearance are clearly observable by others. BDD, in contrast, is diagnosed when the defects or flaws in appearance are nonexistent or only slight (even though the individual with BDD thinks—inaccurately—that the defects/flaws are clearly observable by others). The appearance flaws of body dysmorphic–like disorder with actual flaws may have any number of causes, such as a medical illness or treatment for an illness (e.g., chemotherapy), surgery, an accident, or a congenital deformity. In some cases the appearance "flaws" may reflect a normal variation of appearance (such as baldness due to aging). As is the case for all types of other specified OCRD, the symptoms must be excessive (the concept of "excessiveness" is inherent to all OCRDs) and must cause clinically significant distress or impairment in psychosocial functioning.

Body Dysmorphic–Like Disorder Without Repetitive Behaviors

Body dysmorphic–like disorder without repetitive behaviors is similar to BDD except that the individual has not performed repetitive behaviors (such as mirror checking, excessive grooming, skin picking, or reassurance seeking) or mental acts (such as comparing) in response to preoccupation with nonexistent or slight appearance defects at any point during the course of the disorder. For the diagnostic criteria for BDD to be met, DSM-5 requires the presence of such repetitive behaviors (Criterion B), whereas DSM-IV did not. Virtually all individuals who meet DSM-5 Criteria A, C, and D for BDD also meet Criterion B, but a very small proportion do not; such individuals should be diagnosed with this form of other specified OCRD.

Body-Focused Repetitive Behavior Disorder

Body-focused repetitive behavior disorder is characterized by recurrent behaviors (e.g., nail biting, lip biting, cheek chewing, nose picking) and repeated attempts to decrease or stop the behaviors. This disorder is similar to trichotillomania (hair-pulling disorder) and excoriation (skin-picking) disorder in that the symptoms are purely motoric; they are not triggered by a cognition. As with all "other specified" OCRDs, the diagnosis requires that the symptoms cause clinically significant distress or impairment in social, occupational, or other important areas of functioning. This criterion helps to ensure that normal habits that are not clinically significant are not diagnosed as a mental disorder. For this diagnosis to be made, the behaviors also must not be better explained by another DSM-5 mental disorder such as trichotillomania (hair-pulling disorder), excoriation (skin-picking) disorder, or stereotypic movement disorder.

Obsessional Jealousy

Obsessional jealousy is characterized by nondelusional preoccupation with a partner's perceived infidelity. The preoccupations may lead to repetitive behaviors or mental acts in response to the infidelity concerns, such as repeatedly searching for "evidence" of infidelity, repeatedly checking on the whereabouts of the partner, or seeking reassurance that the infidelity is not occurring. Furthermore, the symptoms must cause clinically significant distress or impairment in social, occupational, or other important areas of functioning. Finally, these preoccupations are not better explained by another mental disorder such as delusional disorder, jealous type or paranoid personality disorder. It is also important to exclude medical factors that may precipitate jealous preoccupations, such as cerebral infarcts or brain tumors (Kuruppuarachchi and Seneviratne 2011).

Shubo-Kyofu

Shubo-kyofu is characterized by excessive fear of having a bodily deformity. It is very similar to BDD. According to the traditional Japanese diagnostic system, *shubo-kyofu* is considered a subtype of *taijin kyofusho,* a cultural syndrome characterized by interpersonal fear and avoidance that overlaps with—but is broader than—social anxiety disorder (social phobia). Many presentations of *shubo-kyofu* are likely the same disorder as BDD, although *taijin kyofusho* is more prominently characterized by concerns about offending others, whereas BDD typically focuses more on fear of being rejected by others because of the perceived appearance defects.

Koro

Koro is another culturally bound syndrome, one that occurs primarily in men in epidemics in Southeast Asia. *Koro* is characterized by an acute fear that the penis (labia, nipples, or breasts in women) is shrinking or retracting and will disappear into the abdomen. This fear is often accompanied by a belief that death will result from these symptoms. *Koro* has some similarities to BDD but also differs from it in a number of ways: *koro* involves a fear that disappearance of the penis will result in death; is usually brief in duration; usually occurs, as epidemic, in a particular geographical area; and often responds to reassurance. Concerns that do not involve these characteristics and that instead focus on the appearance of the penis (e.g., its "small" size) may be more appropriately diagnosed as BDD.

Jikoshu–Kyofu

Jikoshu-kyofu is a subtype of *taijin kyofusho* that denotes fear of emitting a foul or offensive body odor that cannot, however, be detected by others. DSM-5 notes that *jikoshu-kyofu* is also termed *olfactory reference syndrome* (ORS). DSM-5 emphasizes the Japanese cultural variant of this syndrome, perhaps because this condition has been better recognized in Japanese psychiatry than in non-Japanese psychiatry. However, ORS has been reported around the world, and nearly as many cases have been reported from Canada and Nigeria as from Japan (Feusner et al. 2010). Other sizable case series are from the United States and Saudi Arabia (Feusner et al. 2010; Phillips and Menard 2011).

The most common concerns focus on emitting bad breath or a sweaty odor, and the most common sources of body odor are the mouth, armpits, genitals, anus, and feet (Phillips and Menard 2011). The false belief that one emits a foul or offensive body odor usually leads to repetitive behaviors or mental acts in response to the odor concerns. The most common behaviors are smelling oneself to check for body odor, excessive showering, excessive clothes changing, seeking reassurance about the perceived body odor, eating unusual diets (e.g., to minimize perceived halitosis or flatulence), and excessive tooth brushing (to decrease perceived halitosis) (Phillips and Menard 2011). The preoccupation must cause clinically significant distress or impairment in social, occupational, or other important areas of functioning. Furthermore, although not specified by DSM-5, the body odor concerns should not be better explained by another medical condition (e.g., frontal tumors and temporal lobe seizures may be associated with olfactory hallucinations). According to DSM-5, the clinical presentation of individuals with ORS who have absent insight may meet diagnostic criteria for delusional disorder. However, it seems likely that the delusional and nondelusional forms of ORS actually constitute the same disorder (although research is needed to determine whether this is actually the case).

Assessment and Treatment

The literature on the prevalence, psychobiology, and treatment of other specified OCRDs varies by the type of other specified OCRD. Body dysmorphic–like disorder with actual flaws can be assessed with some existing measures for BDD (those that focus on preoccupation with appearance flaws as well as resulting distress or impairment in functioning, but do not require that the appearance defect[s] are nonexistent or only slight). However, there is a dearth of treatment literature for this clinical presentation. It is unknown whether SRIs might be useful, although it is reasonable to think that they might be, because SRIs decrease obsessions/preoccupations in both BDD and OCD. CBT approaches for BDD would probably need to be modified, however. Cognitive restructuring and other cognitive techniques, response prevention for rituals if present, and certain other components of CBT for BDD might be useful; however, exposure exercises would probably need to be modified. For example, when designing exposures, the clinician would need to keep in mind that other people might actually take special notice of or mock an individual with clearly observable physical flaws, whereas in BDD this does not actually occur (even though most patients with BDD think it does).

The literature on DSM-IV-defined BDD is applicable to body dysmorphic–like disorder without repetitive behaviors, because this disorder was diagnosed as BDD in DSM-IV. Screening, diagnostic, and symptom severity measures for DSM-IV BDD, as well as treatments that are recommended for BDD (see Chapter 3, "Body Dysmorphic Disorder"), should be used for these patients.

Although the treatment of body-focused repetitive behavior disorder has not been studied, until such evidence becomes available these patients should be approached similarly to those with trichotillomania (hair-pulling disorder) or excoriation (skin-picking) disorder. Clinical experience suggests that such patients may respond to standard behavioral interventions developed for these conditions (i.e., habit reversal training).

There is an accumulating case literature on obsessional jealousy (Agarwal et al. 2008; Parker and Barrett 1997). It is reasonable to use standard OCD symptom severity scales, such as the Yale-Brown Obsessive Compulsive Scale, to assess jealous preoccupations and accompanying repetitive behaviors or mental acts. Anecdotal reports suggest that patients with obsessional jealousy may respond to SRIs or to cognitive-behavioral interventions (Cobb and Marks 1979; Stein et al. 1994). With individuals with no insight (who are convinced that their belief about infidelity is true), it may be useful to begin with an approach that conceptualizes obsessional jealousy as lying on the

OCRD spectrum, which may be useful in assessing and treating patients. However, clinicians should have a relatively low threshold for replacing or augmenting SRIs with antipsychotic agents, which clinical experience suggests may also be useful for such patients.

Similar considerations may apply to olfactory reference syndrome. Measures that assess ORS are available (www.bodyimageprogram.com). Multiple case reports that focus on treatment have been published, many of which suggest that SRI monotherapy may improve ORS symptoms; others describe response to non-SRI antidepressants, antipsychotics, or a combination of an antidepressant and an antipsychotic (Feusner et al. 2010; Phillips et al. 2006). Our clinical practice is to begin treatment with an SRI, even for patients with delusional beliefs. If response is inadequate after dosages typically used for BDD and OCD are reached, we consider adding an antipsychotic. Indeed, because the majority of individuals with ORS have no insight (i.e., they are completely convinced that they really do smell bad; Phillips and Menard 2011), it would seem reasonable for clinicians to have a low threshold for augmenting SRIs with antipsychotic agents.

There are also anecdotal reports of individuals with ORS responding to cognitive-behavioral interventions, with a focus on exposure and response prevention (Stein et al. 1998). In our clinical experience, because the majority of patients with ORS have delusional beliefs about body odor, motivational interviewing and cognitive approaches are often needed in addition to behavioral interventions. Thus, we suggest a CBT approach that is more similar to that used for BDD than OCD. However, research on the most effective treatment approach for these very ill patients is greatly needed.

A substantial proportion of patients with ORS seek and receive treatment from nonpsychiatric health professionals for their perceived body odor—for example, tonsillectomy, gastrointestinal medication, or electrolysis of the axillae (Phillips and Menard 2011). Available data (while limited), as well as case reports and series, suggest that such treatment is not effective for ORS (Phillips et al. 2006).

Unspecified OCRD

The category of "unspecified OCRD" is similar to the other specified OCRD category except that the clinician chooses not to specify the reason diagnostic criteria for an OCRD are not met—that is, the clinician does not note one of the examples discussed here or another reason. Thus, this diagnosis is used when patients have symptoms characteristic of an OCRD that cause clinically significant distress or impairment in social, occupational, or other important areas of functioning, the symptoms do not meet the full diagnostic criteria for any disorder in the DSM-5 chapter on OCRDs, and the clinician does not note information about presenting symptoms. Unspecified OCRD includes presentations in which there is insufficient information to make a more specific diagnosis (e.g., in emergency room settings).

Key Points

- All patients who present with symptoms characteristic of an obsessive-compulsive and related disorder (OCRD) should be evaluated for the presence of substances/medications that may cause or exacerbate these symptoms.

- All patients who present with symptoms characteristic of an OCRD should be evaluated for the presence of nonpsychiatric medical conditions that may cause or exacerbate these symptoms.

- When an underlying substance/medication or nonpsychiatric medical disorder is found to cause or exacerbate an OCRD-like presentation, an appropriate assessment and management plan, based on clinical judgment, should be put in place.

- For body dysmorphic–like disorder without repetitive behaviors, treatments that are used for body dysmorphic disorder should be implemented. However, the treatment literature is relatively sparse for other examples of other specified OCRD. In such cases, the assessment and treatment suggestions in this chapter may be helpful, in combination with clinical judgment and knowledge of the most relevant similar OCRD, when formulating an assessment and treatment plan.

References

Agarwal AL, Sharma V, Biswas D: Obsessional jealousy: unusual presentation (letter). Aust NZ J Psychiatry 42(12):1068, 2008 19016096

American Psychiatric Association: Diagnostic and Statistical Manual of Mental Disorders, 4th Edition. Washington, DC, American Psychiatric Association, 1994

American Psychiatric Association: Diagnostic and Statistical Manual of Mental Disorders, 5th Edition. Arlington, VA, American Psychiatric Association, 2013

Cobb JP, Marks IM: Morbid jealousy featuring as obsessive-compulsive neurosis: treatment by behavioral psychotherapy. Br J Psychiatry 134:301–305, 1979 509011

Feusner JD, Phillips KA, Stein DJ: Olfactory reference syndrome: issues for DSM-V. Depress Anxiety 27(6):592–599, 2010 20533369

Fried RG: Evaluation and treatment of "psychogenic" pruritus and self-excoriation. J Am Acad Dermatol 30(6):993–999, 1994 8188895

Kuruppuarachchi KA, Seneviratne AN: Organic causation of morbid jealousy. Asian J Psychiatr 4(4):258–260, 2011 23051158

Laplane D, Levasseur M, Pillon B, et al: Obsessive-compulsive and other behavioural changes with bilateral basal ganglia lesions: a neuropsychological, magnetic resonance imaging and positron tomography study. Brain 112 (Pt 3):699–725, 1989 2786440

Madruga-Garrido M, Mir P: Tics and other stereotyped movements as side effects of pharmacological treatment. Int Rev Neurobiol 112:481–494, 2013 24295631

Martin A, Scahill L, Vitulano L, et al: Stimulant use and trichotillomania. J Am Acad Child Adolesc Psychiatry 37(4):349–350, 1998 9549952

Mataix-Cols D, Frost RO, Pertusa A, et al: Hoarding disorder: a new diagnosis for DSM-V? Depress Anxiety 27(6):556–572, 2010 20336805

Parker G, Barrett E: Morbid jealousy as a variant of obsessive-compulsive disorder. Aust NZ J Psychiatry 31(1):133–138, 1997 9088498

Phillips KA, Menard W: Olfactory reference syndrome: demographic and clinical features of imagined body odor. Gen Hosp Psychiatry 33(4):398–406, 2011 21762838

Phillips KA, Gunderson C, Gruber U, et al: Delusions of body malodour: the olfactory reference syndrome, in Olfaction and the Brain. Edited by Brewer W, Castle D, Pantelis C. Cambridge, United Kingdom, Cambridge University Press, 2006, pp 334–353

Ridley RM: The psychology of perseverative and stereotyped behaviour. Prog Neurobiol 44(2):221–231, 1994 7831478

Salib EA: Subacute sclerosing panencephalitis (SSPE) presenting at the age of 21 as a schizophrenia-like state with bizarre dysmorphophobic features. Br J Psychiatry 152:709–710, 1988 3167453

Singer HS, Gilbert DL, Wolf DS, et al: Moving from PANDAS to CANS. J Pediatr 160(5):725–731, 2012 22197466

Stein DJ, Hollander E, Josephson SC: Serotonin reuptake blockers for the treatment of obsessional jealousy. J Clin Psychiatry 55(1):30–33, 1994 8294389

Stein DJ, Le Roux L, Bouwer C, et al: Is olfactory reference syndrome an obsessive-compulsive spectrum disorder? Two cases and a discussion. J Neuropsychiatry Clin Neurosci 10(1):96–99, 1998 9547473

Stein DJ, Grant JE, Franklin ME, et al: Trichotillomania (hair pulling disorder), skin picking disorder, and stereotypic movement disorder: toward DSM-V. Depress Anxiety 27(6):611–626, 2010 20533371

Swedo SE, Grant PJ: Annotation: PANDAS: a model for human autoimmune disease. J Child Psychol Psychiatry 46(3):227–234, 2005 15755299

Swedo SE, Leonard HL, Garvey M, et al: Pediatric autoimmune neuropsychiatric disorders associated with streptococcal infections: clinical description of the first 50 cases. Am J Psychiatry 155(2):264–271, 1998 9464208

Recommended Readings

Ecker W: Non-delusional pathological jealousy as an obsessive-compulsive spectrum disorder: cognitive-behavioural conceptualization and some treatment suggestions. J Obsessive Compuls Relat Disord 1:203–210, 2012

Feusner JD, Phillips KA, Stein DJ: Olfactory reference syndrome: issues for DSM-V. Depress Anxiety 27:592–599, 2010

Phillips KA, Menard W Olfactory reference syndrome: demographic and clinical features of imagined body odor. Gen Hosp Psychiatry 33:398–406, 2011

CHAPTER 8

Tic Disorders

Michelle Tricamo, M.D.
Tara Mathews, Ph.D.
John T. Walkup, M.D.

In 1884, working under the neurologist Jean-Martin Charcot, Gilles de la Tourette identified nine patients with unusual movements and vocalizations. He called their condition "convulsive tic disorder." However, without much medical treatment available, the condition was considered a psychological disorder by Freud and others. Not until the 1960s did the syndrome begin to be attributed to a neurological process, after Dr. Arthur Shapiro from New York and others had successfully treated patients with tics using antipsychotic medications. Today, patients with tics are considered to have a neuropsychiatric disorder, given that psychiatric comorbidity is an important feature of the tic disorders. Tic disorders may have a particularly close relationship with obsessive-compulsive disorder (OCD), as detailed in this chapter.

Diagnostic Criteria and Symptomatology

Tic disorders are neuropsychiatric conditions defined by the presence of motor and/or vocal tics (Box 8–1). A tic is a sudden-onset, nonrhythmic, staccato-like repetitive movement, gesture, sound, or utterance that typically mimics some fragment of normal behavior and is by definition nonpurposeful in nature. Tics can be simple or complex, are distinguished by duration and complexity, and can be classified as either a motor or a vocal tic. *Simple motor tics* are typically brief (less than 1 second in duration), rapid movements involving a single muscle group. Examples include eye blinking, head jerks, and shoulder shrugging. *Complex motor tics* involve multiple muscle groups and can be of longer duration (typically between 1 and 3 seconds). These involve a combination of concurrent simple tics and may appear to be more rhythmic, elaborate, and even purposeful in nature. Examples include repetitive touching or rubbing, simultaneous eye blinking with a facial grimace, and, less frequently, obscene gestures (copropraxia). *Simple vocal tics* are brief (less than 1 second), meaningless sounds or utterances involving contraction of the diaphragm or muscles of the oropharynx, such as throat clearing, humming, sniffing, or grunting. *Complex vocal tics* are meaningful words or phrases that are without purpose and are often not appropriate or related to context. These may occur over several seconds. Complex vocal tics include *palilalia*, defined as the repetition of one's own words; *echolalia*, which involves repetition of the words of others, usually the last heard words or phrases; and *coprolalia*, characterized by obscene words or slurs often having ethnic, religious, or racial connotations (American Psychiatric Association 2013). Although highlighted by popular media and often considered common by the general public, coprolalia, it should be noted, is in fact a relatively infrequent symptom among individuals with tic disorders and is not required for diagnosis.

BOX 8–1. DSM-5 Diagnostic Criteria for Tic Disorders

Note: A tic is a sudden, rapid, recurrent, nonrhythmic motor movement or vocalization.

Tourette's Disorder
A. Both multiple motor and one or more vocal tics have been present at some time during the illness, although not necessarily concurrently.
B. The tics may wax and wane in frequency but have persisted for more than 1 year since first tic onset.
C. Onset is before age 18 years.
D. The disturbance is not attributable to the physiological effects of a substance (e.g., cocaine) or another medical condition (e.g., Huntington's disease, postviral encephalitis).

Persistent (Chronic) Motor or Vocal Tic Disorder
A. Single or multiple motor or vocal tics have been present during the illness, but not both motor and vocal.
B. The tics may wax and wane in frequency but have persisted for more than 1 year since first tic onset.

C. Onset is before age 18 years.

D. The disturbance is not attributable to the physiological effects of a substance (e.g., cocaine) or another medical condition (e.g., Huntington's disease, post-viral encephalitis).

E. Criteria have never been met for Tourette's disorder.

Specify if:
 With motor tics only
 With vocal tics only

Provisional Tic Disorder
A. Single or multiple motor and/or vocal tics.
B. The tics have been present for less than 1 year since first tic onset.
C. Onset is before age 18 years.
D. The disturbance is not attributable to the physiological effects of a substance (e.g., cocaine) or another medical condition (e.g., Huntington's disease, post-viral encephalitis).
E. Criteria have never been met for Tourette's disorder or persistent (chronic) motor or vocal tic disorder.

Reprinted from American Psychiatric Association: *Diagnostic and Statistical Manual of Mental Disorders*, 5th Edition. Arlington, VA, American Psychiatric Association. Copyright 2013, American Psychiatric Association. Used with permission.

Tics typically wax and wane—that is, particular tics may come and go and/or may vary in frequency and intensity over time. For example, one may experience a simple vocal tic such as a sniff; several months later, the sniff may stop but a blinking tic may begin to occur. Increases in frequency or intensity of a particular tic may be influenced by environmental factors such as increased stress or excitement.

Tics are often preceded by an uncomfortable sensation referred to as a "premonitory sensation" or "premonitory urge." The sensation can be described as a feeling of tension, pressure, or discomfort prior to occurrence of the tic, with resolution of the sensation after the tic is completed. Furthermore, many individuals report the ability to resist premonitory urges and suppress resultant tics for a specified period of time or activity. A majority of adults with a tic disorder describe premonitory sensations, whereas fewer than half of youths report such sensations (Banaschewski et al. 2003). The lower prevalence of sensation reporting in youths may be attributed to developmental considerations, the onset of sensations later during development, the child's unawareness of the sensation (children and adults are also often unaware of their tic movements—even those movements readily observed by others), or the child's inability to describe the sensation (i.e., language limitations in describing the sensation).

Tics may be mistakenly perceived as being volitional. Although it has been proposed that volitional suppression of tics may lead to a rebound, this proposal has not been supported by research evidence (American Psychiatric Association 2013; Meidinger et al. 2005; Verdellen et al. 2007).

Tic disorders are categorized by DSM-5 into four diagnostic categories: 1) Tourette's disorder, 2) persistent (chronic) motor or vocal tic disorder, 3) provisional tic disorder, and 4) other specified and unspecified tic disorders. Because tics tend to wax and wane, the presence of the 1-year duration criterion for Tourette's disorder and persistent motor/vocal tic disorder ensures that individuals who receive one of these diagnoses have more persistent symptoms (American Psychiatric Association 2013).

Several changes were made in DSM-5 because some of the criteria in DSM-IV (American Psychiatric Association 1994) were awkward and difficult to operationalize. DSM-5 continues the minimum duration criterion of 1 year for the chronic tic disorders (including Tourette's disorder). Transient tic disorder was eliminated, and provisional tic disorder was added. A reference in DSM-IV to "stimulants" as an example of a substance that causes tics was removed for DSM-5 and replaced with "cocaine." This change was based on data from controlled trials suggesting that stimulant medication is effective for attention-deficit/hyperactivity disorder (ADHD) in children with tic disorders and does not predictably worsen tics. The inclusion of stimulant medication as an example of a medication that worsens tics would perpetuate a concern that has little scientific support at this time (see Walkup and colleagues' review of key issues for DSM-5 for further explanation [Walkup et al. 2010]).

Strong consideration was given to categorizing tic disorders in the chapter on obsessive-compulsive and related disorders (OCRDs) in DSM-5. Indeed, family history data, high comorbidity between tics disorders and OCD, and similarities between complex tics and OCD compulsions suggest a close relationship between these two disorders. Ultimately, however, for a number of reasons, tic disorders were categorized as neurodevelopmental disorders. The tic disorders share many features with other neurodevelopmental disorders with early childhood onset. They also have an evolving course over development that typically includes a marked reduction of symptoms in late adolescence, unlike OCD. In addition, genetic studies indicate a complex relationship between OCD and the tic disorders, with some forms of OCD likely more related to tic disorders than others (e.g., OCD that is largely characterized by physical sensation [not obsessions] and simple motor behavior may be more genetically related to tic disorders). There is limited internal distress associated with tics, which is also distinct from OCD. Finally, although their behavioral approaches to treatment have some similarities, their pharmacological approaches are relatively distinct.

Case Example: Marcus

Marcus is a 19-year-old man who presents with Tourette's disorder. He reports experiencing movements of the face and upper extremities and producing a number of meaningless sounds since age 6. When the movements began, they consisted of eye blinking and shoulder shrugs. Marcus' parents attempted to help by pointing out the movements and encouraging him to stop, but this seemed to worsen the problem. By age 9, the eye blinking was accompanied by a facial grimace. Marcus also began to experience unwanted vocalizations, including throat clearing, coughing, and sniffing. He reports having had a brief period of relief from these symptoms during fifth grade, but when he entered middle school, the movements and vocalizations returned and worsened in frequency and intensity. Marcus reported that an uncomfortable sensation preceded the movements and sounds. Specifically, he described the sensation as feeling similar to the urge to sneeze. He felt a pressure behind his eyes prior to blinking. His vocalizations were preceded by a feeling in his throat similar to having an urge to clear his throat. Marcus felt embarrassed by his symptoms at school and often attempted to suppress the movements and sounds; however, he found this quite difficult. The urge to tic built as he attempted to suppress it and was associated with significant discomfort. Currently, Marcus reports that his vocal tics have disappeared, and he now experiences only occasional eye blinking during stressful periods. This is typical of the improvement most older adolescents will likely experience.

Epidemiology

Tics are common throughout early childhood and less prevalent in adults. Tics commonly present in childhood, with as many as 20% of children experiencing tics at any point in time. The current best estimate of persistent motor and vocal tics is between 0.5% and 1% (Scahill et al. 2009). Because of the transient nature of tics, changing diagnostic criteria, and differing methodologies, wide ranges of prevalence rates have been reported (Bloch and Leckman 2009). Tourette's disorder has been found to occur in approximately 1% of the general population and approximately 4% of children (Robertson 2011).

Comorbidity

Co-occurring psychiatric disorders are common in children and adults with tic disorders, occurring in approximately 80% of cases (Scahill et al. 2009). The most prevalent comorbid disorder is ADHD, which affects about 50%–60% of individuals with tic disorders (Stewart et al. 2006). ADHD is seven or eight times more common in people with a tic disorder than in the general population (Walkup et al. 1996). Because there is an increased prevalence of learning disorders in children with ADHD, it is not surprising that the prevalence of learning disorders is also higher in those with tics, with a prevalence of 23% (Burd et al. 2005). Burd et al. (2005) found that factors including male gender and complications during pregnancy or delivery increased the risk of a comorbid learning disorder. Because ADHD and learning disorders are prevalent in this population, academic difficulties are common among children with a tic disorder. However, most individuals with tic disorders are of average intelligence (Chappell et al. 1995).

There is an especially strong association between tic disorders and OCD. This association is bidirectional, with 20%–60% of patients with a tic disorder having OCD or subthreshold OCD-related symptoms, and 20%–38% of children with OCD reporting comorbid tics (Lewin et al. 2010). In adults (but not children) with tics and OCD, the severity of both disorders is often worse than when only one of these disorders is present. In addition, this form of comorbidity is often associated with an increase in comorbid anxiety, substance use, and DSM-IV mood disorders (Lewin et al. 2010).

Anxiety disorders—in particular, separation anxiety disorder—are highly associated with greater tic severity. One study found that those with tic disorders are 3.5 times more likely to have more severe tics in the presence of multiple anxiety disorders (Coffey et al. 2000). The importance of assessing comorbid anxiety disorders was implied by Gilles de la Tourette in 1899, when he described fears and phobias as common features of Tourette's disorder.

Burd et al. (2009) found that about 5% of patients with Tourette syndrome also have a comorbid pervasive developmental disorder (currently autism spectrum disorder; the presence of Tourette's disorder increases the risk for a comorbid autism spectrum disorder 13-fold). Children with this comorbidity are mostly male and have an increase in other co-occurring psychiatric disorders.

Course and Prognosis

Tics typically begin in childhood; the average age at onset is 7 years. In rare cases, tics have been identified in infants only a few months old (Zinner 2006). Over time, tics tend to wax and wane in severity, and the type of tic tends to change over time as well. Tics involving the head usually begin at an earlier age than those involving the lower extremities—that is, tics typically proceed in a rostral to caudal direction (i.e., head to toe). In addition, simple motor or vocal tics tend to begin at an earlier age than complex tics. Although types of tics tend to vary within an individual, the course described here remains consistent between age groups and across the lifespan.

Between the ages of 10 and 12 years, tics are usually at their peak severity; they begin to decrease in prevalence starting in the middle to late teenage years. At age 18–20, most individuals with a tic disorder (about two-thirds) have experienced reduced tics or reduced tic severity (Leckman et al. 2006). By young adulthood, most individuals with tic disorders have experienced an improvement in their symptoms, whereas only a small proportion experience severe or worsening symptoms in adulthood (American Psychiatric Association 2013; Leckman et al. 1998).

Psychosocial Impairment

Many individuals with tic disorders experience little to no functional impairment. In fact, when impairment is reported, it is most often the result of comorbid conditions such as ADHD or OCD (see section "Comorbidity" earlier in the chapter). However, those with a more severe course of tic disorder report more distress. For example, some patients experience tics that are particularly disruptive or bothersome to themselves or others, become painful with repetition, or cause embarrassment or conflict in peer groups or families. For example, children with highly disruptive tics may become victims of bullying by peers or suffer criticism by parents and teachers. Children with tics may become self-conscious and experience lower self-confidence and develop tic-related avoidance behavior.

Gender–Related Issues

The large majority of prevalence studies have found that tics are more common in males than in females; estimates of the gender ratio are 2:1 to 4:1. There are no gender differences in terms of types of tics, onset, or course.

Cultural Aspects of Phenomenology

Tics have been identified in every racial and ethnic group, yet little is known about whether some racial or ethnic groups have a greater predilection toward tics than other groups. African American youths were found to have lower rates of tics than Caucasians in both the Great Smoky Mountains Study of Youth (Costello et al. 1996) and the Centers for Disease Control and Prevention study (Scahill et al. 2009), but it is unknown whether these differences in prevalence are real or are related to problems with ascertainment. Importantly, race, ethnicity, and culture may influence a family's and community's perception of tics and their approach to help seeking and treatment of tics (American Psychiatric Association 2013).

Assessment and Differential Diagnosis

Assessment

Although tics are considered neurological in etiology, no medical test is available to diagnose tics or tic disorders. A good assessment relies upon clinical interviews, observation of the patient, and self- or caregiver-report instruments. A clinical interview with an adult patient—or, in the case of a child, with both the child and caregiver(s)—should be conducted. Details including age at onset, topography, complexity, frequency, and intensity of tics, as well as subjective distress caused by tics, should be gathered. It is important to obtain any history of waxing and waning of tics as well as a description of ways in which the tics interfere with the patient's functioning. Assessment of the presence of premonitory urges should be included, along with detailed description of the patient's experience of the urge (Murphy et al. 2013). Sample screening questions are presented in Table 8–1.

TABLE 8–1.　Screening questions to assess tic disorders

When was the first time you noticed the tic?

How often does the tic occur?

Under what circumstances is the tic most likely to occur?

Do you feel anything immediately before the movement occurs? If so, please describe.

Does the tic ever interfere with your ability to engage in volitional behavior?

How much are you bothered by the tic?

How much do others seem to be bothered by the tic?

Note.　These questions should be asked with regard to all current tics or tic-like movements. Depending on the age, insight, and verbal abilities of a child with tics, parents may provide the bulk of this information.

Several self-report and parent-report instruments have been developed and can usefully supplement clinical reports and observations. These instruments are quite useful in quantifying tic severity, interference, and intensity of urges and can be used to guide treatment as well as measure improvement. The most widely used instrument is the Yale Global Tic Severity Scale (YGTSS; Leckman et al. 1989). The YGTSS is a semistructured interview that comprises three domains. First, symptom checklists are used to determine topography of any past and current tics the patient has experienced. Next, severity ratings are generated on the basis of the number, frequency, intensity, and complexity of a patient's tics, in addition to the amount of day-to-day interference the patient reports as a result of the tic(s). Each of these dimensions is rated on a Likert scale of 0–5, and the combination yields a severity score for motor tics and a separate severity score for vocal tics. Scores for motor and vocal tics are summed, yielding the total tic severity score, ranging from 0 to 50. Finally, the YGTSS includes a total impairment score, also ranging from 0 to 50, based on the amount of subjective tic-related distress and functional impairment reported by the patient and family. The YGTSS takes approximately 15–30 minutes to administer (Leckman et al. 1989).

The Premonitory Urge for Tics Scale (PUTS) is another instrument that may be used during assessment of tic disorders (Woods et al. 2005). The PUTS is a brief, nine-item self-report scale that can aid in a clinician's understanding of a patient's experiences with premonitory urges. The measure can be particularly helpful in gathering information about the presence of premonitory sensations in younger children. It is also an especially helpful aid to clinicians who are less experienced in identifying tic-related urges (Woods et al. 2005).

Assessment of comorbid conditions—especially attentional and learning issues as well as OCD and other anxiety disorders in children and depression in older teens and adults—is critical to a thorough evaluation of tic disorders, not only for the sake of comprehensive diagnosis but also for treatment planning (see "General Approaches to Treatment and Special Considerations").

Differential Diagnosis

Tic disorders must be differentiated from stereotypies and compulsive behaviors, other neurological conditions, movement disorders, and substance-related disorders (Table 8–2).

TABLE 8–2.   Tic differential diagnosis

If the behavior is purposeful and preceded by an obsessive thought, diagnose as obsessive-compulsive disorder.

If the behavior is rhythmic, bilateral, and redirectable, diagnose as stereotypy.

If a tic originated after substance use, diagnose as substance-induced tic disorder.

If a tic originated with other neurological symptoms, diagnose as tic disorder due to a general medical condition.

Stereotypies

Like tics, *stereotypies* are involuntary repetitive motor movements or vocalizations, such as repeated humming. They can be distinguished from tics by their rhythmicity, lack of change over time, constant form and location, and lack of premonitory sensation. As such, stereotypies appear less random than tics because they tend to occur in a regular, repeated pattern, such as constant repeated hand-flapping behavior. Stereotypies tend to have an earlier onset than tics, often in children as young as 3 years old. They are often exacerbated when the patient is engrossed in an activity and cease with distraction. Stereotypies often occur as a symptom of autism spectrum disorder and stereotypic movement disorder, but they can occur in typically developing children too.

Obsessive-Compulsive Disorder Compulsions

Compulsions may be difficult behaviors to distinguish from complex tics, in that both are repetitive and seemingly meaningless activities. Still, a clinical interview typically reveals that individuals with compulsive behaviors can explain the meaning of their behavior. Compulsions typically consist of behaviors that serve a purpose, although the patient with compulsions may engage in this purposeful behavior in an unreasonable fashion. For example, repeated hand washing, repeatedly opening and closing a door until it feels "just right," and repeatedly counting in one's head each reflect a "real-world" behavior that has a purpose. Tics, on the other hand, rarely resemble real-world purposeful behaviors. Moreover, compulsions can be distinguished from tics in that they comprise more complex behaviors, lasting longer than a few seconds in duration. Finally, a compulsion is typically performed in response to a thought-based drive to engage in a behavior in a particular way (an obsession), and it may be performed a certain number of times or until the individual feels "just right." Both tics and compulsions may be accompanied by a preceding urge, but the urge associated with a compulsion is typically cognitive in nature (i.e., an obsession), whereas tics are preceded by physical sensations (e.g., pressure, discomfort in a particular part of the body). The most difficult compulsive behaviors to differentiate from tics are those that are simple and brief in nature and those with a vague thought-based drive (e.g., repeatedly tapping on one's knee until it "feels right") or a physical sensation–based drive. Still, the purposeful nature of the tapping, combined with a drive to achieve a just-right feeling (as opposed to the removal of an unpleasant physical urge), can differentiate the two.

Neurological and Movement Disorders

In rare cases, tics may manifest as symptoms of a neurological condition—such as central nervous system trauma, tumors, or anoxia—or an effect of medication. Likewise, movement abnormalities can occur as a symptom of neurological diseases such as Wilson's disease, Huntington's syndrome, neuroacanthocytosis, and a variety of fronto-subcortical brain lesions. However, symptoms of these conditions are relatively distinct from tics (McAbee et al. 1999). The history of onset and course of tic-like movements can be helpful with this differential; as previously described, tics have a very specific pattern of onset and course. In addition, tic-like movements that present in a dissimilar fashion, are severe at onset, begin during adulthood, or have their onset in the setting of other medical conditions are likely to reflect other pathologies.

Substance-Related Disorders

Cocaine—and, in the past, other stimulants—have been thought to contribute to new onset or worsening of tics (Brust 2010). However, new onset or worsening of tics may co-occur with medication use by chance or may develop over time unrelated to medication use; in addition, reporting of such change may be impacted by the subjective nature of retrospective reporting. Only randomized placebo-controlled trials that do a sensitive assessment of adverse effects of medication can prove that tic worsening is caused by the medication. In a comparison of methylphenidate, clonidine, and placebo for ADHD in children with tics, there were similar rates (20%–25%) of tic worsening with both medications and placebo, suggesting that stimulants do not worsen tics (Tourette's Syndrome Study Group 2002).

Case Example: Keith

Keith is a 13-year-old boy with a history of inattention, impulsivity, involuntary motor movements, ritualistic behaviors, and persistent vocal tic disorder. Keith was diagnosed with ADHD in kindergarten and has used stimulant medication since age 7. At age 10, Keith washed his hands repeatedly throughout the day. His teacher reported that Keith became irritable and argumentative when requests to use the bathroom were refused. Over the next several months, his parents noted several concerning behaviors indicative of a fear of dirt and contamination; for example, Keith avoided public restrooms, refused to eat foods that had touched countertops, and refused to touch his shoes, insisting that his parents put them on for him. Keith's psychiatrist diagnosed OCD and recommended that Keith begin cognitive-behavioral therapy (CBT). During the course of treatment, Keith's CBT therapist observed occasional sniffing and throat clearing. Keith's parents had not noticed these behaviors, but Keith reported that they had been bothering him for some time but that he was embarrassed to tell anyone about them. Keith cannot control these noises and does not describe a premonitory urge. The noises are worse when he is tired, excited, or anxious.

Etiology and Pathophysiology

The etiology and pathophysiology of tic disorders are complex and remain poorly understood. Family studies have consistently shown that Tourette's disorder is familial, and twin studies have clearly indicated a strong hereditary basis and a genetic contribution to its etiology. Among monozygotic twins, concordance rates for Tourette's disorder range from 53% to 56%, according to two major studies (Hyde et al. 1992; Price et al. 1985). Price et al. (1985) reported a 77% concordance rate for chronic motor tics in monozygotic twins. In contrast, dizygotic twins exhibited only an 8% concordance rate for Tourette's disorder and a 23% rate for chronic motor tics (Price et al. 1985). Multiple studies show that having a first-degree relative with Tourette's disorder increases the risk of having the disorder by 10%–15%; this risk is increased to 15%–20% when one has a first-degree relative with any tics at all (Hebebrand et al. 1997a, 1997b; Pauls et al. 1991; Walkup et al. 1996). An individual is 10–100 times more likely to develop Tourette's disorder when a first-degree relative carries the diagnosis (Pauls et al. 1991).

Tic disorders are considered to have polygenic origins. Researchers have identified some potential genetic variants that may contribute to the development of tic disorders, but they account for a limited amount of risk. Whereas early segregation studies of Tourette's disorder suggested a single-gene autosomal dominant disorder, later studies have pointed to more complex models, including additive and multifactorial inheritance and likely interaction with environmental factors.

Neurotransmitters are often considered to be etiologically relevant for a variety of reasons, including drug response. Early treatment success with particular psychotropics led to an increased interest in the role of related neurotransmitter systems. Thus, dopamine/acetylcholine and norepinephrine and serotonin metabolism have at times been considered important due to the positive drug effects of dopamine blockers and α-agonists as well as the beneficial effects of selective serotonin reuptake inhibitors (SSRIs) on OCD. Although the exact cellular and molecular base of Tourette's disorder is still elusive, neurophysiological studies have pointed to abnormalities in dopamine, glutamate, γ-aminobutyric acid (GABA), and serotonin neurotransmitter systems (Leckman et al. 2010). The most consistent evidence implicates involvement of dopamine-related abnormalities—that is, a reduction in tonic extracellular dopamine levels along with hyperresponsive spike-dependent dopamine release following stimulation. Genetic and gene expression findings very much support involvement of these neurotransmitter systems.

Findings regarding dopamine are consistent with the view that Tourette's disorder is mediated by the basal ganglia. Among children and adults with tic disorders, neuroimaging studies have discovered decreased activity in the basal ganglia (Rickards 2009), smaller volumes of the caudate, and decreased cells in the striatum (Paschou 2013). It is theorized that faulty regulation in this circuit—namely, poor inhibitory control and excessive motor activity—causes an individual to respond to a sensation or urge and the associated involuntary motor movement (Wang et al. 2011).

The common co-occurrence of anxiety disorders in tic disorder has implicated the GABAergic system. The occurrence of self-injurious behavior and postmortem brain studies have also implicated the endorphin system, whereas the male preponderance of the persistent tic disorders has implicated male sex hormones. The availability of glutamatergic modulating agents and the interplay of glutamate and dopamine systems have led to research on the glutaminergic system and pilot clinical trials of glutamine modulators.

Moreover, intriguingly, genetic work on a two-generation pedigree has opened new research pointing to a role for histamine, a rather neglected neurotransmitter, with the potential for the development of new treatment options. Lastly, the efficacy of behavioral strategies to reduce tic severity suggests that other neurotransmitters might have an etiological role, including those neurotransmitter systems that enhance cognition or support extinction learning. Nonetheless, the most evidence supports a pivotal role for dopamine in Tourette's disorder. Future studies should be aimed at directly linking neurotransmitter-related genetic and gene expression findings to imaging studies (imaging genetics), which may enable a better understanding of the pathways and mechanisms through which the dynamic interplay of genes, brain, and environment shapes the Tourette's disorder phenotype (Paschou et al. 2013).

Neuropsychological studies have not led to a specific pattern of neuropsychological dysfunction in patients with tic disorders. Early studies suggested a variety of abnormalities but failed to control for the presence of co-occurring conditions. More recent studies that have better controlled for co-occurring conditions suggest that the majority of neuropsychological deficits in those with tic disorder are likely due to co-occurring conditions such as ADHD. Nonetheless, a number of observational studies have suggested that children and adults with tic disorder are vulnerable to problems with inhibitory control, executive functioning, sensory integration, verbal and auditory processing, sustained attention, and handwriting. Given the complexity of clinical presentations of those with the tic disorders and the lack of a specific and consistent neuropsychological deficit attributable to the tic disorders, the presence of functional impairment should drive any clinical neuropsychological evaluation.

Finally, although tics are considered to be involuntary in nature, both individual and environmental factors can affect their expression. Tics are most commonly exacerbated by stress, excitement, and fatigue. In some cases, tics can be triggered by another person's speech or behavior, resulting in a tic characterized by a similar gesture or sound. Tics can be mitigated by engagement in calming, focused activities as well as during sleep. Many children experience a reduction in tic severity while at school, due to engagement in calming, structured activities, and a resurgence after school. The increased frequency of tics that often occurs following school or work is most likely due to less-focused activities and fatigue.

Treatment

General Approaches to Treatment and Special Considerations

Behavioral treatment should be considered the first-line treatment for all tic disorders (see subsection "Psychosocial Treatments" later in this section). However, behavioral treatment is not readily available to all; thus, psychopharmacological treatments remain the most widely used interventions (see subsection "Somatic Treatments").

Psychoeducation should be provided to the patient and family when a tic disorder is diagnosed. This should include discussion of general course and prognosis, exacerbating and alleviating factors, and options for treatment. Development of a treatment plan for tic disorders must first include consideration of comorbid conditions. In most cases, psychosocial and/or pharmacological treatment of comorbid conditions should take priority in treating an individual with a tic disorder. Co-occurring conditions such as ADHD, anxiety disorders, and autism spectrum disorder are typically associated with more distress and impairment than the tic disorder itself. Moreover, treatment of tic disorders is more likely to be effective when other conditions are well managed.

Both psychopharmacological and behavioral treatment can be effective in treating individuals with tics. Several factors should be considered in determining whether formal treatment should be pursued. For individuals with mild symptom severity and low to no interference from the tic disorder, psychoeducation alone may suffice, and formal treatment may not be necessary. To determine whether treatment is warranted, clinicians and families should consider the extent to which an individual experiences functional impairment at home, work, or school as the result of tic symptoms. Individuals who have moderate to severe tics or tics that interfere with their ability to complete tasks or interfere with social interactions, are disruptive to others, or cause the patient subjective pain or distress are considered appropriate candidates for treatment.

Age and developmental level are other factors to be considered when determining whether to treat tics. There is no recommendation for a specific age at which a child would be a good candidate for behavioral treatment. Children may present with tics at a very young age, before they have the capacity to learn from behavioral therapy, and in such cases behavioral therapy may be limited to family-based work. Especially among children, the awareness of a premonitory urge can predict one's likelihood of success with behavioral therapy. Because of their greater difficulty in gaining awareness of premonitory urges, less-developed language abilities, and poorer executive control, younger children may be less able to engage in habit reversal training, which is the hallmark of behavioral treatments for tic disorders (see subsection "Psychosocial Treatments" later in this section). Thus, consideration of an individual child's cognitive capacity, language base, and social maturity determines approach to treatment. Although parents and practitioners may be wary of using medication due to concerns about side effects, psychopharmacological use is approved for young children and is warranted when severity and functional impairment from tics are high.

Somatic Treatments

Pharmacological treatment is used when tics are severe enough to cause impairment in school, at work, in social relationships, or in activities of daily living. Most frequently, comorbid disorders are treated first. There are very few data from randomized controlled trials to support psychopharmacological approaches, so most of the evidence is from open-label studies, case studies, or case series. Data from pharmacotherapy studies for tic disorders are summarized in Table 8–3, which also includes dosing information.

The first-line pharmacological treatment for tic disorders at this time (although agreement is not universal) comprises the α_2-adrenergic agonists, including clonidine and guanfacine. Clonidine reduces norepinephrine release by acting primarily on presynaptic autoreceptors in the locus coeruleus. Guanfacine is longer acting and thought to be more selective to postsynaptic receptors in the prefrontal cortex. Both were found to be effective in suppressing tics in children and adults; however, improvement was greatest when comorbid ADHD was present. These medications can cause sedation, which frequently leads to poor compliance or discontinuation. Blood pressure and pulse should be monitored at baseline and with every dosage increase. Most studies suggest that the α agonists, although often used as a first-line approach, are less efficacious than antipsychotics; nonetheless, α agonists tend to be tried first due to their milder side-effect profile. If guanfacine is used, long-acting guanfacine is recommended when initiating treatment; a 6-week trial at the most effective dosage is adequate to determine efficacy.

Antipsychotic medications have the most extensive evidence for efficacy in the treatment of tics. Because dysfunction in the dopamine system has been implicated in the etiology of tics, this provides a rationale for the use of these agents, which decrease dopamine input to the basal ganglia and ventral tegmentum. Haloperidol and pimozide are the only two medications with U.S. Food and Drug Administration approval for use in tic disorders. Both

TABLE 8–3. Most common and important medication for pharmacological treatment of Tourette's disorder and other chronic tic disorders

Medication	Indication	Starting dosage (mg)	Therapeutic range (mg)	Frequent adverse reactions	Physical examination—at start and at control	Level of evidence
Alpha-adrenergic agonists						
Clonidine	ADHD/TS	0.05	0.1–0.3	Orthostatic hypotension, sedation, sleepiness	Blood pressure, ECG	A
Guanfacine	ADHD/TS	0.5–1.0	1.0–4.0	Orthostatic hypotension, sedation, sleepiness	Blood pressure, ECG	A
Typical neuroleptics						
Haloperidol	TS	0.25–0.5	0.25–15.0	EPS, sedation, increased appetite	Blood count, ECG, weight, transaminases, neurological status, prolactin	A
Pimozide	TS	0.5–1.0	1.0–6.0	EPS, sedation, increased appetite	Blood count, ECG, weight, transaminases, neurological status, prolactin	A
Atypical neuroleptics						
Aripiprazole	TS	2.5	2.5–30.0	Sedation, akathisia, EPS, headache, increased appetite (less than with other neuroleptics), orthostatic hypotension	Blood count, blood pressure, weight, ECG, transaminases, blood sugar	C
Olanzapine	TS/OCB	2.5–5.0	2.5–20.0	Sedation, increased appetite, akathisia	Blood count, blood pressure, ECG, weight, electrolytes, transaminases, prolactin, blood lipids and sugar	B

TABLE 8–3. Most common and important medication for pharmacological treatment of Tourette's disorder and other chronic tic disorders *(continued)*

Medication	Indication	Starting dosage (mg)	Therapeutic range (mg)	Frequent adverse reactions	Physical examination—at start and at control	Level of evidence
Atypical neuroleptics *(continued)*						
Quetiapine	TS	100–150	100–600	Sedation, increased appetite, agitation, orthostatic hypotension	Blood count, blood pressure, ECG, weight, electrolytes, transaminases, prolactin, blood lipids and sugar	C
Risperidone	TS/DBD	0.25	0.25–6.0	EPS, sedation, increased appetite, orthostatic hypotension	Blood count, blood pressure, ECG, weight, electrolytes, transaminases, prolactin, blood lipids and sugar	A
Ziprasidone	TS	5.0–10.0	5.0–10.0	EPS, sedation	Blood count, ECG, weight, transaminases, prolactin	A
Benzamides						
Sulpiride	TS/OCB	50–100 (2 mg/kg)	2–10 mg/kg	Problems with sleep, agitation, increased appetite	Blood count, ECG, weight, transaminases, prolactin, electrolytes	B
Tiapride	TS	50–100 (2 mg/kg)	2–10 mg/kg	Sedation, increased appetite	Blood count, ECG, weight, transaminases, prolactin, electrolytes	B

Note. Evidence level: A (>2 controlled randomized trials); B (1 controlled randomized trial); C (case studies, open trials). DBD=disruptive behavior disorder; ECG=electrocardiogram; EPS=extrapyramidal symptoms; OCB=obsessive-compulsive behavior; TS=Tourette's syndrome.
Source. Reprinted from Roessner V, Plessen KJ, Rothenberger A, et al.; ESSTS Guidelines Group: "European Clinical Guidelines for Tourette Syndrome and Other Tic Disorders, Part II: Pharmacological Treatment." *European Child and Adolescent Psychiatry* 20(4):173–196, 2011. Copyright 2011, Springer. Used with permission.

have robust empirical support (in randomized clinical trials and a placebo-controlled crossover trial that tested the two medications); however, there is no clear evidence confirming the superiority of one over the other. Both medications antagonize the D_2 receptor, but pimozide also blocks calcium channels. Pimozide has frequently been cited as having less risk of extrapyramidal symptoms and thus is more tolerable to patients. However, it can prolong the QTc interval, and electrocardiographic monitoring is therefore recommended. Pimozide cannot be combined with certain medications (macrolide antibiotics, azole antifungals, and other drugs that prolong the QT interval), and consultation with a cardiologist should be considered when treating patients with a personal or family history of cardiac arrhythmias or cardiomyopathy. Low dosages of both medications are often sufficient and encouraged.

The atypical antipsychotic risperidone was found to have efficacy similar to that of both pimozide and haloperidol in several randomized controlled trials. The mechanism of action is slightly different, however, as atypical antipsychotics also act as antagonists to serotonin $5-HT_2$ receptors. Thus, the side-effect profile is reportedly better. However, risperidone and other atypical antipsychotics have a higher risk of metabolic syndrome and weight gain.

Other atypical antipsychotics are used clinically, although there is a relative lack of evidence from well-designed trials. Aripiprazole is one such atypical agent that is thought to have promise, and it is the most often used in clinical settings. Although to date there have been no blinded placebo-controlled trials in patients with tic disorders, aripiprazole has been reported to reduce tics in both open-label and observational studies. The most common side effects were sedation, akathisia, and insomnia. As for the other atypical agents, two studies have established the effectiveness of ziprasidone in children. Although tic reduction has been shown with use of olanzapine, the high risk of weight gain has diminished its use. There are only case reports suggesting quetiapine's usefulness. Overall, we recommend that fluphenazine or risperidone be the first antipsychotic that is tried. A 2- to 3-week trial is usually sufficient to determine efficacy at an appropriate dosage.

Two medications not available in the United States for treatment of tic disorders, tiapride and sulpiride, act as more selective D_2 and D_3 antagonists. They have less propensity to cause extrapyramidal symptoms, thus explaining one of the reasons tiapride is recommended as a first-line treatment for Tourette's disorder in Europe. Evidence from a randomized controlled trial supports its efficacy; many open-label and retrospective studies provide additional support for the use of these medications. Tetrabenazine has long been used in treating hyperkinetic movement disorders. This medication blocks monoamine transporters, thereby depleting presynaptic storage of catecholamines, and also antagonizes postsynaptic dopamine receptors.

More recently, studies have shown improvement in tics as well as a mild side-effect profile with minimal weight gain. Because it may possibly worsen depressive symptoms, tetrabenazine must be used with caution.

Other medications have received attention for their potential in reducing tics as well, although they are less frequently used. Studies have examined the use of GABA-modulating agents such as clonazepam, topiramate, and baclofen, which have shown varied efficacy in improving tics. A randomized, double-blind, placebo-controlled study of tetrahydrocannabinol (THC) (the active substance in marijuana) showed a significant decrease in tic severity over a 6-week period (Müller-Vahl et al. 2003). However, clinicians must be cautious, because marijuana can increase anxiety, psychotic symptoms, panic, insomnia, and depression. Although patients report a sense of calm, not enough studies have been done to determine its efficacy and thus it is not recommended at this time.

Botox (botulinum toxin) has also received attention in the literature. Its mechanism of action includes inhibiting the release of acetylcholine from the presynaptic terminal at the neuromuscular junction. There are a number of case reports and case series and one randomized, double-blind, controlled clinical trial that support its use in the treatment of isolated or focal motor tics that may be painful, such as neck twitches. Preliminary evidence also suggests that botulinum toxin may decrease vocal tics when injected into the laryngeal folds. It has also been shown to reduce premonitory urges. Side effects include muscle weakness, erythema, and pain or rash at the injection site. Botulinum toxin should be considered when tics are unresponsive to other pharmacotherapies. It is best used for single, large debilitating tics that occur frequently or are dystonic in nature.

If tics are severe and refractory to medication, deep brain stimulation can be considered. This surgical approach has proposed benefits due to its effects on the cortico-striato-thalamo-cortical circuit, which may be involved in tic development. Case reports have shown reduction of tics, and a small number of cases have shown persistent reduction in tic frequency. At this time, more definitive evidence is lacking, and strict criteria have not been developed regarding which patients would potentially benefit, but in general, individuals under 25 years old are not considered eligible. Of note, the Tourette's Syndrome Association has developed a registry to include the experiences of all cases worldwide using deep brain stimulation for tics.

As previously stated, most clinical guidelines emphasize the treatment of comorbidities prior to treatment of tics. ADHD is the most commonly comorbid condition, and thus much attention has been placed on its treatment in the context of tic disorders. Early studies asserted that stimulants used to treat ADHD could actually increase tics. However, new evidence refutes this finding. The Tourette's Syndrome Study Group performed a multicenter, randomized, double-blind controlled clinical trial that compared placebo, clonidine, methylphenidate, and a combination of the two drugs in a sample of children with both tics and ADHD. The combination of the two medications had the greatest benefit in improving ADHD symptoms. In addition, there was no difference in the rates of tics worsening between the groups; tics increased an average of 20%–25% (Tourette's Syndrome Study Group 2002). To date, no data exist to suggest that among children without prior tics, use of stimulants leads to the development of a tic disorder. Stimulants are the most effective treatment for ADHD and are therefore the first-line treatment for ADHD; thus they should not be avoided. The side-effect profile is relatively mild and most commonly includes appetite suppression, insomnia, and increased blood pressure and pulse. In children with a tic disorder and comorbid ADHD, alternatives such as clonidine and guanfacine, as well as atomoxetine, can be used. Atomoxetine, a selective norepinephrine-reuptake inhibitor used as second-line treatment for ADHD, reduces tics and ADHD in children and adolescents with both disorders. Adverse effects include nausea, appetite suppression, and insomnia. On the basis of the findings described above, choice of a psychopharmacological agent for individuals with both tics and ADHD should depend upon the severity of the ADHD symptoms.

OCD, another common comorbidity, is often treated with both CBT and serotonin reuptake inhibitors (SRIs). However, OCD in a patient with a co-occurring tic disorder tends not to respond as robustly to an SRI as OCD in the absence of a comorbid tic disorder. Thus, an antipsychotic may need to be added to an SRI. Risperidone or other atypical augmentation has been shown to be efficacious in these situations.

Psychosocial Treatments

Psychopharmacological treatment remains the most commonly used intervention for tic disorders. However, ample evidence supports the efficacy of behavioral therapy, and this approach is gaining popularity among clinicians and patients. A variety of behavioral psychotherapy approaches have been used to treat tics over the past several decades, including functional analysis, management of environmental contingencies, positive reinforcement for tic reduction, awareness training, and habit reversal training.

Comprehensive behavioral intervention for tics (CBIT), which incorporates all of the approaches mentioned with a particular emphasis on habit reversal training, is currently considered the most comprehensive and effective psychotherapeutic treatment. Habit reversal training was initially described by Azrin and Nunn in 1973. Several studies, although many with methodological limitations, supported habit reversal training's effectiveness in tic reduction over the three decades that followed. Later, two well-controlled trials provided additional support for the efficacy of habit reversal training in samples of both children and adults (for a review, see Piacentini and Chang 2005). In 2010, a larger randomized controlled trial demonstrated the efficacy of the combined approach known as CBIT in treating children with Tourette's disorder and chronic tic disorders. Not only did study participants experience reduction in tic severity, but most continued to report benefit at 6-month follow-up (Piacentini et al. 2010).

CBIT is a short-term behavioral intervention for use with both children and adults that targets the reduction of tics and related impairment. CBIT should not be considered a cure for tic disorders but rather an approach to managing the disorder; under ideal circumstances, this treatment may eliminate the presence of particular tics. CBIT has been manualized for clinicians' use (Woods et al. 2008) and comprises several components that are applied in a systematic fashion. Once a thorough assessment of tics and psychoeducation have been completed, a tic hierarchy is created. The tic hierarchy lists tics in the order in which they are most bothersome to the patient. This guides the priority with which tics will be addressed. In most cases, the most bothersome tic is targeted first. When patient motivation or confidence is in question, clinicians can begin with a less bothersome tic that may be more easily reduced with treatment. For example, facial and vocal tics are more difficult to treat, whereas simple motor tics tend to respond most readily to habit reversal training.

Another component of CBIT is the functional assessment; a functional behavioral analysis of each tic is conducted to identify antecedents (e.g., provoking experiences or contexts) and consequences (e.g., social responses). Functional interventions are then implemented to modify any environmental factors that worsen tics. For example, a functional analysis may reveal that when a parent repeatedly tells a child to "stop" in response to a tic, the frequency of the tic tends to increase. In this case, the functional intervention would include working with parents to eliminate this response.

Tic awareness training, another component of CBIT, consists of maximizing the patient's understanding of the exact sequence of movements that constitute a given tic, as well as his or her awareness of and ability to identify the premonitory urge. Awareness training begins in session with the therapist asking the patient to signal each time he or she experiences an urge or tic. Patients are assigned homework to practice awareness training during predetermined time intervals, usually with the assistance of a parent (or, in the case of an adult patient, a spouse or other support person).

Once awareness of a given tic and its urge has been established, patients can begin to generate and practice competing responses, the hallmark of habit reversal training (Table 8–4). A competing response is generated based on several key principles, with the goal of replacing the tic with a different behavior: The competing response must be physically incompatible with the tic; the competing response should be less noticeable than the tic; the competing response can continue for at least a minute or until the urge to tic subsides (whichever is longer); and engagement in the competing response must be feasible across different situations and physical positions. Two hypotheses have been proposed to explain how the competing response produces change. First, it is possible that the competing response engages the basal ganglia in shifting the signal from producing the tic to producing the alternative behavior. A second hypothesis involves the notion that repeated engagement in the competing response leads to gradual habituation to and improved tolerance of the premonitory urge. The competing response is implemented after a patient becomes aware of an urge to tic, to interrupt a tic in progress, or after a tic has finished. In many cases, repeated use of a competing response can lead to the complete elimination of the premonitory urge and the tic itself.

TABLE 8–4. Examples of tics and competing responses

Tic	Competing response
Vocal tics	Use diaphragmatic breathing.
Eye blinking	Use controlled blinking maintained at a predetermined rate.
Leg movements	Place feet flat on floor and tense muscles in the leg.
Mouth movements	Clench jaw while engaging in controlled breathing.
Shoulder shrugs	Tense shoulder and upper arm muscles and push toward chest.

Children are most often the recipients of CBIT; thus, parental involvement throughout treatment is critical. Parents, and at times school personnel, are usually involved in implementing functional interventions. Moreover, treatment includes behavioral reward plans for maximizing children's cooperation with sessions and completion of homework (e.g., practicing awareness training and competing responses at home and at school). For adults who participate in CBIT, a support person should be designated to provide assistance and encouragement as needed.

As behavioral therapy progresses, patients move through the tic hierarchy, creating and practicing competing responses for each individual tic. Ideally, by the conclusion of CBIT, patients and families will have achieved the ability to utilize what they have learned in order to generalize habit reversal training to new tics that may arise in the future.

Key Points

- A diagnosis of Tourette's disorder requires both motor and vocal tics that occur for more than 1 year.
- About 80% of individuals with tic disorders have symptoms that meet diagnostic criteria for another mental disorder (attention-deficit/hyperactivity disorder, obsessive-compulsive disorder, and learning disabilities are most common).
- Tics most typically have their onset during childhood and remit by late adolescence.
- Tics tend to wax and wane and can be exacerbated by stress, fatigue, excitement, and focus on the tics themselves.
- The most widely used assessment tool is the Yale Global Tic Severity Scale.
- Numerous pharmacological approaches may be used to effectively treat tic disorders. The first-line pharmacological treatment for tic disorders at this time (although agreement is not universal) comprises the α_2-adrenergic agonists, including clonidine and guanfacine.
- A manualized treatment known as comprehensive behavioral intervention for tics, or CBIT, is an efficacious treatment for all tic disorders.

References

American Psychiatric Association: Diagnostic and Statistical Manual of Mental Disorders, 4th Edition. Arlington, VA, American Psychiatric Association, 1994

American Psychiatric Association: Diagnostic and Statistical Manual of Mental Disorders, 5th Edition. Arlington, VA, American Psychiatric Association, 2013

Azrin NH, Nunn RG: Habit-reversal: a method of eliminating nervous habits and tics. Behav Res Ther 11(4):619–628, 1973 4777653

Banaschewski T, Woerner W, Rothenberger A: Premonitory sensory phenomena and suppressibility of tics in Tourette syndrome: developmental aspects in children and adolescents. Dev Med Child Neurol 45(10):700–703, 2003 14515942

Bloch MH, Leckman JF: Clinical course of Tourette syndrome. J Psychosom Res 67(6):497–501, 2009 19913654

Brust JC: Substance abuse and movement disorders. Mov Disord 25(13):2010–2020, 2010 20721928

Burd L, Freeman RD, Klug MG, et al: Tourette syndrome and learning disabilities. BMC Pediatr 5:34, 2005 16137334

Burd L, Li Q, Kerbeshian J, et al: Tourette syndrome and comorbid pervasive developmental disorders. J Child Neurol 24(2):170–175, 2009 19182154

Chappell PB, Riddle MA, Scahill L, et al: Guanfacine treatment of comorbid attention-deficit hyperactivity disorder and Tourette's syndrome: preliminary clinical experience. J Am Acad Child Adolesc Psychiatry 34(9):1140–1146, 1995 7559307

Coffey BJ, Biederman J, Smoller JW, et al: Anxiety disorders and tic severity in juveniles with Tourette's disorder. J Am Acad Child Adolesc Psychiatry 39(5):562–568, 2000 10802973

Costello EJ, Angold A, Burns BJ, et al: The Great Smoky Mountains Study of Youth: goals, design, methods, and the prevalence of DSM-III-R disorders. Arch Gen Psychiatry 53(12):1129–1136, 1996 8956679

Hebebrand J, Klug B, Fimmers R, et al: Rates for tic disorders and obsessive compulsive symptomatology in families of children and adolescents with Gilles de la Tourette syndrome. J Psychiatr Res 31(5):519–530, 1997a 9368194

Hebebrand J, Nöthen MM, Ziegler A, et al: Nonreplication of linkage disequilibrium between the dopamine D4 receptor locus and Tourette syndrome. Am J Hum Genet 61(1):238–239, 1997b 9246007

Hyde TM, Aaronson BA, Randolph C, et al: Relationship of birth weight to the phenotypic expression of Gilles de la Tourette's syndrome in monozygotic twins. Neurology 42(3 Pt 1):652–658, 1992 1549232

Leckman JF, Riddle MA, Hardin MT, et al: The Yale Global Tic Severity Scale: initial testing of a clinician-rated scale of tic severity. J Am Acad Child Adolesc Psychiatry 28(4):566–573, 1989 2768151

Leckman JF, Zhang H, Vitale A, et al: Course of tic severity in Tourette syndrome: the first two decades. Pediatrics 102(1 Pt 1):14–19, 1998 9651407

Leckman JF, Bloch MH, King RA, et al: Phenomenology of tics and natural history of tic disorders. Adv Neurol 99:1–16, 2006 16536348

Leckman JF, Bloch MH, Smith ME, et al: Neurobiological substrates of Tourette's disorder. J Child Adolesc Psychopharmacol 20(4):237–247, 2010 20807062

Lewin AB, Chang S, McCracken J, et al: Comparison of clinical features among youth with tic disorders, obsessive-compulsive disorder (OCD), and both conditions. Psychiatry Res 178(2):317–322, 2010 20488548

McAbee GN, Wark JE, Manning A: Tourette syndrome associated with unilateral cystic changes in the gyrus rectus. Pediatr Neurol 20(4):322–324, 1999 10328286

Meidinger AL, Miltenberger RG, Himle M, et al: An investigation of tic suppression and the rebound effect in Tourette's disorder. Behav Modif 29(5):716–745, 2005 16046662

Müller-Vahl KR, Schneider U, Prevedel H, et al: Delta 9-tetrahydrocannabinol (THC) is effective in the treatment of tics in Tourette syndrome: a 6-week randomized trial. J Clin Psychiatry 64(4):459–465, 2003 12716250

Murphy TK, Lewin AB, Storch EA, et al: Practice parameter for the assessment and treatment of children and adolescents with tic disorders. J Am Acad Child Adolesc Psychiatry 52(12):1341–1359, 2013 24290467

Paschou P: The genetic basis of Gilles de la Tourette syndrome. Neurosci Biobehav Rev 37(6):1026–1039, 2013 23333760

Paschou P, Fernandez TV, Sharp F, et al: Genetic susceptibility and neurotransmitters in Tourette syndrome. Int Rev Neurobiol 112:155–177, 2013 24295621

Pauls DL, Raymond CL, Stevenson JM, et al: A family study of Gilles de la Tourette syndrome. Am J Hum Genet 48(1):154–163, 1991 1985456

Piacentini J, Chang S: Habit reversal training for tic disorders in children and adolescents. Behav Modif 29(6):803–822, 2005 16204417

Piacentini J, Woods DW, Scahill L, et al: Behavior therapy for children with Tourette disorder: a randomized controlled trial. JAMA 303(19):1929–1937, 2010 20483969

Price RA, Kidd KK, Cohen DJ, et al: A twin study of Tourette syndrome. Arch Gen Psychiatry 42(8):815–820, 1985 3860194

Rickards H: Functional neuroimaging in Tourette syndrome. J Psychosom Res 67(6):575–584, 2009 19913661

Robertson MM: Gilles de la Tourette syndrome: the complexities of phenotype and treatment. Br J Hosp Med (Lond) 72(2):100–107, 2011 21378617

Scahill L, Bitsko RH, Visser SN, et al: Prevalence of diagnosed Tourette syndrome in persons aged 6–17 years—United States, 2007. MMWR Morb Mortal Wkly Rep 58(21):581–585, 2009 19498335

Stewart SE, Illmann C, Geller DA, et al: A controlled family study of attention-deficit/hyperactivity disorder and Tourette's disorder. J Am Acad Child Adolesc Psychiatry 45(11):1354–1362, 2006 17075358

Tourette's Syndrome Study Group: Treatment of ADHD in children with tics: a randomized controlled trial. Neurology 58(4):527–536, 2002 11865128

Verdellen CW, Hoogduin CA, Keijsers GP: Tic suppression in the treatment of Tourette's syndrome with exposure therapy: the rebound phenomenon reconsidered. Mov Disord 22(11):1601–1606, 2007 17534958

Walkup JT, LaBuda MC, Singer HS, et al: Family study and segregation analysis of Tourette syndrome: evidence for a mixed model of inheritance. Am J Hum Genet 59(3):684–693, 1996 8751870

Walkup JT, Ferrão Y, Leckman JF, et al: Tic disorders: some key issues for DSM-V. Depress Anxiety 27(6):600–610, 2010 20533370

Wang Z, Maia TV, Marsh R, et al: The neural circuits that generate tics in Tourette's syndrome. Am J Psychiatry 168(12):1326–1337, 2011 21955933

Woods DW, Piacentini J, Himle MB, et al: Premonitory Urge for Tics Scale (PUTS): initial psychometric results and examination of the premonitory urge phenomenon in youths with tic disorders. J Dev Behav Pediatr 26(6):397–403, 2005 16344654

Woods DW, Piacentini JC, Chang SW, et al: Managing Tourette Syndrome: A Behavioral Intervention for Children and Adults, Therapist Guide. New York, Oxford University Press, 2008

Zinner S: Tourette syndrome in infancy and early childhood. Infants Young Child 19:353–370, 2006

Recommended Readings

McKinlay D: Nix Your Tics! Eliminate Unwanted Tic Symptoms: A How-To Guide for Young People. London, ON, Canada, Life's a Twitch Publishing, 2012

Murphy TK, Lewin AB, Storch EA, et al: Practice parameter for the assessment and treatment of children and adolescents with tic disorders. J Am Acad Child Adolesc Psychiatry 52(12):1341–1359, 2013

National Tourette Syndrome Association: http://www.tsa-usa.org/

Woods DW, Piacentini JC, Chang SW, et al: Managing Tourette Syndrome: A Behavioral Intervention for Children and Adults, Therapist Guide. New York, Oxford University Press, 2008

CHAPTER 9

Illness Anxiety Disorder

Lillian Reuman, M.A.
Jonathan S. Abramowitz, Ph.D.

In DSM-5 (American Psychiatric Association 2013), illness anxiety disorder (IAD), characterized by preoccupation with having or acquiring a serious medical condition, is a reconceptualized version of DSM-IV hypochondriasis (American Psychiatric Association 1994). Although changes from DSM-IV are notable, the signs and symptoms of IAD were included in the DSM-IV diagnosis of hypochondriasis, a term that was considered by some to have pejorative connotations. Over the past quarter century, the application of conceptual models and treatment techniques used for anxiety disorders has greatly improved the prognosis for what is now labeled IAD. In this chapter, we review key features of this disorder, including symptomatology, epidemiology, and comorbidity of IAD, based upon existing research regarding hypochondriasis, as research to date has not yet examined IAD according to DSM-5 criteria. In addition, we include two case examples to illustrate the disorder's presentation. We also consider developmental, gender-related, and cross-cultural issues and then turn to a discussion of conceptual models and their implications for the assessment and treatment of IAD.

Diagnostic Criteria and Symptomatology

According to DSM-5, the essential feature of IAD entails a preoccupation with the (unsubstantiated) belief that one has, or is in danger of developing, a serious undiagnosed medical illness even though no (or minimal) somatic symptoms are present (Box 9–1). For example, IAD may be characterized by the belief that one has latent heart disease despite the absence of cardiac abnormalities.

BOX 9–1. DSM-5 Diagnostic Criteria for Illness Anxiety Disorder

---

A. Preoccupation with having or acquiring a serious illness.

B. Somatic symptoms are not present or, if present, are only mild in intensity. If another medical condition is present or there is a high risk for developing a medical condition (e.g., strong family history is present), the preoccupation is clearly excessive or disproportionate.

C. There is a high level of anxiety about health, and the individual is easily alarmed about personal health status.

D. The individual performs excessive health-related behaviors (e.g., repeatedly checks his or her body for signs of illness) or exhibits maladaptive avoidance (e.g., avoids doctor appointments and hospitals).

E. Illness preoccupation has been present for at least 6 months, but the specific illness that is feared may change over that period of time.

F. The illness-related preoccupation is not better explained by another mental disorder, such as somatic symptom disorder, panic disorder, generalized anxiety disorder, body dysmorphic disorder, obsessive-compulsive disorder, or delusional disorder, somatic type.

Specify whether:

   Care-seeking type: Medical care, including physician visits or undergoing tests and procedures, is frequently used.

   Care-avoidant type: Medical care is rarely used.

Reprinted from American Psychiatric Association: *Diagnostic and Statistical Manual of Mental Disorders*, 5th Edition. Arlington, VA, American Psychiatric Association. Copyright 2013, American Psychiatric Association. Used with permission.

The illness-related preoccupations are typically accompanied by excessive health-related anxiety as well as excessive behaviors or maladaptive avoidance that has the aim of reducing fear and protecting one's health. Common examples include excessively seeking reassurance from medical professionals regarding good health (e.g., medical tests to confirm healthy blood pressure), checking one's body for signs of illness (e.g., frequent breast self-examinations for cancer), reviewing published sources of information on the feared illness (e.g., searching the Internet), and trying various remedies such as herbal preparations. Avoidance of situations and stimuli perceived to be associated with the feared malady (e.g., avoidance of airport security checkpoints for fear of radiation) and avoidance of illness-related stimuli, such as doctor visits and hospitals, may occur.

Individuals with IAD usually do not conceptualize their concerns as being psychological in origin and therefore may reject the suggestion that they seek consultation or treatment from a mental health professional. Instead, they typically seek treatment in primary care and specialty medical settings. Additionally, although individuals with IAD may admit to being overly concerned about their feared illness, they frequently remain dissatisfied until they receive a medical explanation for their fears or symptoms. For this reason, many individuals with IAD "shop" for physicians who can provide a concrete explanation. Many individuals with IAD feel their complaints are quickly dismissed and not taken seriously by medical professionals. These behaviors can be costly, strain the doctor-patient relationship, lead to care from an excessive number of health care providers, and cause patients to undergo potentially harmful testing procedures despite having good health.

DSM-5 contains two specifiers for IAD: care-seeking type and care-avoidant type. Individuals with the care-seeking specifier engage in frequent physician visits and medical testing. They attempt to gain reassurance regarding the feared medical problem. In contrast, the care-avoidant type is characterized by a lack of interaction with physicians. Such individuals appear to avoid reminders of illness as a way of controlling their levels of anxiety and distress. Others might avoid doctors because they dread receiving the feared diagnosis. Although this dichotomy seems intuitively accurate from a clinical perspective, to our knowledge no empirical studies have been conducted to validate these diagnostic specifiers.

Both IAD and somatic symptom disorder have replaced hypochondriasis in DSM-5. Unlike DSM-IV hypochondriasis, IAD focuses on a patient's preoccupation with his or her own health regardless of whether medical symptoms are present. Most individuals with DSM-IV hypochondriasis are now classified as having somatic symptom disorder; however, the diagnosis of IAD may apply in certain cases. Somatic symptom disorder is diagnosed when one's preoccupation with an illness leads to excessive health concerns—more than would be expected to arise from the physical illness alone. Somatic symptom disorder differs from IAD in that somatic symptom disorder entails the presence of significant somatic symptoms, whereas somatic symptoms are absent or only mild in intensity in IAD. The DSM-5 diagnoses of IAD and somatic symptom disorder, which focus on the positive symptoms of the disorder (e.g., preoccupation, high levels of anxiety), represent a shift from DSM-IV's focus on medically unexplained symptoms. The DSM-IV and DSM-5 diagnoses both recognize that psychological symptoms and concerns may exist with or without the presence of an actual nonpsychiatric medical condition that explains the symptoms; however, DSM-5 emphasizes medically unexplained symptoms to a lesser extent. A reason for changing the name of this condition is that the term *hypochondriasis* was often considered pejorative toward patients.

We base our discussion of IAD on existing research on DSM-IV hypochondriasis, because to our knowledge, published research to date has not yet examined IAD according to DSM-5 criteria. We include research from studies about illness worry, health worry, and illness anxiety, because these synonymous terms have been used by researchers to define similar phenomena, based upon different scales and assessment measures. Additionally, health-related worry may exist along a continuum, with normal illness worry at one end and hypochondriasis at the other; as such, illness worry, health worry, and illness anxiety may characterize individuals who fall somewhere along the spectrum. The terms collectively refer to excessive preoccupation about one's health. In many instances, the extreme focus on general health and tendency to be easily alarmed by health-related information disrupt social, occupational, and family functioning. Moreover, preoccupations persist despite appropriate medical evaluation and reassurance of good health from qualified clinicians using valid and reliable diagnostic tests. Patients' preoccupation may be symptom based, with a focus on specific bodily functions (e.g., belching), actual mild physical sensations that merit little concern (e.g., a small sore), or vague physical sensations (e.g., "twisted, tightening stomach"). The person ascribes these relatively banal signs and sensations to a feared perilous or undetected medical disease (e.g., colon cancer) and remains preoccupied with determining their meaning, authenticity, and underlying etiology.

Case Example: Sam

Sam, a 28-year-old Caucasian student, was referred to our clinic by his primary care physician for psychological assessment and treatment because of Sam's persistent fear that he had a serious heart condition. He occasionally felt mild dizziness, shortness of breath, and a rapid heart rate—often following physical exertion. A comprehensive medical evaluation, including a complete cardiac workup, revealed no evidence of a medical condition that might account for his complaints.

Sam reported engaging in a number of precautionary behaviors that he believed would reduce the risks of ill health. First, he moved from his home in Florida to Rochester, Minnesota, in order to be closer to the Mayo Clinic—the only place he believed could accurately detect and save him from his "misunderstood" physical problems. He demanded that his fiancée, Melanie, stay with him at all times in the event he needed transportation to the hospital. Because of his fear that physical exertion would strain his "delicate" heart, Sam abstained from many athletic activities he had previously enjoyed, including jogging, biking, and playing basketball. He used a portable heart rate monitor to monitor whether immediate medical attention was warranted. He spent hours each day searching the Internet for information about cardiovascular and other medical diseases.

Various medical providers told Sam that the "symptoms" he experienced upon exertion were common and not serious and that he "had nothing to worry about." Yet Sam was not satisfied with these doctors because they were not interested in trying to determine what was *causing* his symptoms. Sam believed he was not being taken seriously enough and that his doctors thought his problems were "all in his head." When Sam was initially encouraged to seek consultation from a psychologist, he became angry and felt "cast off." He strongly maintained that he was in danger of developing a serious medical condition.

Case Example: Julia

Julia, a 43-year-old married, Asian American, full-time (i.e., stay-at-home) mother of two children, was referred to our clinic by her husband, who cited increased dissatisfaction with their relationship because of his wife's incessant fear of falling ill with cancer. Despite being at low risk (e.g., negative family history) for breast cancer, Julia maintained that she "had a gut feeling" that she would develop cancer. Consequently, she led a rigid lifestyle regarding her health by following a strict organic, plant-based diet and excessively exercising (i.e., more than 2 hours daily). She also conducted extensive online searches (sometimes lasting hours) and questioning of "experts" about food and makeup products so that she could avoid all possible carcinogens (e.g., makeup containing parabens and plastic water bottles containing bisphenol A).

This preoccupation, rigid behavior, and extensive information gathering became increasingly problematic, as it caused arguments regarding family meal plans, diverted time from family activities, and prevented her from attending events that would make her anxious about her health status. For example, Julia resisted visits to the doctor out of fear that her physician would uncover a malignant tumor. Furthermore, she avoided visiting her ailing grandmother in the hospital, attending funerals, and taking her young daughters to doctors' appointments because these activities reminded her of cancer. Such behaviors strained her marriage, and Julia's husband insisted that she seek help for her "ridiculous" behavior and "unfounded fears." Julia maintained that such precautions were "smart and savvy" and that she was "in no way overreacting."

Epidemiology

Prevalence estimates of IAD are based on estimates of the prevalence of hypochondriasis as defined in DSM-IV. A systematic review of population-based surveys cited a low prevalence of hypochondriasis (median rate of 0.4%) in the general population; this low prevalence made it difficult to study associated features of the disorder (Creed and Barsky 2004). Taken together, studies suggest that the 1- to 2-year prevalence of illness anxiety (although not necessarily DSM-5-defined IAD) in population-based samples ranges from 1.3% to 10% (American Psychiatric Association 2013). Available lifetime prevalence rate estimates also vary widely and range from 0.8% to 8.5% depending on the setting (Barsky et al. 1990; Faravelli et al. 1997).

Among patients in medical settings, where prevalence rates of hypochondriasis seem to be higher than in the community or in psychiatric settings, studies estimated a range of 0.8% to 10.3% (Kellner et al. 1983–1984; Noyes 2001). Such estimates were higher still among medical specialty populations (e.g., 13% of otolaryngology patients; Schmidt et al. 1993). The prevalence of hypochondriasis among psychiatric patients, although difficult to ascertain (given individuals' reluctance to seek mental health consultation), was even higher (up to 49%); however, it was rarely their primary diagnosis, and studies used DSM-III and earlier criteria (American Psychiatric Association 1980; Noyes 2001).

These rates must be interpreted with caution, because hypochondriasis is not typically diagnosed on the basis of reliable and valid structured interviews. In addition, as previously noted, no studies to our knowledge have examined the prevalence of DSM-5 IAD. Subthreshold illness preoccupations are likely more common than DSM-IV hypochondriasis or DSM-5 IAD. For example, Noyes et al. (2005) found that 6.9% of their surveyed population had illness worry for at least 6 months, but almost none of the worried study participants met full criteria for hypochondriasis. This distinction may be relevant to prevalence rates for IAD. In addition, the change in diagnostic criteria and division of hypochondriasis into somatic symptom disorder and IAD might sharply reduce the number of IAD diagnoses.

Comorbidity

Comorbidities for IAD are unknown because available studies have used diagnostic criteria for hypochondriasis. Therefore, we address comorbidity as previously documented with regard to hypochondriasis and illness worry. Research suggests that individuals with DSM-III-R hypochondriasis (American Psychiatric Association 1987) have elevated rates of mood and anxiety disorders (e.g., obsessive-compulsive disorder [OCD], panic disorder, generalized anxiety disorder) relative to individuals without concerns about their health (Barsky et al. 1992).

Approximately two-thirds of individuals with DSM-III-R hypochondriasis have at least one current comorbid mental disorder (Barsky et al. 1992). Depression among individuals with illness worry is common; studies suggest that 28%–43% of individuals with hypochondriasis also have symptoms that meet criteria for major depressive disorder across an array of settings (Barsky et al. 1992). Conversely, pathological concerns about health and illness are prevalent among outpatients with DSM-III-R depression, although the temporal relationship between the conditions is unclear.

In one study, 85.7% of individuals with hypochondriasis also met diagnostic criteria for a lifetime anxiety disorder (Barsky et al. 1992). Panic disorder in particular appears to be associated with hypochondriasis. In one study, 85% of individuals with panic attacks reported that illness anxiety preceded such events (Fava et al. 1988). Furer et al. (1997) found that hypochondriasis was more prevalent among individuals with panic disorder than among those with social phobia or without any diagnosed anxiety disorder. Additionally, patients with panic disorder displayed significantly more hypochondriacal concerns than those with generalized anxiety disorder (Starcevic et al. 1994). Lifetime prevalence of OCD among individuals with hypochondriasis is about 10% (Barsky et al. 1992).

Research suggests that personality disorders commonly co-occur with hypochondriasis; one study found that approximately 40% of individuals with hypochondriasis had features that met criteria for a personality disorder (Fallon et al. 2012). The most common personality disorder diagnoses among individuals with hypochondriasis include paranoid, avoidant, and obsessive-compulsive personality disorders. Although personality disorders may complicate the presentation and treatment of hypochondriasis, they should not be assumed to be the source of hypochondriasis or IAD.

Course and Prognosis

There are no data on the average age at onset or the prevalence of illness anxiety among children. As with many other mental disorders, onset appears especially likely in early adulthood as the individual faces increased responsibility, including the maintenance of his or her own health. Other potential onset triggers include increased life stress, personal experience with illness, illness or death of a loved one, and exposure to media coverage of illnesses.

In a longitudinal study of patients with hypochondriasis recruited from a medical outpatient setting, Barsky et al. (1998) found that 63.5% ($n=54$) still met diagnostic criteria 4–5 years later. Although these patients exhibited some improvement in their functional status, level of fear, disease conviction, and bodily preoccupations, they remained significantly more symptomatic and functionally impaired compared with a control group of individuals without hypochondriasis at follow-up.

Psychosocial Impairment and Suicidality

Individuals with hypochondriasis report poor physical functioning and impaired work performance (Noyes et al. 1993). Hypochondriasis has also been related to the presence of general medical conditions (e.g., fibromyalgia, coronary artery disease, chronic fatigue) and is a strong predictor of pain due to osteoarthritis, disability in patients with coronary artery disease, and breathlessness among individuals with chronic lung disease. Symptoms associated with the aforementioned diseases may aggravate illness-related concerns, and vice versa.

Additionally, individuals with IAD may experience a contentious relationship with the health care system and providers. Individuals with IAD may acquire excessive financial burden due to frequent medical appointments/testing and accompanying costs, although they are typically dissatisfied with the care they receive. Individuals with pervasive illness worry are more likely to feel that their health problems are not taken seriously compared with individuals without illness worry. Furthermore, they have been found to miss more scheduled health care appointments than their healthier counterparts (Kellner 1990).

There are no large studies of suicide in hypochondriasis or illness-related anxiety. Bebbington (1976) published two case studies of individuals with hypochondriasis who committed suicide and suggested that this outcome may be more common among individuals with hypochondriasis who also have severe comorbid depressive symptoms. Although individuals with severe illness anxiety tend to view their health as worse than the general population's (Gureje et al. 1997) and might feel as though their symptoms are a sign of impending death, clinical observations and available case reports suggest early mortality is extremely low.

Developmental Considerations

To date, no research regarding developmental considerations for IAD exists, and research regarding developmental considerations for hypochondriasis is limited. Findings from a population-based survey suggested that health anxiety was strongly age dependent, with older participants endorsing hypochondriacal symptoms more frequently and scoring higher on an index designed to measure hypochondriacal features; however, they do not necessarily seek more medical care (Rief et al. 2001).

Gender-Related Issues

Findings regarding gender-related issues in hypochondriasis are equivocal. Multiple studies suggest that illness anxiety presents equally in males and females (Barsky et al. 1990; Gureje et al. 1997). In contrast, Noyes et al. (1993) found that individuals with hypochondriasis were more often women, and Rief et al. (2001) found that women had more hypochondriacal features than did men. These findings might be explained by differences in help-seeking behavior between men and women.

Cultural Aspects of Phenomenology

Although there may be cross-cultural differences in manifestations of illness anxiety and hypochondriasis, scant research exists regarding cultural aspects of the phenomenology of hypochondriasis. The World Health Organization characterized patients with hypochondriasis across 15 sites in 14 countries. This cross-national study (Gureje et al. 1997) found that rates of hypochondriasis in patients in a primary care setting, as diagnosed by ICD-10 criteria, did not differ across sites. Compared with individuals without hypochondriasis, patients with hypochondriasis (across sites) tended to utilize more health care services and reported more disagreement with physicians regarding their health. These findings are limited by the fact that data collection was confined to cities in developed countries; individuals in rural areas and developing societies that may rely more heavily on traditional medicine and accompanying beliefs were excluded. It is unclear to what extent the primarily Western DSM-5 definition of IAD is appropriate cross-culturally, given that attitudes toward defining illness, seeking help, and trusting doctors/healers may vary.

Cultural factors can influence the perception of bodily sensations, reflecting variability in cultural views of the relationship between body and mind. In Western cultures, for example, the predominant view is a *psychosomatic* perspective, in which psychological distress is expressed as physical complaints. Physical complaints often occur in reaction to stress among Asian Americans (Sue and Sue 1990). In many other cultures, however, the dominant view is the *somatopsychic* perspective, in which physical problems are thought to produce emotional symptoms.

In addition, culture appears to influence the presentation of somatization and illness anxiety (i.e., the types of bodily concerns). Among some African groups, somatic complaints (e.g., hot flashes, numbness and tingling sensations) differ from those expressed in Western cultures. These differences may reflect variability in cultural views of the relationship between body and mind. Germanic cultures tend to emphasize cardiopulmonary symptoms such as poor circulation, whereas in the United Kingdom, health concerns often focus on constipation and other gastrointestinal concerns. In the United States and Canada, concerns about environmental viruses and diseases (e.g., AIDS; severe acute respiratory syndrome, or SARS) are highly prominent.

Cultural differences also exist in the propensity to seek medical attention for bodily concerns. Compared with other groups, for example, Asian Americans, African Americans, and Latino groups living in the United States show a stronger tendency to report medically unexplained symptoms to their physicians. It is therefore important to attend to contextual factors when working with individuals who have health anxiety and are from diverse ethnic and cultural backgrounds.

Assessment and Differential Diagnosis

Assessment

Important steps in the assessment of IAD include diagnosing any nonpsychiatric medical conditions that may be responsible for presenting problems and in need of treatment, establishing that the presenting illness concerns that are associated with IAD are clearly excessive if another nonpsychiatric medical disorder could explain the symptoms, and ruling in the presence of IAD. It is important to recognize that according to DSM-5, someone could have a clinical presentation that meets criteria for IAD even with a bona fide medical disorder that manifests with symptoms similar to the patient's concerns (Box 9–1).

A variety of self-report questionnaires are available to facilitate assessment of the severity of various symptoms of IAD, including the Illness Behavior Questionnaire (Pilowsky and Katsikitis 1994), Illness Attitudes Scale (Kellner 1987), and Health Anxiety Inventory (Salkovskis et al. 2002). The Yale-Brown Obsessive Compulsive Scale (Y-BOCS; Goodman et al. 1989), a semistructured clinical interview developed to assess the severity of obsessions and compulsions in OCD, was modified to assess hypochondriasis (Greeven et al. 2009a) and therefore can likely be used to assess illness-related preoccupation, safety behaviors and reassurance-seeking, and illness-related avoidance, all of which are included as diagnostic criteria for IAD. Use of clinician-administered measures with sound psychometric properties expands opportunities for in-depth inquiry about IAD-related concerns and behaviors that self-report assessments may not capture. Suggested screening questions for IAD are presented in Table 9–1.

Differential Diagnosis

The symptoms of IAD overlap to some extent with those of OCD and some anxiety, psychotic, and DSM-IV mood disorders, as well as symptoms of somatic symptom disorder, a diagnosis that is new to DSM-5. In this section, we discuss these overlaps as well as strategies for differentiating IAD from these other diagnoses. Key considerations for differential diagnosis are presented in Table 9–2.

Obsessive-Compulsive Disorder

The persistent illness preoccupation in hypochondriasis (and now in IAD) has similarities to obsessions in OCD because both involve intrusive preoccupations and provoke subjective distress. Furthermore, the repetitive checking and reassurance seeking observed in IAD are functionally similar to compulsions in OCD; both serve to reduce distress in the short run but

TABLE 9–1. Screening questions for illness anxiety disorder
Do you often worry that you have a serious illness?
What symptoms (if any) do you experience?
How strongly do you believe that you are ill?
Is there any evidence you can think of that might suggest that you are not ill?
Have your doctors told you that you are ill? How do you feel about your doctors' assessment of your health?
To what extent do your worries about illness get in the way of your daily functioning (e.g., work, family)?
What do you do on your own to try to figure out if you have a serious illness (e.g., checking your blood pressure)?

paradoxically end up maintaining the illness-related fears in the long run (Abramowitz and Deacon 2005). On the basis of the overlaps in psychological mechanisms that maintain these problems, it may be useful to conceptualize IAD as an obsessive-compulsive and related disorder, an approach that was considered but not adopted during the development of DSM-5.

There are two important differences between OCD and IAD that have relevance for assessment and treatment. First, whereas individuals with OCD tend to have multiple types of obsessions and compulsions (e.g., contamination, harm, religion-focused), some of which may be concerned with health and illness, those with IAD tend to be "singly obsessed" with health/illness-related preoccupations. Second, on the whole, individuals with IAD appear to evidence less insight into the senselessness of their fears as compared with individuals with OCD, whose insight often varies (Neziroglu et al. 2000).

Panic Disorder

Individuals with panic disorder often attribute their panic attacks (and related body sensations, such as shortness of breath and racing heart) to medical illnesses, such as a cardiac or neurological condition. Accordingly, patients with panic disorder often seek extensive medical examinations and consult numerous specialists (e.g., cardiologists) in the hope of obtaining a medical explanation for their panic symptoms. They also typically resort to avoidance strategies (e.g., of strenuous activity, caffeine) and safety-seeking behaviors (e.g., keeping medication, cell phone, or a water bottle nearby at all times) to help manage health-related worries. Clinical observations indicate that many individuals with illness anxiety also experience occasional panic at-

TABLE 9–2. Key considerations for differential diagnosis for illness anxiety disorder (IAD)

Obsessive-compulsive disorder (OCD)	In OCD, the obsessions may be more heterogeneous (e.g., contamination, harm, religion), whereas in IAD, the focus is exclusively on health and illness.
	Patients with IAD tend to have poorer insight into the senselessness of their fears than do those with OCD.
Panic disorder	Panic attacks are typically associated with immediate medical emergencies (e.g., heart attack, stroke, fainting), whereas the concerns in IAD are more future oriented (e.g., cancer, dementia, degenerative diseases).
	Panic attacks are characterized by a fear of acute and episodic arousal-related body sensations, whereas illness anxiety may be associated with arousal and nonarousal sensations or with thoughts and images of becoming ill.
Generalized anxiety disorder	In generalized anxiety, the excessive worries are many and varied, and illness concerns are typically vague; in IAD, the focus is exclusively on one or more specific feared illnesses.
Somatic symptom disorder	Whereas individuals with IAD are primarily preoccupied with the notion of becoming ill, and may or may not exhibit mild physical symptoms, those with somatic symptom disorder experience significant somatic symptoms.

tacks. Thus, there appears to be a significant overlap between panic disorder and IAD.

Despite these similarities, the sense of doom experienced during panic attacks arises from fears of *immediate* life-threatening physical catastrophe (e.g., a heart attack, aneurysm) resulting from the sensations associated with anxious arousal. In contrast, patients with IAD experience a more incipient fear of delayed or protracted consequences (e.g., "I am slowly dying from lung cancer"), and the sorts of bodily sensations and variations that cue such concerns may or may not be arousal related (e.g., rashes, dull pain). Put another way, patients with panic disorder often fear they *are dying*, whereas patients with IAD fear their *eventual death.*

Generalized Anxiety Disorder

Persistent and uncontrollable worrying, which is a main symptom of generalized anxiety disorder, is also a prominent feature of IAD. Individuals may worry excessively about interpersonal relationships, work or school, finances, the future, and their own and significant others' health (American Psychiatric Association 2013). However, health-related worries in generalized anxiety disorder are less frequent and less intrusive than those observed in IAD. Individuals with generalized anxiety also report fewer somatic symptoms, fewer fears and misinterpretations of specific bodily sensations, and less fear of death relative to those with anxiety about illnesses (Starcevic et al. 1994).

Somatic Symptom Disorder

Both IAD and somatic symptom disorder involve health concerns. However, individuals with IAD are primarily preoccupied with the possibility of becoming ill, rather than the presence of physical symptoms. On the other hand, those with somatic symptom disorder experience significant somatic symptoms, which are the primary focus of concern. Whereas somatic symptoms are required in somatic symptom disorder, they may or may not be present in IAD, and if they are present they are only mild in intensity.

Depression

Individuals with unipolar depression might present with somatic complaints (e.g., stomach pain, low energy). However, anhedonia and other symptoms, such as worthlessness, low self-esteem, and depressed mood, are features of depressive disorders that are not present in IAD.

Delusional Disorder, Somatic Type

In contrast to individuals with delusional disorder, somatic type, those with IAD are able to acknowledge the possibility that the feared medical disease is not present. Moreover, beliefs typical of IAD are more realistic (e.g., "a tumor is slowly growing") than those in true somatic delusions, which tend to be more bizarre (e.g., "the organ is rotting"). However, it is possible that these two disorders are actually the same disorder, varying along a dimension of insight (like OCD and body dysmorphic disorder); research is needed to investigate this possibility.

Etiology, Pathophysiology, and Risk Factors

The cause of IAD is unknown, and it is most likely multifactorial. Contemporary psychological models have the most consistent support, emphasizing environmental and learning factors and cognitive and behavioral mechanisms (i.e., cognitive-behavioral models; Abramowitz and Braddock 2008). Specifically, dysfunctional beliefs about bodily symptoms and illness (e.g., "My body is weak, and I am vulnerable to illnesses") are thought to play a significant role in the development of IAD. Such beliefs as well as ambiguous health-related information increase the likelihood of catastrophic misinterpretations of benign bodily sensations and perturbations. Once concerned about illness, the person becomes vigilant for signs of being ill and is motivated to reduce anxiety by trying to gain reassurance about his or her health. According to this model, the mistaken beliefs are maintained (despite contradictory information and repeated reassurance of good health from medical professionals) by maladaptive strategies used to cope with illness-related anxiety. These strategies include attempts to prevent the feared illness, avoidance, and attempts to attain certainty about health status. These safety behaviors prevent individuals with hypochondriasis from acquiring information that would disconfirm their mistaken beliefs about illnesses.

From this cognitive-behavioral perspective, potential vulnerability factors for IAD include personal experience with illness (either in oneself or in a close friend or relative), observing how others cope with illness, and a history of childhood abuse (Noyes et al. 2002). More specific cognitive factors include anxiety sensitivity—the tendency to fear the sensations of anxious arousal based on the belief that they are dangerous—which is a known risk factor for the development of panic disorder (Abramowitz and Braddock 2008; Olatunji and Wolitzky-Taylor 2009). The cognitive-behavioral model of IAD, which is partially derived from conceptualizations of the development of anxiety disorders, has been empirically supported and has important clinical implications (as we discuss later in this chapter).

Some researchers have examined possible genetic factors and interactions with the environment with respect to understanding illness-related anxiety. Anxiety sensitivity, for example, appears to be moderately heritable (Stein et al. 1999). Moreover, various features of illness anxiety (e.g., disease

conviction, fear of diseases, interference in functioning) appear to be influenced by a common set of genes and feature-specific environmental influences
(Taylor et al. 2006). Few imaging studies on hypochondriasis exist; however,
available data suggest that individuals with hypochondriasis may exhibit
volumetric abnormalities in the orbitofrontal cortex, thalamus, and pituitary (Atmaca et al. 2010a, 2010b).

Treatment

General Approaches to Treatment and Special Considerations

Individuals with IAD typically resist the notion that their complaints represent anything other than a nonpsychiatric medical illness, making it difficult
to engage them in appropriate psychological or psychiatric treatment. However, several evidence-based cognitive-behavioral treatments are available for
those who can be motivated to consider alternatives to disease-based explanations. Details of these treatments are described by Taylor and Asmundson
(2004) and Abramowitz and Braddock (2010) and summarized in the following discussion. Effective pharmacotherapies are also discussed.

Motivational interviewing techniques may be helpful in encouraging patients to accept mental health treatment. Motivational interviewing explores
ambivalence regarding change rather than attempting to confront or persuade the patient into making changes. In IAD, this approach is introduced
early in treatment to increase motivation to change and weaken the patient's
conviction regarding the presence of the feared illness. Components of motivational interviewing include examining the advantages and disadvantages
of maintaining the status quo (versus trying a new approach), helping the
patient to observe discrepancies between his or her current levels of functioning and goals and values, and reinforcing self-efficacy statements. These
strategies have the goal of helping patients resolve their ambivalence in the
direction of a commitment to treatment and becoming their own advocates
for change (Miller and Rollnick 2002).

Psychoeducation

Psychoeducation programs provide an individual with information about the
nature of his or her presenting concerns and potential strategies for addressing these concerns. This approach has the advantage of being relatively simple
to administer to either individuals or groups. It also contrasts with the provi-
sion of reassurance in that the individual is presented with new information,
rather than the repeated presentation of old information (e.g., repeating mes-

sages assuring the individual of good health, unnecessary medical tests to placate concerns). Emotion regulation strategies (e.g., relaxation training) are often used in psychoeducation, but systematic exposure exercises are usually not included.

Studies examining the merits of group psychoeducation as the main component of treatment suggest that it is superior to a wait-list control in reducing illness anxiety, with a corresponding reduction in frequency of medical service utilization and gains maintained at follow-up periods of up to 1 year (Bouman 2002). Participants in psychoeducation also value the opportunity to share their concerns, and most are relieved to learn that they are not suffering alone. However, psychoeducation alone is often not a sufficient treatment; more often, it is used early in the treatment to set the stage for treatment and to help engage the patient in psychotherapy or pharmacotherapy.

Pharmacotherapy

There is a limited database of studies of the pharmacotherapy of hypochondriasis, and to date no medication has been U.S. Food and Drug Administration–approved for the treatment of this disorder. Nevertheless, early case studies and a small number of open-label trials (all with sample sizes of less than 20) indicated that clomipramine (25–225 mg/day), imipramine (125–150 mg/day), fluoxetine (20–80 mg/day), fluvoxamine (300 mg/day), paroxetine (60 mg/day), and nefazodone (200–500 mg/day) may be effective in reducing illness fears and related beliefs, pervasive anxiety, somatic complaints, avoidance, and reassurance seeking (Fallon et al. 2003). This work gave impetus to a small number of subsequent randomized controlled trials of the selective serotonin reuptake inhibitors (SSRIs) in hypochondriasis, although the evidence base remains very limited with regard to key questions, such as predictors of pharmacotherapy response, pharmacotherapy of hypochondriasis subtypes (e.g., poor insight), and management of refractory cases.

A first placebo-controlled pharmacotherapy trial for hypochondriasis (Fallon et al. 2008) indicated that among treatment completers, but not in the intent-to-treat sample, fluoxetine is superior to placebo, in terms of outcome after 12 weeks and at 24-week follow-up. At follow-up, among treatment completers, 54.2% (13/24) of fluoxetine patients and 23.8% (5/21) of placebo patients were classified as responders on the Clinical Global Impression Scale (i.e., "much or very much improved"). A second trial ($N=112$) comparing 16 weeks of cognitive-behavioral therapy (CBT), paroxetine, and placebo (Greeven et al. 2007) found that both CBT and paroxetine were effective in reducing hypochondriacal symptoms as well as in reducing symptoms of comorbid anxiety, depressive, and somatoform disorders. The treatment effect of both CBT and paroxetine was sustained at 18 months (Greeven et al. 2009b).

In practice, clinical consensus is that any SSRI may be used in the first-line pharmacotherapy of this disorder. These agents are also useful for many of the most frequent comorbid disorders seen in patients with hypochondriasis, including major depressive disorder and panic disorder. Clinical consensus is that the principles of pharmacotherapy are similar to those established for OCD: relatively higher dosages of SSRIs may be required (in the study by Fallon et al. [2008], the mean fluoxetine dosage was 51.4 mg/day); SSRI use should be attempted even when insight is poor; treatment should be continued for at least 12 weeks before a decision is made to switch medicine (e.g., to another SSRI or to clomipramine) or to augment (e.g., with a low dosage of an atypical antipsychotic); and maintenance pharmacotherapy should last at least 1 year (with very gradual decrease in dosage when attempting to discontinue pharmacotherapy). Given that many patients with hypochondriasis have heightened somatic awareness or comorbid panic attacks, it may be prudent to initiate SSRI pharmacotherapy with relatively low dosages (e.g., fluoxetine 5 mg/day).

Psychotherapy

On the basis of clinical observations of the lack of positive responses to early psychodynamic interventions, hypochondriasis and illness anxiety have historically been considered resistant to treatment. Emergence of the cognitive-behavioral model described previously paved the way for the application of a more effective treatment approach. This approach emphasizes the role of dysfunctional beliefs in maintaining illness anxiety and suggests that avoidance and escape behaviors prevent these beliefs from being disconfirmed. This functional analysis framework indicates that CBT, based on the idea that emotional disorders are maintained by faulty cognitions and maladaptive behaviors, should be effective.

Exposure and Response Prevention

People with IAD are often fearful and avoidant of stimuli associated with their feared illness. Accordingly, clinicians have used various forms of exposure therapy to reduce severe illness anxiety, including in vivo exposure (e.g., visiting cancer units, reading about feared medical conditions), interoceptive exposure (e.g., inducing body sensations that trigger illness fear), and imaginal exposure (e.g., imagining that one has developed the feared illness). Clinical experience suggests that imaginal exposure may be less helpful with patients who have poor insight. Exposure is conducted in treatment sessions and also as homework assignments. Response prevention (preventing repetitive behaviors such as seeking reassurance about one's health) is combined with exposure to encourage the patient to delay or refrain from behaviors that maintain illness fears (e.g., seeking reassurance). Uncontrolled trials (Visser and Bouman 1992) indicate that exposure and response prevention might effectively reduce hypochondriasis and illness anxiety. In a controlled study of patients with hypochondriasis (Visser and Bouman 2001), this treatment was found to be effective and superior to a wait-list control, with gains maintained at 7-month follow-up.

Behavioral Stress Management

Behavioral stress management emphasizes the role of stress in producing harmless but unpleasant bodily sensations and changes. It involves training the patient in various stress management exercises (e.g., relaxation training, time management, effective problem solving) as well as reintroducing regularly scheduled pleasurable activities that promote a healthy lifestyle, as a means of managing stress (Taylor and Asmundson 2004). These strategies may collectively reduce the subtle bodily sensations that can fuel illness worry, and they may increase a sense of well-being. Behavioral stress management was originally developed as a control condition in a randomized controlled study for hypochondriasis comparing CBT, behavioral stress management, and a wait-list control (Clark et al. 1998). However, it proved to be effective at reducing illness-related anxiety. When this form of therapy is used, it is important to ensure that patients understand that the rationale for using stress management is to reduce unpleasant but *harmless* bodily sensations, rather than to avoid sensations believed to be dangerous.

Cognitive–Behavioral Therapy

CBT for illness anxiety incorporates psychoeducation and exposure and response prevention along with cognitive restructuring and behavioral exercises. Cognitive restructuring is used to examine beliefs about the meaning of bodily sensations and changes. Behavioral exercises are used to further test the consequences of these beliefs and to examine the effects of behavior patterns that maintain and exacerbate illness anxiety. For example, patients may be asked to test the effects of seeking reassurance versus living with uncertainty, or to test the effects of directing attention *toward* versus *away* from bodily sensations. The goal is for patients to learn that they can manage and tolerate illness-related worry and distress without the need to seek reassurance. Patients often discover that their patterns of dysfunctional behaviors and their excessive attention to bodily sensations drive their fears and feelings of vulnerability.

Numerous uncontrolled trials (Martínez and Botella 2005) have suggested that CBT can effectively reduce hypochondriasis. Trials comparing CBT to wait-list control groups, other treatment conditions (e.g., progressive muscle relaxation), and medical treatment as usual (e.g., routine reassurance from providers) have also produced results suggesting the superiority of CBT (Barsky and Ahern 2004; Clark et al. 1998). CBT studies have most often used individual treatment protocols (see clinician manual by Abramowitz and Braddock 2010), but several researchers have reported that group treatment for hypochondriasis is also effective (Bouman 2002).

Treatment Preference

Given that CBT-based psychological treatments and SSRIs may be roughly equivalent, patients may be given the opportunity to choose their preferred method of treatment. One study found that 74% (17) of a sample of 23 treatment-seeking individuals with severe health anxiety selected CBT as their preferred treatment (with 48% [11] indicating they would accept only CBT, whereas only 4% [1] preferred medication) (Walker et al. 1999). The availability of choice might enhance treatment acceptability and adherence and, in cases where patients fail to benefit from one intervention, provides alternative courses of action.

Key Points

- Illness anxiety is a common presentation in medical settings, more so than in psychiatric settings.
- The symptoms of illness anxiety disorder (IAD) overlap in numerous ways with the symptoms of obsessive-compulsive disorder, anxiety disorders, and somatic symptom disorder.
- A cognitive-behavioral framework for conceptualizing, assessing, and treating IAD is recommended. Serotonin reuptake inhibitors may also be effective.
- Effective treatment techniques for IAD include psychoeducation, cognitive restructuring, exposure and response prevention, other assorted anxiety-management techniques, and pharmacotherapy.
- Patients often have difficulty accepting a psychological explanation for their somatic concerns; they commonly believe that a medical explanation is more adequate. Motivational interviewing may help engage patients in treatment.
- It is important to consider cultural factors when working with patients from diverse backgrounds.

References

Abramowitz JS, Braddock AE: Psychological Treatment of Health Anxiety and Hypochondriasis: A Biopsychosocial Approach. Boston, MA, Hogrefe, 2008

Abramowitz JS, Braddock AE: Hypochondriasis and Health Anxiety: Advances in Psychotherapy—Evidence Based Practice. Cambridge, MA, Hogrefe and Huber, 2010

Abramowitz JS, Deacon BJ: Obsessive-compulsive disorder: essential phenomenology and overlap with other anxiety disorders, in Concepts and Controversies in Obsessive-Compulsive Disorder. Edited by Abramowitz JS, Houts AC. New York, Springer, 2005, pp 119–149

American Psychiatric Association: Diagnostic and Statistical Manual of Mental Disorders, 3rd Edition. Washington, DC, American Psychiatric Association, 1980

American Psychiatric Association: Diagnostic and Statistical Manual of Mental Disorders, 3rd Edition Revised. Washington, DC, American Psychiatric Association, 1987

American Psychiatric Association: Diagnostic and Statistical Manual of Mental Disorders, 4th Edition. Washington, DC, American Psychiatric Association, 1994

American Psychiatric Association: Diagnostic and Statistical Manual of Mental Disorders, 5th Edition. Arlington, VA, American Psychiatric Association, 2013

Atmaca M, Sec S, Yildirim H, et al: A volumetric MRI analysis of hypochondriac patients. Bulletin of Clinical Psychopharmacology 20:293–299, 2010a

Atmaca M, Yildirim H, Sec S, et al: Pituitary volumes in hypochondriac patients. Prog Neuropsychopharmacol Biol Psychiatry 34(2):344–347, 2010b 20026150

Barsky AJ, Ahern DK: Cognitive behavior therapy for hypochondriasis: a randomized controlled trial. JAMA 291(12):1464–1470, 2004 15039413

Barsky AJ, Wyshak G, Klerman GL, et al: The prevalence of hypochondriasis in medical outpatients. Soc Psychiatry Psychiatr Epidemiol 25(2):89–94, 1990 2336583

Barsky AJ, Wyshak G, Klerman GL: Psychiatric comorbidity in DSM-III-R hypochondriasis. Arch Gen Psychiatry 49(2):101–108, 1992 1550462

Barsky AJ, Fama JM, Bailey ED, et al: A prospective 4- to 5-year study of DSM-III-R hypochondriasis. Arch Gen Psychiatry 55(8):737–744, 1998 9707385

Bebbington PE: Monosymptomatic hypochondriasis, abnormal illness behaviour and suicide. Br J Psychiatry 128:475–478, 1976 1276552

Bouman TK: A community-based psychoeducational group approach to hypochondriasis. Psychother Psychosom 71(6):326–332, 2002 12411767

Clark DM, Salkovskis PM, Hackmann A, et al: Two psychological treatments for hypochondriasis: a randomised controlled trial. Br J Psychiatry 173:218–225, 1998 9926097

Creed F, Barsky A: A systematic review of the epidemiology of somatisation disorder and hypochondriasis. J Psychosom Res 56(4):391–408, 2004 15094023

Fallon BA, Qureshi AI, Schneier FR, et al: An open trial of fluvoxamine for hypochondriasis. Psychosomatics 44(4):298–303, 2003 12832595

Fallon BA, Petkova E, Skritskaya N, et al: A double-masked, placebo-controlled study of fluoxetine for hypochondriasis. J Clin Psychopharmacol 28(6):638–645, 2008 19011432

Fallon BA, Harper KM, Landa A, et al: Personality disorders in hypochondriasis: prevalence and comparison with two anxiety disorders. Psychosomatics 53(6):566–574, 2012 22658329

Faravelli C, Salvatori S, Galassi F, et al: Epidemiology of somatoform disorders: a community survey in Florence. Soc Psychiatry Psychiatr Epidemiol 32(1):24–29, 1997 9029984

Fava GA, Kellner R, Zielezny M, et al: Hypochondriacal fears and beliefs in agoraphobia. J Affect Disord 14(3):239–244, 1988 2898492

Furer P, Walker JR, Chartier MJ, et al: Hypochondriacal concerns and somatization in panic disorder. Depress Anxiety 6(2):78–85, 1997 9451549

Goodman WK, Price LH, Rasmussen SA, et al: The Yale-Brown Obsessive Compulsive Scale, I: development, use, and reliability. Arch Gen Psychiatry 46(11):1006–1011, 1989 2684084

Greeven A, van Balkom AJ, Visser S, et al: Cognitive behavior therapy and paroxetine in the treatment of hypochondriasis: a randomized controlled trial. Am J Psychiatry 164(1):91–99, 2007 17202549

Greeven A, Spinhoven P, van Balkom AJ: Hypochondriasis Y-BOCS: a study of the psychometric properties of a clinician-administered semi-structured interview to assess hypochondriacal thoughts and behaviours. Clin Psychol Psychother 16(5):431–443, 2009a 19618479

Greeven A, van Balkom AJ, van der Leeden R, et al: Cognitive behavioral therapy versus paroxetine in the treatment of hypochondriasis: an 18-month naturalistic follow-up. J Behav Ther Exp Psychiatry 40(3):487–496, 2009b 19616195

Gureje O, Ustün TB, Simon GE: The syndrome of hypochondriasis: a cross-national study in primary care. Psychol Med 27(5):1001–1010, 1997 9300506

Kellner R: A symptom questionnaire. J Clin Psychiatry 48(7):268–274, 1987 3597327

Kellner R: Somatization: theories and research. J Nerv Ment Dis 178(3):150–160, 1990 2407806

Kellner R, Abbott P, Pathak D, et al: Hypochondriacal beliefs and attitudes in family practice and psychiatric patients. Int J Psychiatry Med 13(2):127–139, 1983–1984 6642874

Martinez MP, Botella C: An exploratory study of the efficacy of a cognitive-behavioral treatment for hypochondriasis using different measures of change. Psychother Res 15:392–408, 2005

Miller WR, Rollnick S: Motivational Interviewing: Preparing People to Change, 2nd Edition. New York, Guilford, 2002

Neziroglu F, McKay D, Yaryura-Tobias JA: Overlapping and distinctive features of hypochondriasis and obsessive-compulsive disorder. J Anxiety Disord 14(6):603–614, 2000 11918094

Noyes R Jr: Epidemiology of hypochondriasis, in Hypochondriasis: Modern Perspectives on an Ancient Malady. Edited by Starcevic V, Lipsitt D. New York. Oxford University Press, 2001, pp 127–154

Noyes R Jr, Kathol RG, Fisher MM, et al: The validity of DSM-III-R hypochondriasis. Arch Gen Psychiatry 50(12):961–970, 1993 8250682

Noyes R Jr, Stuart S, Langbehn DR, et al: Childhood antecedents of hypochondriasis. Psychosomatics 43(4):282–289, 2002 12189253

Noyes R Jr, Carney CP, Hillis SL, et al: Prevalence and correlates of illness worry in the general population. Psychosomatics 46(6):529–539, 2005 16288132

Olatunji BO, Wolitzky-Taylor KB: Anxiety sensitivity and the anxiety disorders: a meta-analytic review and synthesis. Psychol Bull 135(6):974–999, 2009 19883144

Pilowsky I, Katsikitis M: A classification of illness behaviour in pain clinic patients. Pain 57(1):91–94, 1994 8065802

Rief W, Hessel A, Braehler E: Somatization symptoms and hypochondriacal features in the general population. Psychosom Med 63(4):595–602, 2001 11485113

Salkovskis PM, Rimes KA, Warwick HMC, et al: The Health Anxiety Inventory: development and validation of scales for the measurement of health anxiety and hypochondriasis. Psychol Med 32(5):843–853, 2002 12171378

Schmidt AJM, van Roosmalen R, van der Beek JM, et al: Hypochondriasis in ENT practice. Clin Otolaryngol Allied Sci 18(6):508–511, 1993 8877231

Starcevic V, Fallon S, Uhlenhuth EH, et al: Generalized anxiety disorder, worries about illness, and hypochondriacal fears and beliefs. Psychother Psychosom 61(1–2):93–99, 1994 8121980

Stein MB, Jang KL, Livesley WJ: Heritability of anxiety sensitivity: a twin study. Am J Psychiatry 156(2):246–251, 1999 9989561

Sue DW, Sue D: Counseling the Culturally Different: Theory and Practice. New York, Wiley, 1990

Taylor S, Asmundson GJ: Treating Health Anxiety: A Cognitive-Behavioral Approach. New York, Guilford, 2004

Taylor S, Thordarson DS, Jang KL, et al: Genetic and environmental origins of health anxiety: a twin study. World Psychiatry 5(1):47–50, 2006 16757996

Visser S, Bouman TK: Cognitive-behavioural approaches in the treatment of hypochondriasis: six single case cross-over studies. Behav Res Ther 30(3):301–306, 1992 1586367

Visser S, Bouman TK: The treatment of hypochondriasis: exposure plus response prevention vs cognitive therapy. Behav Res Ther 39(4):423–442, 2001 11280341

Walker J, Vincent N, Furer P, et al: Treatment preference in hypochondriasis. J Behav Ther Exp Psychiatry 30(4):251–258, 1999 10759322

Recommended Readings

Abramowitz JS, Braddock AE: Psychological Treatment of Health Anxiety and Hypochondriasis: A Biopsychosocial Approach. Boston, MA, Hogrefe, 2008

Barsky AJ, Ahern DK: Cognitive behavior therapy for hypochondriasis: a randomized controlled trial. JAMA 291(12):1464–1470, 2004

Deacon B, Abramowitz JS: Is hypochondriasis related to obsessive-compulsive disorder, panic disorder, or both? An empirical evaluation. J Cogn Psychother 22(2):115–127, 2008

Furer P, Walker JR, Stein MB: Treating Health Anxiety and Fear of Death: A Practitioner's Guide. New York, Springer, 2007

Taylor S, Asmundson GJ: Treating Health Anxiety: A Cognitive-Behavioral Approach. New York, Guilford, 2004

CHAPTER 10

Obsessive–Compulsive Personality Disorder

Naomi A. Fineberg, M.B.B.S., M.A., M.R.C.Psych.
Sukhwinder Kaur, M.B.B.S., M.R.C.Psych.
Sangeetha Kolli, M.B.B.S., M.R.C.Psych.
Davis Mpavaenda, Dip.C.B.T., B.A.B.C.P. Accred.,
    Masters Health Law
Samar Reghunandanan, M.B.B.S., M.D., M.R.C.Psych.

Obsessive-compulsive personality disorder (OCPD), as defined by DSM-5 (American Psychiatric Association 2013), is a disorder characterized by a preoccupation with orderliness, perfectionism, and mental and interpersonal control, at the expense of flexibility, openness, and efficiency. Typically appearing in late childhood or adolescence and continuing in a relatively stable form through adulthood, OCPD is responsible for considerable personal and social disruption (Skodol et al. 2005).

OCPD is a relatively poorly researched and underrecognized disorder. Notably, there are few studies that have investigated "pure" OCPD in the absence of other major psychiatric comorbidity. This may be attributed, at least in part, to its current classification within the personality disorder grouping, as current research in that field has tended to focus on personality disorders with high overt risks, such as borderline personality disorder. In this chapter we outline what is known about OCPD, including symptomatology, developmental considerations, epidemiology, comorbidity, course, impairment, suicidality, etiology, and treatment response. We include two vignettes to demonstrate the disorder's psychopathology and its impact.

Historically, OCPD has been conceptualized as bearing a close relationship with obsessive-compulsive disorder (OCD). Indeed, the validity of separating a "personality trait" from a "mental state" disorder remains controversial. In light of the recent establishment of an obsessive-compulsive and related disorder (OCRD) category in DSM-5, this chapter also touches on the relationship between OCPD, OCD, and other disorders currently thought to bear a close relationship with OCD, including other disorders in the DSM-5 OCRD chapter. In addition, we discuss the potential clinical utility of conceptualizing OCPD as an OCRD.

Diagnostic Criteria and Symptomatology

DSM conceptualizes personality disorders as qualitatively distinct clinical syndromes characterized by the failure to develop an adaptive self-concept and interpersonal relations. They represent an enduring pattern of inner experience and behavior that deviate markedly from the expectations of the individual's culture. They are also pervasive and inflexible, have an onset in adolescence or early adulthood, tend to be stable over time, and lead to clinically significant distress or impairment in functioning. Within this framework, OCPD is described as an excessively rigid self-concept, to the extent that the ability to respond adaptively to environmental contingencies, such as unexpected change in routines or the need to prioritize timeliness over perfection, is impaired.

In the early DSM editions (DSM-I, DSM-II, and DSM-III), OCPD was defined as a "persistence of an adolescent pattern of behavior" or a "regression from more mature functioning as a result of stress" (American Psychiatric Association 1952, 1968, 1980). Diagnostic traits included "affective constriction" and difficulty expressing warm and tender emotions, reminiscent of autistic disorders. However, in the transition from DSM-III to DSM-III-R (American Psychiatric Association 1987), affective constriction was deleted and other criteria, including excessive preoccupation with details and rules, overconscientiousness, scrupulousness, inflexibility about matters of morality, ethics, or values, lack of generosity, and inability to discard worthless objects, were amplified.

In DSM-III, DSM-III-R, DSM-IV, and DSM-IV-TR (American Psychiatric Association 1994, 2000), personality disorders were placed on a separate axis of classification (Axis II). DSM-IV OCPD was classified alongside avoidant personality disorder and dependent personality disorder under the "anxious-fearful" (Cluster C) category of personality disorder, on the basis that fear and anxiety about interpersonal situations represented a common characteristic of the three disorders. The criteria for diagnosing OCPD in DSM-5 have not changed from those in DSM-IV. However, in DSM-5, the multiaxial approach to personality disorder has been abandoned. For a DSM-5 diagnosis, the general criteria for a personality disorder must be met, including clinically significant distress or impairment in social, occupational, or other areas of functioning as a result of the personality disorder. Four or more of the eight listed items are also required (see Box 10–1).

BOX 10–1. Diagnostic Criteria for Obsessive-Compulsive Personality Disorder

---

A pervasive pattern of preoccupation with orderliness, perfectionism, and mental and interpersonal control, at the expense of flexibility, openness, and efficiency, beginning by early adulthood and present in a variety of contexts, as indicated by four (or more) of the following:

1. Is preoccupied with details, rules, lists, order, organization, or schedules to the extent that the major point of the activity is lost.
2. Shows perfectionism that interferes with task completion (e.g., is unable to complete a project because his or her own overly strict standards are not met).
3. Is excessively devoted to work and productivity to the exclusion of leisure activities and friendships (not accounted for by obvious economic necessity).
4. Is overconscientious, scrupulous, and inflexible about matters of morality, ethics, or values (not accounted for by cultural or religious identification).
5. Is unable to discard worn-out or worthless objects even when they have no sentimental value.
6. Is reluctant to delegate tasks or to work with others unless they submit to exactly his or her way of doing things.
7. Adopts a miserly spending style toward both self and others; money is viewed as something to be hoarded for future catastrophes.
8. Shows rigidity and stubbornness.

Reprinted from American Psychiatric Association: *Diagnostic and Statistical Manual of Mental Disorders,* 5th Edition. Arlington, VA, American Psychiatric Association. Copyright 2013, American Psychiatric Association. Used with permission.

Weaknesses in the conceptualization and assessment of the DSM-IV OCPD construct have been recognized, including questionable psychometric strength and diagnostic efficiency (sensitivity, specificity, predictive power). Studies have also called into question the utility of some of the criteria. For example, in the large multisite Comprehensive Longitudinal Personality Study, four of the DSM-IV OCPD criteria (preoccupation with details, perfectionism, reluctance to delegate, rigidity and stubbornness) were found to be useful for making the diagnosis, whereas two criteria (miserly spending style and excessive devotion to work and productivity) performed so poorly that their removal was recommended (Grilo et al. 2001). Analysis of the course and stability of DSM-IV personality disorders in the Comprehensive Longitudinal Personality Study similarly found that perfectionism, reluctance to delegate, and rigidity were the most prevalent and stable OCPD criteria over a 2-year follow-up period (McGlashan et al. 2005).

Nevertheless, in DSM-5, all eight DSM-IV criteria are retained (in fact, no changes were made to the diagnostic criteria of any of the personality disorders in DSM-5). In addition, in recognition of ongoing uncertainties about the diagnostic criteria and the need for further research on personality disorders, an alternative approach to diagnosis of the personality disorders was developed, which is included in DSM-5's Section III. The alternative conceptualizations in Section III do not constitute official diagnostic criteria; rather, they are provided to stimulate further research on the definition of and diagnostic criteria for personality disorders. The alternative OCPD diagnosis that is included in Section III hinges on the presence of general impairment in personality functioning (Criterion A) and a set of specific pathological personality traits (Criterion B). The model emphasizes the degree of impairment in personality functioning; at least a moderate level of impairment is required for the diagnosis. This alternative approach also allows personality functioning and personality traits to be assessed, whether or not the individual fulfills criteria for a personality disorder (American Psychiatric Association 2013).

Categorical Versus Dimensional Models of OCPD

The diagnostic approach used in DSM-IV and DSM-5 follows a categorical perspective (although the alternative conceptualization in DSM-5's Section III includes an assessment of dimensional traits). However, the existing categorical model of personality disorder has been criticized because it has the capacity to produce considerable intragroup variability in terms of psychopathology. The categorical model also assumes that personality disorders are unidimensional, whereas the empirical literature and clinical opinion suggest that a multifactorial model may be a more appropriate way to understand them (Grilo 2004). From a dimensional perspective, studies of patients with OCPD with and without mental state disorder comorbidity support the following two models for the disorder: One model incorporates two factors, "perfectionism" (including constructs such as preoccupation with details, perfectionism, excessive devotion to work and productivity) and "rigidity" (including rigidity, reluctance to delegate, hypermorality), which reflect underlying intrapersonal and interpersonal control, respectively (Ansell et al. 2008). The second model, a three-factor model, comprises "rigidity," "perfectionism," and "miserliness" (miserly spending styles, inability to discard) (Grilo 2004).

Maladaptive personality traits can be identified in the general population in those without a diagnosis of personality disorder. Indeed, most of the OCPD criteria could be considered maladaptive variants of general personality functioning. Another dimensional model of personality disorder proposes a continuous spectrum of maladaptive variants of personality traits that merge imperceptibly into normality and into one another. Several such models—for example, the Five Factor Model (Costa and McCrae 1992) and the DSM-5 alternative personality disorder model in Section III—have been proposed to cover disordered personality function in a dimensional way. Their integration, clinical utility, and relationship with the DSM and ICD personality disorder diagnostic categories are under active investigation (American Psychiatric Association 2013).

Case Example: Melinda

Melinda is an 18-year-old female college student of Greek ethnicity who was referred by her mother for a consultation. Her mother reports that her daughter has always been an excellent student—well-organized, conscientious, and dedicated to doing her best. Since starting college, however, she has been excessively focused on a number of concerns and as a consequence has been having difficulty sleeping. She also reports that Melinda spends long periods of time working in her room instead of with friends. Melinda reports a variety of fears, including not performing well enough in college, not being a good enough friend, and not being a loyal daughter. For example, she believes that her grades should be better and that her report cards should be perfect, because she wishes to bring success to the family. When asked about her grades, Melinda reveals that she is receiving As in all of her classes. She is quick to point out her errors on previous examinations; she is able to recall a surprising number of questions she answered incorrectly on a test taken several weeks ago. Melinda says that she has difficulty prioritizing important issues over minor ones, is easily distracted by details and rules, and feels a strong urge to ensure that she has completed any task perfectly. She checks over her work excessively and takes several hours longer than she should to complete assignments. She has started to miss deadlines because it takes so long to get her work exactly right. She would like to socialize but cannot find the time. She does not wish others to help her because she believes she has a duty to do the work herself and does not trust others to do it properly. Doubts enter her mind frequently, such as "Am I smart enough?" She responds by attempting to work harder.

Epidemiology

Individual traits of OCPD, which do not meet the diagnostic threshold for the disorder, are commonly found in the general population (Nestadt et al. 1991). These traits can be advantageous, especially in situations that reward high performance. In contrast, syndromal OCPD is generally disadvantageous. Depending on the definition of OCPD that is used, estimated point prevalence rates vary from 1% or 2% (Nestadt et al. 1991; Torgersen et al. 2001) to around 8% (B.F. Grant et al. 2004; J.E. Grant et al. 2012) in large community samples. Indeed, OCPD is thought by some authors to have the highest prevalence of all personality disorders in the general population (B.F. Grant et al. 2004), including among older adults (Schuster et al. 2013). OCPD is especially common in psychiatric outpatient groups, affecting up to approximately one-quarter of individuals in some studies. For example, the point prevalence of OCPD in outpatients with OCD (22.9%) and panic disorder (17.1%) significantly exceeded that in a comparison sample of individuals with no history of mental disorder (3.0%) (Albert et al. 2004). OCPD is equally common in males and females, both in community-based (B.F. Grant et al. 2004; J.E. Grant et al. 2012; Torgersen et al. 2001) and clinical (Albert et al. 2004) samples.

Comorbidity

The coexistence of two or more illnesses, at a rate exceeding that expected from the population frequency, indicates the possibility of a shared etiology (environmental and/or genetic; discussed later). OCPD has high comorbidity with many psychiatric disorders, particularly those characterized by compulsive behavior, including OCD (25%–32% of patients with OCD have OCPD; Coles et al. 2008; Pinto et al. 2006), body dysmorphic disorder (BDD; 14%–28% of patients with BDD have OCPD; Phillips and McElroy 2000), and eating disorder (20%–61% of patients with an eating disorder have OCPD; Karwautz et al. 2003). In a large longitudinal study of OCD, 25% of case subjects were diagnosed with comorbid DSM-IV OCPD compared with 15% who were diagnosed with avoidant personality disorder (Pinto et al. 2006). The presence of comorbid OCPD may be associated with a different presentation of the mental state disorder; in the study by Coles et al. (2008), OCD patients with OCPD reported an earlier onset of OCD symptoms, more symmetry and hoarding obsessions, and more cleaning, ordering, repeating, and hoarding compulsions. They were also more globally impaired compared to the noncomorbid group. One interpretation is that comorbid OCPD represents a marker of increased OCD severity.

OCPD is the most frequent personality disorder in patients with anorexia nervosa—restricting type, binge-eating disorder (Sansone et al. 2005), and bipolar disorder (Rossi et al. 2001), and it occurs in approximately one-third of patients with major depressive disorder (Rossi et al. 2001) and 17% of patients with panic disorder (Albert et al. 2004). These disorders also have high comorbidity with OCD.

Conversely, the most common lifetime comorbid disorders affecting individuals with OCPD include illnesses for which considerable comorbidity with OCD has been reported. For example, it is not uncommon for OCPD to occur with anxiety, depression, anorexia nervosa, hypochondriasis, and Parkinson's disease, but further research is necessary to understand the implications of these links (Starcevic and Brakoulias 2014). Thus, although OCPD is not uniquely or preferentially associated with OCD and OCRDs, its comorbidity profile is similar to theirs. In contrast, data on comorbidity between OCPD and other personality disorders is inconsistent. For example, in one study, only comorbidity with paranoid personality disorder occurred at a rate that was significantly higher than expected (Hummelen et al. 2008). On the other hand, Costa et al. (2005) calculated average comorbidity scores for each of the Axis II disorders from three published studies and noted a considerable overlap between OCPD and other Cluster C disorders (avoidant [43%], dependent [28%]), and also with paranoid (30%), passive-aggressive (27%), and schizoid (25%) personality disorder.

Course and Prognosis

By definition, OCPD has an onset relatively early in life and follows a chronic course, although the severity of symptoms may vary over time. However, the lack of stability of the signs and symptoms of OCPD, as demonstrated in some follow-up studies, raises questions as to whether it should be classified as a personality disorder. For example, in a follow-up study of adolescents with a personality disorder, only 32% of those initially diagnosed with OCPD still had features that met the diagnostic criteria 2 years later (Bernstein et al. 1993), suggesting that the disorder may appear in adolescence but not necessarily progress into adulthood as generally thought. In the Collaborative Longitudinal Personality Study, only about half of the adults with OCPD at baseline continued to have the diagnosis after 2 years (Grilo et al. 2004). Nonetheless, in this study, personality disorders, including OCPD, were more stable than major depressive disorder. They also constituted a significant and long-term health problem with respect to associated functional impairment (Skodol et al. 2005). In the Collaborative Longitudinal Personality Study, the most stable OCPD criteria (perfectionism, reluctance to delegate, and rigidity) were trait-like or attitudinal in nature, whereas the most unstable (miserliness) were considered symptomatic behaviors. Consequently, the authors proposed a "hybrid" model for OCPD, consisting of stable personality traits that are linked to less stable, or intermittently expressed, discrete (either people adopt them or they do not) dysfunctional behaviors. It is thought that these dysfunctional behaviors are used to compensate for the pathological traits and that they fluctuate because they are susceptible to life events and stress (McGlashan et al. 2005).

Psychosocial Impairment and Suicidality

Studies of OCPD have demonstrated long-standing disability at 1- and 2-year follow-up, sometimes to an extent exceeding that found in major mental disorders such as OCD (Grilo et al. 2004; Skodol et al. 2005). Recent studies have shown high levels of treatment utilization by individuals with OCPD, even after controlling for comorbid psychiatric disorders, with high rates of primary healthcare use (Sansone et al. 2003). Indeed, individuals with OCPD are estimated to be three times more likely to receive psychotherapy than patients with major depressive disorder (Bender et al. 2006).

The presence of comorbid OCPD has negative prognostic significance for the course of anxiety disorders (Ansell et al. 2011) and is associated with poorer treatment outcomes in OCD (Pinto et al. 2011) as well as accelerated relapse after remission in OCD (Eisen et al. 2013) and major depressive disorder (Grilo et al. 2010). OCPD also appears to increase the risk for nonfatal suicidal behavior, independent of the risk conferred by depression. In a large cross-sectional study, depressed patients with comorbid OCPD reported significantly increased current and lifetime suicidal ideation and an increased frequency of suicide attempts, which often consisted of multiple attempts, compared with patients with depression alone, patients without depression, and patients with a personality disorder (Diaconu and Turecki 2009).

Developmental Considerations

Personality disorders can be traced to childhood emotional and behavioral disturbances, suggesting that these problems have both general and specific relationships to adolescent personality functioning. In a large community-based sample of adolescents (Bernstein et al. 1993), the prevalence of personality disorders peaked at age 12 in boys and at age 13 in girls and declined thereafter. OCPD was the most prevalent "moderate" personality disorder, based on both moderate and severe diagnostic thresholds. All moderate personality disorders were associated with significantly greater odds for at least

5 of 12 DSM-III-R diagnostic validators. Longitudinal follow-up revealed that although most personality disorders did not persist over a 2-year period, subjects with disorders identified earlier remained at elevated risk for receiving a diagnosis again at follow-up, suggesting that an early onset of OCPD traits predicts continuation into adulthood.

Gender Issues and Cultural Aspects

OCPD appears to be equally common in males and females, both in community-based (B.F. Grant et al. 2004; J.E. Grant et al. 2012) and in clinical (Albert et al. 2004) samples. Little is known about the cross-national population prevalence or correlates of personality disorders. A review of DSM-IV personality disorders in the WHO World Mental Health Surveys showed a consistent pattern of between-country differences for all three personality disorder clusters, with the lowest prevalence estimates in Nigeria and Western Europe for Cluster C (0.9%–1.2%) compared with other regions (Huang et al. 2009). In a U.S. study, OCPD was significantly less common in those of Asian and Hispanic ethnicity (Grant et al. 2012). In general, a personality disorder diagnosis is more common among those who are single and those with lower educational achievement (Torgersen et al. 2001). In contrast, studies have shown OCPD to be significantly more common among employed individuals with at least a high school education (Grant et al. 2012; Nestadt et al. 1991).

Assessment and Differential Diagnosis

Assessment

OCPD tends to be overlooked in clinical settings. Better awareness of the diagnosis could be expected to lead to improved treatment outcomes. Studies have criticized the low level of agreement between the various methods of personality disorder assessment. A recent large study compared two clinical interviews for DSM-IV personality disorder: the Personality Disorder Schedule of the Standardized Psychiatric Examination (Romanoski et al. 1988) and the International Personality Disorder Examination (Loranger et al. 1994). Although there was low concordance in the raw measurement of the individual personality disorder criteria between the two clinical methods, and OCPD ranked among those disorders with the lowest concordance, suggesting the disorder is comparatively difficult to assess reliably, the authors concluded that DSM-IV personality disorders could be measured with a moderate degree of confidence regardless of the clinical approach used (Nestadt et al. 2012). Other, older structured interviews for diagnosis (Spitzer et al. 1987; Pfohl et al. 1982), such as the Structured Clinical Interview for DSM-IV Axis

II Personality Disorders and Structured Interview for DSM-III Personality Disorders, have been shown to possess reasonably good interrater reliability for DSM-IV OCPD ($\kappa > 0.70$), although the test-retest reliability over even short-term intervals is lower (0.50 for the former, and 0.66 for the latter) (Clark and Harrison 2001).

There are no established rating instruments for assessing the severity of OCPD. Some studies have computed the number of positively scored OCPD criteria as a proxy measure of severity (Ansseau 1996; Pinto et al. 2006). In a treatment study by Ansseau (1996), each of the eight DSM-IV criteria was rated for severity on a five-point scale. The scale was sensitive enough to discriminate active from inactive treatment over just 12 weeks. These findings support the likely utility of this scale. The Compulsive Personality Assessment Scale (Fineberg et al. 2007) was devised to simulate this model (see Table 10–1) and is easily applied in the clinical setting. It uses eight simple screening questions to evaluate each DSM-5 criterion and produces a composite score. Its reliability, discriminant validity (to differentiate DSM-IV and DSM-5 OCPD from personality functioning in the normal population), and sensitivity to change remain to be confirmed.

There are also a few self-report questionnaires that have not been systematically validated—such as the self-rated Obsessive-Compulsive Personality Inventory (Stein et al. 1992). Other self-rated scales have been devised to measure specific attitudes or beliefs that resemble OCPD traits such as perfectionism, doubts about actions, and concern over mistakes—for example, the Multidimensional Perfectionism Scale (Frost et al. 1994). These scales also have not been validated against DSM-IV or DSM-5 OCPD, but they have shown some evidence of sensitivity to change in treatment studies.

Differential Diagnosis

Obsessive–Compulsive Disorder

Differentiating OCPD from OCD may be a major clinical challenge. OCPD and OCD overlap in the expression of inflexible and stereotyped patterns of thinking and behavior, including, in some cases, preoccupation with orderliness, perfectionism, and scrupulosity as well as behavioral or cognitive rigidity (Nelson et al. 2006; Rhéaume et al. 1995). Moreover, aspects of self-directed perfectionism that characterize OCPD, such as believing a perfect solution is commendable, discomfort if things are sensed to have been done incompletely, and doubting that one's actions were performed correctly, have also been proposed as enduring features of some forms of OCD (Rhéaume et al. 1995). The overlap between the phenomenology of OCPD and OCD is further highlighted by the work of Eisen et al. (2006). Three OCPD criteria—preoccupation with details, perfectionism, and hoarding—were found to oc-

TABLE 10–1. Compulsive Personality Assessment Scale

Items refer to a stable pattern of enduring traits dating back to adolescence or early adulthood. Use the questions listed as part of a semistructured interview.

For each item, circle the appropriate score: 0=absent; 1=mild; 2=moderate; 3=severe; 4=very severe.

Item	Rating				
1. Preoccupation with details Are you preoccupied with details, rules, lists, order, organization, or schedules to the extent that the major aim of the activity is lost?	0	1	2	3	4
2. Perfectionism Would you describe yourself as a perfectionist who struggles with completing the task at hand?	0	1	2	3	4
3. Workaholism Are you excessively devoted to work to the exclusion of leisure activities and friendships?	0	1	2	3	4
4. Overconscientiousness Would you describe yourself as overconscientious and inflexible about matters of morality, ethics, or values?	0	1	2	3	4
5. Hoarding Are you unable to discard worn-out or worthless objects even when they have no sentimental value?	0	1	2	3	4

TABLE 10–1. Compulsive Personality Assessment Scale *(continued)*

Item		Rating			
6. Need for control Are you reluctant to delegate tasks or to work with others unless they submit to exactly your way of doing things?	0	1	2	3	4
7. Miserliness Do you see money as something to be hoarded for future catastrophes?	0	1	2	3	4
8. Rigidity Do you think you are rigid or stubborn?	0	1	2	3	4
Total:					

Source. Adapted from Fineberg NA, Sharma P, Sivakumaran T, et al.: "Does Obsessive-Compulsive Personality Disorder Belong Within the Obsessive-Compulsive Spectrum?" *CNS Spectrums* 12(6):467–482, 2007. Copyright 2007, Cambridge University Press. Used with permission.

cur significantly more frequently in OCPD subjects with comorbid OCD than in subjects without OCD, suggesting that these OCPD traits may be related to OCD. In addition, compulsive-type behaviors (i.e., intentional, repetitive, time consuming, difficult to resist or control, not pleasurable, and associated with distress or disability) such as checking may occur in OCPD. These behaviors may be differentiated from OCD by their being considered desirable and not resisted or unwanted. However, the clinician may also bear in mind that in the DSM-IV field trials, a majority of OCD patients reported being unsure whether their obsessive-compulsive symptoms really were unreasonable (Foa et al. 1995), and in DSM-5, OCD has an insight specifier that includes "delusional beliefs/absent insight" as well as poor insight.

Table 10–2 compares OCPD with OCD in terms of some of these clinical features. Unlike patients with OCD, patients with OCPD do not describe obsessions and compulsions, as strictly defined in DSM-IV or DSM-5. For example, whereas in OCD obsessions are intrusive, distressing, and often ego-dystonic—that is, recognized as alien to the individual's values and sense of self—in OCPD the problematic traits and symptomatic behaviors are considered ego-syntonic, in that they are viewed as correct or desirable (Fineberg et al. 2007). In addition, OCPD is not usually associated with morally repugnant urges. Thus, to differentiate OCPD from OCD, it can be helpful to determine the extent to which the patient approves of or values the compulsive-type behavior.

The symptom of incompleteness has particular relevance to both OCD and OCPD. Summerfeldt (2004) proposed the existence of two core dimensions in OCD, "incompleteness" and "harm avoidance," each of which has unique affective, cognitive, and motivational characteristics. Incompleteness, representing an inner sense of imperfection or the uncomfortable subjective state that one's actions or experiences are not "just right," was proposed as a temperament-like motivational variable within OCD that results in symmetry, counting, repeating, and slowness compulsions. However, a sense of incompleteness also characterizes OCPD, and it contributes to key diagnostic traits such as pathological perfectionism and indecisiveness. High incompleteness scores in patients with OCD are predictive of meeting criteria for comorbid OCPD (Summerfeldt 2004). Thus, symptoms of OCD that are motivated by feelings of incompleteness may be linked to the presence of OCPD (as opposed to those motivated by harm avoidance).

Hoarding Disorder

Hoarding behavior is another potential source of overlap between OCPD, OCD, and OCRDs and has been found to correlate with perfectionism (Pertusa et al. 2010). The nosological status of hoarding and its relationship with OCPD

TABLE 10–2. A comparison of obsessive-compulsive personality disorder (OCPD) and obsessive–compulsive disorder (OCD) using nosological factors

Factor	OCPD	OCD
Presence of obsessions or compulsions	+	+++
	Tend to be experienced as integral and compatible with personal values (e.g., checking for perfection, completeness, fairness, symmetry)	Tend to be experienced as alien and incompatible with personal values (e.g., intrusive taboo thoughts, contamination fears)
Gender	Male and female approximately equal	Male and female approximately equal
Early age at onset	+++	+++
Chronic course	++	++
Functional impairment	++	+++
Highly comorbid with depression	+++	+++
Highly comorbid with eating disorder	+++	+++
Highly comorbid with obsessive-compulsive spectrum disorder	+++	+++
Highly comorbid with anxiety disorder	+++	+++
Both disorders cluster in the same families	+++	+++

TABLE 10–2. A comparison of obsessive-compulsive personality disorder (OCPD) and obsessive-compulsive disorder (OCD) using nosological factors *(continued)*

Factor	OCPD	OCD
Neurocognitive inflexibility (impaired performance on extra-dimensional set-shift task)	++	+++
Response to serotonin reuptake inhibitor	+	+++
Response to cognitive-behavioral therapy	+	+++

Note. + = limited evidence or small effect size; ++ = strong evidence or large effect size; +++ = strong evidence and large effect size.

remain complex and controversial. In DSM-5, it is included as a diagnostic item for OCPD and also as a separate disorder within the OCRD grouping. Clinicians should look for the presence of OCPD in patients presenting with problematic hoarding. The diagnosis of hoarding disorder is appropriate if hoarding behavior represents the predominant source of distress or disability and meets all diagnostic criteria for hoarding disorder.

Autism Spectrum Disorder

Autism spectrum disorder is an early-onset neurodevelopmental disorder that also shares overlapping phenomenology with OCPD, including rigid and inflexible thinking patterns, preoccupation with details, a desire for completeness, and a narrow/restricted repertoire of interests. However, autism spectrum disorder is additionally characterized by social communication problems and repetitive, stereotyped behaviors, which differentiate this disorder from OCPD.

Case Example: Alan

Alan is a 45-year-old accountant of Indian ethnicity. His wife has brought him for a consultation because he is depressed. He is not sleeping or eating, has lost 11 pounds, and is anxious all the time about losing his job. He reports he has recently been struggling at work, since the firm was taken over by new employers who are expecting him to complete more auditing work in less time, and he is highly anxious about making mistakes. He says that he has always been extremely conscientious and notes difficulties delegating his work as well as a tendency to get easily distracted by details. He cites as an example the fact that he finds small discrepancies, such as pennies missing at audit, highly distracting and spends longer than he should searching for the source of insignificant errors. As a result he is slower than most of his colleagues, but he says that the quality of his work is higher than that of many of his colleagues and that previously his meticulousness was not considered a problem. He is angry and critical of his new employers for having a different attitude. He does not see a good reason to change the way he works. He admits to long-standing workaholic tendencies, has almost no social life apart from his relationship with his wife, and holds judgmental attitudes toward others. His wife describes him as obstinate, rigid, and stubborn. During the consultation, he has poor eye contact. He is tearful, and his mood appears irritable and sad. He describes distressing pessimistic ruminations and expresses the wish to die, because he cannot see a way out of his problems.

Etiology and Pathophysiology

Environmental Risk Factors

Few studies have examined the contribution of environmental factors to the development of OCPD. Compared to healthy control subjects and to other psychiatric outpatients, patients with OCPD report significantly lower levels of parental care and significantly higher levels of overprotection (Nordahl and Stiles 1997). Similar findings have been reported for OCD.

Genetic Factors

Twin studies suggest that OCPD has a high degree of heritability and that a common genetic mechanism may underpin obsessive-compulsive symptoms and traits (Taylor et al. 2011). An increased frequency of OCPD traits is found in relatives of patients with OCD. In one family study (Calvo et al. 2009), a higher incidence of DSM-IV OCPD was found in the parents of pediatric OCD probands compared with the parents of healthy control children, even after parents with OCD were excluded. Similarly, another family study (Samuels et al. 2000) found an increased prevalence of OCPD in the first-degree relatives of OCD-affected probands. In a further study, OCPD was the only personality disorder to co-occur significantly more often in the relatives of OCD probands than in relatives of control subjects after adjustment for the occurrence of OCD in the relatives (Bienvenu et al. 2012). Familial aggregation of OCPD traits has also been reported in anorexia nervosa (Lilenfeld et al. 1998), another disorder characterized by compulsive behavior. Taken together, these data suggest that a specific shared heritability exists across OCPD and other compulsive disorders and that they may be related disorders. In contrast, statistical modeling of genetic and familial factors has found only limited shared genetic (11%) and environmental (15%) variance between OCPD and the other Cluster C personality disorders (Reichborn-Kjennerud et al. 2007), suggesting OCPD may be etiologically distinct from avoidant and dependent personality disorder.

Neuropsychological Factors

Brain imaging studies of OCPD have not so far been performed. It is hypothesized that OCPD could be underpinned by specific neurocognitive changes previously identified in some other OCRDs, including hyperactive error responses, a tendency to focus attention on parts of stimuli rather than the whole, and impaired attentional set-shifting (Fineberg et al. 2007), although only the last domain has been subject to controlled investigation. A small controlled study suggested that patients with OCD and comorbid OCPD demonstrated even greater cognitive inflexibility on the extra-dimensional set-shift paradigm (Cambridge Neuropsychological Test Automated Battery [CANTAB]; www.camcog.com)—which is thought to be mediated by prefrontal cortex and associated subcortical brain circuitry—than OCD patients without comorbid OCPD (Fineberg et al. 2007). This abnormality also exists in OCD probands and their unaffected first-degree relatives as well as in patients with schizo-OCD, BDD, and anorexia nervosa and may represent a neurocognitive endophenotype or "vulnerability factor" for compulsive disorders sharing neurocircuitry with OCD (reviewed in Fineberg et al. 2014).

Treatment

General Approaches to Treatment

OCPD is common in the clinical setting and frequently co-occurs with mood disorders, anxiety disorders, and OCRDs. Therefore, clinicians should routinely ask about OCPD traits and symptoms in patients who present with these disorders, because the diagnosis may substantially impact treatment outcome and prognosis. For example, in a 5-year follow-up study of treatment outcomes in patients with OCD, the presence of comorbid OCPD doubled the risk of relapse (Eisen et al. 2013).

The general criteria for a personality disorder require the presence of clinically significant distress or impairment in social, occupational, or other areas of functioning. Although there are situations in which extreme orderliness, perfectionism, and conscientiousness may be useful (see case studies), OCPD traits are generally not adaptive in interpersonal situations. In determining the threshold for diagnosis, the clinician needs to take cultural and social factors into account. It is also important to acknowledge that the "label" of a personality disorder may have a potentially stigmatizing effect and may deter the clinician from making the diagnosis so as not to distress the patient. It is therefore advisable to explain to the patient, with sensitivity and care, the relevance of the diagnosis and its clinical implications.

In a minority of cases, the patient will present for help with the symptoms of OCPD—for example, if he or she is behaving in an excessively rigid way and having relationship problems with family members or colleagues. In most cases, however, the patient will present with a comorbid disorder as the principal clinical problem, such as a depressive disorder, anxiety disorder, eating disorder, or OCD; in these circumstances, the OCPD could easily be overlooked. Moreover, the presence of OCPD may significantly interfere with the outcome of treatment for the mental state disorder. For example, in patients with OCD, underlying OCPD has been reported to predict a poorer outcome to treatments such as exposure and response prevention (Pinto et al. 2011), although patients co-diagnosed with OCPD are not necessarily nonresponders to cognitive-behavioral therapy (CBT). In the study by Pinto et al. (2011), of the individual OCPD criteria that were tested, only perfectionism predicted a poorer treatment outcome. These findings highlight the need for clinicians to pay attention to OCPD-related traits, such as perfectionism, and the importance of a specifically tailored treatment approach based on an individual case formulation in patients with complex symptomatology and comorbid OCPD.

Therefore, we recommend that clinicians actively search for OCPD in patients presenting with common mental disorders. In such cases, treatment for the presenting disorder should be the priority. However, the clinician may tailor the treatment to take account of the coexisting OCPD by choosing psychological or pharmacological strategies that may also benefit the OCPD. For example, in the case of comorbid depression or OCD, the clinician may choose a selective serotonin reuptake inhibitor (SSRI) as the first-line medication, because this may have a beneficial effect on the OCPD. In our experience, the use of pharmacotherapy with an SSRI may also have a beneficial effect on CBT outcomes in OCPD, although this has not been formally studied.

Cognitive-Behavioral Therapy

Although there is a lack of evidence in the form of randomized controlled trials for the use of CBT in patients with OCPD, for several reasons this form of treatment may be considered well suited to address the varied and long-standing problems associated with OCPD. From a CBT perspective, OCPD is maintained by a combination of maladaptive beliefs about the self and others (e.g., rigid self-concept; need for perfection, completeness, and control), along with skill deficits (cognitive inflexibility, difficulties negotiating unpredictable change). CBT involves a wide range of techniques to modify these factors, including cognitive restructuring, behavior modification, exposure and response prevention, psychoeducation, and skills training.

To be successful, CBT for OCPD depends on a supportive, collaborative, and well-defined therapeutic relationship, which emphasizes the patient's willingness to make changes (Matusiewicz et al. 2010). Because individuals with OCPD may have difficulty with trust and commitment, the therapist should focus on developing the therapeutic alliance, keeping in mind that a long and comprehensive course of treatment may be required. For example, in an open trial that included 16 patients with OCPD (and 24 with avoidant personality disorder), up to 52 weekly sessions of CBT were provided. The results indicated that 53% of patients with OCPD showed clinically significant reductions in depressive symptoms, and 83% exhibited clinically significant reductions in OCPD symptom severity (Strauss et al. 2006).

However, many people with OCPD do not benefit from CBT. One possible explanation is that the interpersonal dysfunction associated with OCPD—often manifested as an overwhelming need to be in control—substantially interferes with the collaborative relationship between the therapist and the patient and hampers the working alliance. Alternatively, the cognitive rigidity associated with OCPD may actively impede the ability to effect enduring adaptive behavioral changes. Therefore, clinicians and researchers continue to examine alternative forms of psychological treatment for this large clinical population.

In recent years, there has been a shift toward strategies that promote the acceptance of symptoms and traits. *Acceptance and commitment therapy* is a cognitive-behavioral treatment model that focuses on awareness and non-judgmental acceptance of all experiences, both positive and negative; iden-tification of valued life directions; and appropriate action toward goals that support those values. Patients are encouraged to invest energy in committed actions, such as actively engaging in leisure, social, or occupational activi-ties, rather than struggling against psychological events. These strategies are simple to apply and review in the outpatient clinic, and although not so far tested in OCPD trials, in our experience they are likely to have practical value for this patient group.

Metacognitive interpersonal therapy is another form of psychological ther-apy aimed at both improving metacognition—the ability to understand men-tal states—and modulating problematic interpersonal representations while building new and adaptive ones. One positive individual case report reported a good outcome when the therapy was used for OCPD. This form of treatment merits study.

Developed for eating disorders, *cognitive remediation therapy* targets at-tention to detail and set-shifting, encourages flexible behavior, and increases motivation and perceived ability to change. It has not thus far been tested in OCPD. However, when combined with treatment as usual, it was shown to provide clinical benefits in patients with an eating disorder and OCD. Inter-estingly, cognitive inflexibility predicted a better response to cognitive re-mediation therapy (Dingemans et al. 2014). Thus, this approach may have promise as an adjunct to CBT in disorders characterized by cognitive inflexi-bility, such as OCPD, although this treatment remains to be studied in OCPD.

Psychodynamic psychotherapy has been utilized in clinical practice over many decades; however, to our knowledge, there is no evidence to suggest that it has a beneficial effect in OCPD.

Somatic Treatments

No randomized controlled trials have evaluated medication treatment for uncomplicated OCPD, stringently defined. However, the available evidence hints that OCPD may respond to serotonin reuptake inhibitors (SRIs). A small randomized placebo-controlled trial suggested OCPD traits may re-spond to SRIs (Ansseau 1996). In this study, 24 outpatients with DSM-IV OCPD were randomly assigned to receive fluvoxamine (50–100 mg/day) or placebo for up to 12 weeks. There was substantially greater improvement in

OCPD severity scores in the group treated with fluvoxamine than in the placebo-treated group. Ekselius and Von Knorring (1999) studied the effects of 24 weeks of sertraline and citalopram in 308 depressed patients with comorbid DSM-III-R personality disorder. A significant reduction in dysfunctional traits was observed in most personality disorder categories, including OCPD, and the improvement did not appear to depend on changes in depressive symptoms.

It is of clinical relevance to consider the effect of comorbid OCPD on response to psychopharmacological treatment in patients with OCD. Cavedini et al. (1997) investigated a group of 30 OCD patients. Those with comorbid OCPD experienced a worse outcome following 10 weeks of SSRI treatment than those without comorbid OCPD. In another study of patients with OCD, clomipramine was more efficacious than imipramine in improving scores on a self-rated OCPD inventory, suggesting that SRIs might be preferentially efficacious for OCPD traits (Volavka et al. 1985); however, the results were not clinically confirmed and were based on a completer analysis rather than the intention-to-treat sample.

A recent neurosurgical study suggested that capsulotomy was effective in reducing compulsive symptoms in OCD patients with and without OCPD (Gouvea et al. 2010). On the other hand, the authors of studies of deep brain stimulation have reported that comorbid OCPD traits may interfere with a good treatment outcome in highly resistant OCD cases. However, no studies of these treatments have reported detailed data on OCPD.

Summary

There is a clear need for further treatment development and evaluation in order to provide clinicians with specific and unambiguous treatment recommendations for OCPD.

Key Points

- Obsessive-compulsive personality disorder (OCPD) is a common and impairing, yet under-researched disorder.
- OCPD tends to be overlooked in clinical practice, yet it may have a major impact on treatment outcome and prognosis.
- Clinicians need to approach the diagnosis with sensitivity, in view of its potentially stigmatizing effect.
- OCPD is frequently confused with obsessive-compulsive disorder.
- Existing evidence suggests nosological overlap with the obsessive-compulsive and related disorders in the domains of phenomenolo-

gy, course of illness, gender ratio, comorbidity, heritability, etiological factors, and aspects of treatment-response. However, it also shares features with other personality disorders.

• As yet, there are no evidence-based treatments, but pharmacotherapy with serotonin reuptake inhibitors and cognitive-behavioral therapy may be helpful.

References

Albert U, Maina G, Forner F, et al: DSM-IV obsessive-compulsive personality disorder: prevalence in patients with anxiety disorders and in healthy comparison subjects. Compr Psychiatry 45(5):325–332, 2004 15332194

American Psychiatric Association: Diagnostic and Statistical Manual: Mental Disorders. Washington, DC, American Psychiatric Association, 1952

American Psychiatric Association: Diagnostic and Statistical Manual of Mental Disorders, 2nd Edition. Washington, DC, American Psychiatric Association, 1968

American Psychiatric Association: Diagnostic and Statistical Manual of Mental Disorders, 3rd Edition. Washington, DC, American Psychiatric Association, 1980

American Psychiatric Association: Diagnostic and Statistical Manual of Mental Disorders, 3rd Edition, Revised. Washington, DC, American Psychiatric Association, 1987

American Psychiatric Association: Diagnostic and Statistical Manual of Mental Disorders, 4th Edition. Washington, DC, American Psychiatric Association, 1994

American Psychiatric Association: Diagnostic and Statistical Manual of Mental Disorders, 4th Edition, Washington, DC, American Psychiatric Association, 2000

American Psychiatric Association: Diagnostic and Statistical Manual of Mental Disorders, 5th Edition. Arlington, VA, American Psychiatric Association; 2013

Ansell EB, Pinto A, Edelen MO, et al: Structure of Diagnostic and Statistical Manual of Mental Disorders, Fourth Edition criteria for obsessive-compulsive personality disorder in patients with binge eating disorder. Can J Psychiatry 53(12):863–867, 2008 19087485

Ansell EB, Pinto A, Edelen MO, et al: The association of personality disorders with the prospective 7-year course of anxiety disorders. Psychol Med 41(5):1019–1028, 2011 20836909

Ansseau M: Serotonergic antidepressants in obsessive personality. Encephale 22:309–310, 1996

Bender DS, Skodol AE, Pagano ME, et al: Prospective assessment of treatment use by patients with personality disorders. Psychiatr Serv 57(2):254–257, 2006 16452705

Bernstein DP, Cohen P, Velez CN, et al: Prevalence and stability of the DSM-III-R personality disorders in a community-based survey of adolescents. Am J Psychiatry 150(8):1237–1243, 1993 8328570

Bienvenu OJ, Samuels JF, Wuyek LA, et al: Is obsessive-compulsive disorder an anxiety disorder, and what, if any, are spectrum conditions? A family study perspective. Psychol Med 42(1):1–13, 2012 21733222

Calvo R, Lázaro L, Castro-Fornieles J, et al: Obsessive-compulsive personality disorder traits and personality dimensions in parents of children with obsessive-compulsive disorder. Eur Psychiatry 24(3):201–206, 2009 19118984

Cavedini P, Erzegovesi S, Ronchi P, et al: Predictive value of obsessive-compulsive personality disorder in antiobsessional pharmacological treatment. Eur Neuropsychopharmacol 7(1):45–49, 1997 9088884

Clark LA, Harrison JA: Assessment instruments, in Handbook of Personality Disorders: Theory, Research and Treatment. Edited by Livesley WJ. New York, Guilford, 2001, pp 277–306

Coles ME, Pinto A, Mancebo MC, et al: OCD with comorbid OCPD: a subtype of OCD? J Psychiatr Res 42(4):289–296, 2008 17382961

Costa PT Jr, McCrae RR: The five-factor model of personality and its relevance to personality disorders. J Pers Disord 6(4):343–359, 1992

Costa P, Samuels J, Bagby M, et al: Obsessive-compulsive personality disorder: a review, in Personality Disorders (World Psychiatric Association Series, Vol 8). Edited by Maj M, Akiskal H, Mezzich J, et al. New York, Wiley, 2005, pp 405–477

Diaconu G, Turecki G: Obsessive-compulsive personality disorder and suicidal behavior: evidence for a positive association in a sample of depressed patients. J Clin Psychiatry 70(11):1551–1556, 2009 19607764

Dingemans AE, Danner UN, Donker JM, et al: The effectiveness of cognitive remediation therapy in patients with a severe or enduring eating disorder: a randomized controlled trial. Psychother Psychosom 83(1):29–36, 2014 24281361

Eisen JL, Coles ME, Shea MT, et al: Clarifying the convergence between obsessive compulsive personality disorder criteria and obsessive compulsive disorder. J Pers Disord 20(3):294–305, 2006 16776557

Eisen JL, Sibrava NJ, Boisseau CL, et al: Five year course of obsessive-compulsive disorder: predictors of remission and relapse. J Clin Psychiatry 74(3):233–239, 2013 23561228

Ekselius L, Von Knorring L: Changes in personality traits during treatment with sertraline or citalopram. Br J Psychiatry 174:444–448, 1999 10616614

Fineberg NA, Sharma P, Sivakumaran T, et al: Does obsessive-compulsive personality disorder belong within the obsessive-compulsive spectrum? CNS Spectr 12(6):467–482, 2007 17545957

Fineberg NA, Chamberlain SR, Goudriaan AE, et al: New developments in human neurocognition: clinical, genetic, and brain imaging correlates of impulsivity and compulsivity. CNS Spectr 19(1):69–89, 2014 24512640

Foa EB, Kozak MJ, Goodman WK, et al: DSM-IV field trial: obsessive-compulsive disorder. Am J Psychiatry 152(1):90–96, 1995 7802127

Frost RO, Martin P, Lahart C, et al: Frost Multidimensional Perfectionism Scale, in Measures for Clinical Practice: A Sourcebook. Edited by Fischer J, Corcoran K. New York, Oxford University Press, 1994, pp 232–235

Gouvea F, Lopes A, Greenberg B, et al: Response to sham and active gamma ventral capsulotomy in otherwise intractable obsessive-compulsive disorder. Stereotact Funct Neurosurg 88(3):177–182, 2010 20431329

Grant BF, Hasin DS, Stinson FS, et al: Prevalence, correlates, and disability of personality disorders in the United States: results from the National Epidemiologic Survey on Alcohol and Related Conditions. J Clin Psychiatry 65(7):948–958, 2004 15291684

Grant JE, Mooney ME, Kushner MG: Prevalence, correlates, and comorbidity of DSM-IV obsessive-compulsive personality disorder: results from the National Epidemiologic Survey on Alcohol and Related Conditions. J Psychiatr Res 46(4):469–475, 2012 22257387

Grilo CM: Factor structure of DSM-IV criteria for obsessive compulsive personality disorder in patients with binge eating disorder. Acta Psychiatr Scand 109(1):64–69, 2004 14674960

Grilo CM, McGlashan TH, Morey LC, et al: Internal consistency, intercriterion overlap and diagnostic efficiency of criteria sets for DSM-IV schizotypal, borderline, avoidant and obsessive-compulsive personality disorders. Acta Psychiatr Scand 104(4):264–272, 2001 11722301

Grilo CM, Sanislow CA, Gunderson JG, et al: Two-year stability and change of schizotypal, borderline, avoidant, and obsessive-compulsive personality disorders. J Consult Clin Psychol 72(5):767–775, 2004 15482035

Grilo CM, Stout RL, Markowitz JC, et al: Personality disorders predict relapse after remission from an episode of major depressive disorder: a 6-year prospective study. J Clin Psychiatry 71(12):1629–1635, 2010 20584514

Huang Y, Kotov R, de Girolamo G, et al: DSM-IV personality disorders in the WHO World Mental Health Surveys. Br J Psychiatry 195(1):46–53, 2009 19567896

Hummelen B, Wilberg T, Pedersen G, et al: The quality of the DSM-IV obsessive-compulsive personality disorder construct as a prototype category. J Nerv Ment Dis 196(6):446–455, 2008 18552621

Karwautz A, Troop NA, Rabe-Hesketh S, et al: Personality disorders and personality dimensions in anorexia nervosa. J Pers Disord 17(1):73–85, 2003 12659548

Lilenfeld LR, Kaye WH, Greeno CG, et al: A controlled family study of anorexia nervosa and bulimia nervosa: psychiatric disorders in first-degree relatives and effects of proband comorbidity. Arch Gen Psychiatry 55(7):603–610, 1998 9672050

Loranger AW, Sartorius N, Andreoli A, et al: The International Personality Disorder Examination. The World Health Organization/Alcohol, Drug Abuse, and Mental Health Administration international pilot study of personality disorders. Arch Gen Psychiatry 51(3):215–224, 1994 8122958

Matusiewicz AK, Hopwood CJ, Banducci AN, et al: The effectiveness of cognitive behavioural therapy for personality disorders. Psychiatr Clin North Am 33(3):657–685, 2010 3138327

McGlashan TH, Grilo CM, Sanislow CA, et al: Two-year prevalence and stability of individual DSM-IV criteria for schizotypal, borderline, avoidant, and obsessive-compulsive personality disorders: toward a hybrid model of Axis II disorders. Am J Psychiatry 162(5):883–889, 2005 15863789

Nelson EA, Abramowitz JS, Whiteside SP, et al: Scrupulosity in patients with obsessive-compulsive disorder: relationship to clinical and cognitive phenomena. J Anxiety Disord 20(8):1071–1086, 2006 16524696

Nestadt G, Romanoski AJ, Brown CH, et al: DSM-III compulsive personality disorder: an epidemiological survey. Psychol Med 21(2):461–471, 1991 1876651

Nestadt G, Di C, Samuels JF, et al: Concordance between personality disorder assessment methods. Psychol Med 42(3):657–667, 2012 21861952

Nordahl HM, Stiles TC: Perceptions of parental bonding in patients with various personality disorders, lifetime depressive disorders, and healthy controls. J Pers Disord 11(4):391–402, 1997 9484698

Pertusa A, Frost RO, Fullana MA, et al: Refining the diagnostic boundaries of compulsive hoarding: a critical review. Clin Psychol Rev 30(4):371–386, 2010 20189280

Pfohl B, Stangl DA, Zimmerman M, et al: Structured Interview for DSM-II Personality Disorders (SIDP). Iowa City, University of Iowa, 1982

Phillips KA, McElroy SL: Personality disorders and traits in patients with body dysmorphic disorder. Compr Psychiatry 41(4):229–236, 2000 10929788

Pinto A, Mancebo MC, Eisen JL, et al: The Brown Longitudinal Obsessive Compulsive Study: clinical features and symptoms of the sample at intake. J Clin Psychiatry 67(5):703–711, 2006 16841619

Pinto A, Liebowitz MR, Foa EB, et al: Obsessive compulsive personality disorder as a predictor of exposure and ritual prevention outcome for obsessive compulsive disorder. Behav Res Ther 49(8):453–458, 2011 21600563

Reichborn-Kjennerud T, Czajkowski N, Neale MC, et al: Genetic and environmental influences on dimensional representations of DSM-IV Cluster C personality disorders: a population-based multivariate twin study. Psychol Med 37(5):645–653, 2007 17134532

Rhéaume J, Freeston MH, Dugas MJ, et al: Perfectionism, responsibility and obsessive-compulsive symptoms. Behav Res Ther 33(7):785–794, 1995 7677716

Romanoski AJ, Nestadt G, Chahal R, et al: Inter-observer reliability of a "Standardized Psychiatric Examination" (SPE) for case ascertainment (DSM-III). J Nerv Ment Dis 176(2):63–71, 1988 3339343

Rossi A, Marinangeli MG, Butti G, et al: Personality disorders in bipolar and depressive disorders. J Affect Disord 65(1):3–8, 2001 11426507

Samuels J, Nestadt G, Bienvenu OJ, et al: Personality disorders and normal personality dimensions in obsessive-compulsive disorder. Br J Psychiatry 177:457–462, 2000 11060001

Sansone RA, Hendricks CM, Sellbom M, et al: Anxiety symptoms and healthcare utilization among a sample of outpatients in an internal medicine clinic. Int J Psychiatry Med 33(2):133–139, 2003 12968826

Sansone RA, Levitt JL, Sansone LA: The prevalence of personality disorders among those with eating disorders. Eat Disord 13(1):7–21, 2005 16864328

Schuster JP, Hoertel N, Le Strat Y, et al: Personality disorders in older adults: findings from the National Epidemiologic Survey on Alcohol and Related Conditions. Am J Geriatr Psychiatry 21(8):757–768, 2013 23567365

Skodol AE, Pagano ME, Bender DS, et al: Stability of functional impairment in patients with schizotypal, borderline, avoidant, or obsessive-compulsive personality disorder over two years. Psychol Med 35(3):443–451, 2005 15841879

Spitzer RL, Williams JB, Gibbon M: Structured Clinical Interview for DSM-III-R Personality Disorders (SCID-II). New York, New York State Psychiatric Institute, 1987

Starcevic V, Brakoulias V: New diagnostic perspectives on obsessive-compulsive personality disorder and its links with other conditions. Curr Opin Psychiatry 27(1):62–67, 2014 24257122

Stein DJ, Hollander E, Mullen LS: Comparison of clomipramine, alprazolam and placebo in the treatment of obsessive compulsive disorder. Hum Psychopharmacol 7(6):389–395, 1992

Strauss J, Hayes A, Johnson S, et al: Early alliance, alliance ruptures, and symptom change in a nonrandomized trial of cognitive therapy for avoidant and obsessive-compulsive personality disorders. J Consult Clin Psychol 74(2):337–345, 2006 16649878

Summerfeldt LJ: Understanding and treating incompleteness in obsessive-compulsive disorder. J Clin Psychol 60(11):1155–1168, 2004 15389620

Taylor S, Asmundson GJ, Jang KL: Etiology of obsessive-compulsive symptoms and obsessive-compulsive personality traits: common genes, mostly different environments. Depress Anxiety 28(10):863–869, 2011 21769999

Torgersen S, Kringlen E, Cramer V: The prevalence of personality disorders in a community sample. Arch Gen Psychiatry 58(6):590–596, 2001 11386989

Volavka J, Neziroglu F, Yaryura-Tobias JA: Clomipramine and imipramine in obsessive-compulsive disorder. Psychiatry Res 14(1):85–93, 1985 3887445

Recommended Readings

Maj M, Akiskal H, Mezzich J, et al (eds): Personality Disorders (World Psychiatric Association Series, Vol 8). New York, Wiley, 2005

Mancebo MC, Eisen JL, Grant JE, et al: Obsessive compulsive personality disorder and obsessive compulsive disorder: clinical characteristics, diagnostic difficulties, and treatment. Ann Clin Psychiatry 17:197–204, 2005

Phillips KA, Stein DJ, Rauch S, et al: Should an obsessive-compulsive spectrum grouping of disorders be included in DSM-V? Depress Anxiety 27(6):528–555, 2010

Pinto A, Eisen JL, Mancebo MC, et al: Obsessive compulsive personality disorder, in Obsessive-Compulsive Disorder: Subtypes and Spectrum Conditions. Edited by Abramowitz JS, McKay D, Taylor S. New York, Elsevier, 2008, pp 246–270

CHAPTER 11

Conclusions

Dan J. Stein, M.D., Ph.D.
Katharine A. Phillips, M.D.

The development process that led to the publication of DSM-5 provided a timely opportunity to review the literature on obsessive-compulsive and related disorders (OCRDs). This process also enabled research published since the early 1990s (when DSM-IV was developed [American Psychiatric Association 1994]) to inform the revision of diagnostic criteria in order to optimize the diagnosis of each of these disorders and enhance the assessment and treatment of this underdiagnosed and undertreated group of conditions. Each of the preceding chapters has focused on the diagnosis, assessment, and treatment of a specific OCRD (or, in the case of Chapter 7, group of OCRDs). In this concluding chapter, we aim to review the clinical take-home messages that emerge from a consideration of the OCRDs as a whole. We include discussion of assessment and treatment, cross-cultural issues, special populations, gender, consumer advocacy, and personalized medicine.

Assessment and Treatment

Awareness of the OCRDs

One key theme that emerges from a consideration of the OCRDs as a whole is a lack of awareness of these disorders and consequent underdiagnosis. Epidemiological data indicate that the OCRDs are highly prevalent and that they are associated not only with individual suffering and disability but also with significant societal costs. Only a few decades ago, these conditions were considered by many to be rare, and even now data indicate that many patients with OCRDs either do not present for treatment or are not appropriately diagnosed if they do. Although this contrast between high burden of disease and low rates of clinical diagnosis is by no means restricted to the OCRDs, it does seem particularly stark in the case of this group of disorders.

Several factors may contribute to the underdiagnosis of OCRDs. First, many of these disorders have only recently gained entry into our psychiatric nomenclature. Although clinical descriptions of body dysmorphic disorder (BDD), hoarding disorder, trichotillomania (hair-pulling disorder), and excoriation (skin-picking) disorder have been available for more than a century, BDD and trichotillomania were first included in DSM in DSM-III-R, published in 1987 (American Psychiatric Association 1987), and hoarding disorder and excoriation (skin-picking) disorder are included for the first time in DSM-5 (American Psychiatric Association 2013). The inclusion of BDD and trichotillomania in DSM-III-R led to increased research on these conditions as well as increased clinician and patient awareness, and we are hopeful that the inclusion of hoarding disorder and excoriation (skin-picking) disorder in DSM-5 will provide a similar impetus for increased research on and recognition of these conditions.

Second, despite some overlap in the phenomenology of these disorders, frequent comorbidity between some of them, and similar assessment methods (e.g., using variations of the Yale-Brown Obsessive Compulsive Scale), those disorders that were included in prior editions of DSM were in different chapters: OCD was classified in the chapter on anxiety disorders, BDD in the chapter on somatoform disorders, and trichotillomania (hair-pulling disorder) in the chapter on impulse-control disorders not elsewhere classified. The lack of a conceptual grouping of these disorders in the nomenclature may have contributed to a failure to train clinicians to think about these conditions in a clear way as well as to a failure by researchers, such as psychiatric epidemiologists, to investigate the prevalence and risk factors associated with this set of conditions.

Third, the nature of the symptoms of these disorders often contributes to delays in care seeking. Many of the intrusive symptoms of OCRDs are associated with high levels of shame. (For example, consider the young woman who has intrusive obsessions about harming her baby or the young man who cannot walk into a room without the thought that people are laughing at the shape of his mouth.) Many of the repetitive behaviors of OCRDs are also associated with similar negative feelings; patients who wash their hands to the point of skin peeling, who pull out their hair to the point of baldness, or who have unsightly lesions of skin picking are often embarrassed that they have been unable to exert control over their symptoms. It is key for clinicians to be aware of the high degree of self-stigmatization associated with the OCRDs.

Fourth, there are a range of other barriers to diagnosis. In recent decades, it would seem that levels of mental health literacy have increased in the community as a whole and among some groups of clinicians. Nevertheless, in general, many patients continue to report immense relief when they learn, after years of treatment seeking, that their symptoms are in fact well described in the medical literature, underscoring the fact that knowledge about these disorders is not widely dispersed. In addition, our impression is that many clinicians continue to have relatively little knowledge of current evidence-based treatment approaches to the OCRDs, underscoring the point that better training of clinicians and increased research on these conditions remain important priorities.

There is an urgent need for increased awareness of these disorders among both patients and clinicians. We hope that the new way in which these disorders are grouped together in DSM-5—in the new chapter of OCRDs—will facilitate greater awareness of these prevalent and sometimes disabling conditions and lead to more frequent treatment seeking. Research to improve recognition of these disorders is greatly needed. For example, the OCRDs need to be included in large international epidemiological studies so their prevalence and clinical correlates can be better understood. In addition, clinicians need more training on how to recognize these disorders, which is the first essential step to providing adequate care. Advocacy efforts that have developed since DSM-IV need to be further increased to even more effectively reach and inform patients with an OCRD and family members.

Assessment and Evaluation

In addition to the high degree of self-stigmatization in the OCRDs, a number of other key assessment and evaluation issues are relevant to this group of disorders.

First, although there are significant differences between each of the OCRDs, there are a number of important uniformities in the structure of symptoms across these disorders, and as a consequence it is possible to develop questions that are useful in screening for a number of different OCRDs, determining whether an OCRD may be present, and assessing symptom severity. As noted in Chapter 1 ("Introduction and Major Changes for the Obsessive-Compulsive and Related Disorders in DSM-5") of this book, in the section on assessment measures, DSM-5 provides a self-rated cross-cutting symptom measure with two questions for OCRDs: 1) "Unpleasant thoughts, urges or images that repeatedly enter your mind?" and 2) "Feeling driven to perform certain behaviors or mental acts over and over again?" These questions performed well in the DSM-5 field trials but require further testing. Patients who score 2 (mild) or higher on these questions should be further assessed for the possible presence of an OCRD.

The DSM-5 subworkgroup on OCRDs also developed brief, self-rated scales for each individual OCRD that are consistent in their structure, reflect DSM-5 criteria, and can be used by clinicians to help generate a dimensional severity rating for the disorders (LeBeau et al. 2013). Questions were drawn from a self-rated symptom severity scale for OCD, the Florida Obsessive-Compulsive Inventory (Storch et al. 2007), and also took into consideration published symptom severity scales for OCRDs. Further work is needed to assess these scales' reliability and validity in clinical samples.

Second, in many of the OCRDs, it is important to assess level of insight. DSM-5 provides analogous specifiers for insight in the diagnostic criteria for OCD, BDD, and hoarding disorder. In OCD and BDD, good or fair insight is specified when the individual recognizes that his or her disorder-related beliefs are definitely or probably not true or that they may or may not be true. In hoarding disorder, good or fair insight is specified when the individual recognizes that his or her hoarding-related beliefs and behaviors are problematic. In OCD and BDD, poor insight is specified when the individual thinks that his or her disorder-related beliefs are probably true, and absent insight/delusional beliefs is specified when the individual is completely convinced that these beliefs are true. In hoarding disorder, poor insight is specified when the individual is mostly convinced that hoarding-related beliefs and behaviors are not problematic, and absent insight/delusional beliefs is specified when the individual is completely convinced that such symptoms are not problematic despite evidence to the contrary.

The insight specifier has important clinical utility. Patients with OCRDs and absent insight are often misdiagnosed as having a psychotic disorder and consequently may be treated inappropriately with high doses of antipsychotic medications. There is a growing evidence base demonstrating that such patients may respond instead to standard pharmacotherapy interventions for OCRDs (e.g., patients with delusional BDD often respond to treatment with serotonin reuptake inhibitor [SRI] monotherapy) and to standard cognitive-behavioral therapy (CBT) interventions for OCRDs (e.g., OCD patients with no insight may respond to exposure and response prevention interventions) (Leckman et al. 2010; Phillips et al. 2014). Thus, the new insight specifier in DSM-5 fixes a problem present in earlier editions of DSM, which encouraged clinicians to diagnose the delusional form of these disorders as a psychotic disorder.

Third, there are a number of key comorbid symptoms and disorders that deserve evaluation in any patient with an OCRD. The OCRDs have high comorbidity with mood and anxiety disorders, and treatment plans need to be configured in order to address such comorbidity. Suicidal thoughts and behaviors are an important consideration in patients with OCRDs, particularly in those with more severe BDD or comorbid depression. In addition, any individual with an OCRD should also be evaluated for the presence of other OCRDs as well as tic disorders, illness anxiety disorder, and obsessive-compulsive personality disorder. Comorbidity with other OCRDs is generally not as frequent as with mood and anxiety disorders (although BDD is an exception; approximately one-third of patients with BDD have comorbid OCD). However, comorbid OCRDs are highly prevalent comorbid disorders, given their relatively lower base rate in the population as a whole (e.g., although comorbid major depressive disorder is more common than comorbid trichotillomania (hair-pulling disorder) in OCD, the latter is much more common in individuals with OCD than in those drawn from the general population) (Lochner and Stein 2010).

Finally, the presence of nonpsychiatric medical disorders and substance use disorders that may be contributing to symptoms should always be considered (e.g., stimulant use in a patient with excoriation [skin-picking] disorder). Although DSM-5 does not yet include the construct *pediatric autoimmune neuropsychiatric disorders associated with streptococcal infections* (PANDAS), research on this putative condition has emphasized the value of assessing a broad range of potential triggers of OCRDs.

A fourth consideration is the patient's explanatory model of the OCRD. This is related in part to mental health literacy; those patients who have greater mental health literacy may offer more sophisticated models of the possible pathogenesis of their disorder. At the same time, sophistication does not necessarily mean that the model is correct; for example, some patients may describe well-formulated models of symptoms that rely on outdated psychoanalytic drive theories or self-blame for having the disorder. Explanatory models are also related in part to cultural factors; patients may attribute their symptoms to particular belief systems that have origins in their religious or ethnic backgrounds.

The DSM-5 section on cultural formulation offers a series of useful probes for assessing such models (American Psychiatric Association 2013). Questions include "Why do you think this is happening to you?" and "What do you think are the causes of your [PROBLEM]?" Further possible prompts include "Some people may explain their problem as the result of bad things that happen in their life, problems with others, a physical illness, a spiritual reason, or many other causes." DSM-5's cultural formulation is an excellent addition to the assessment of any patient, regardless of his or her cultural, ethnic, or religious background.

We believe that it is helpful for clinicians to be aware of a patient's explanatory model for his or her illness, because this understanding may facilitate a better therapeutic alliance with the patient. If the patient's model is inaccurate or unhelpful (e.g., when it involves unwarranted self-blame for having symptoms of a disorder), it may be helpful for the clinician to gently challenge that model using a psychoeducational approach. It is usually useful for clinicians to share their own explanatory models of OCD, which may enhance the patient's willingness to engage in treatment, and then to negotiate a shared approach to the treatment plan. In some cases, understanding the patient's view of how he or she developed the illness may inform implementation of CBT, although the key recommended elements of CBT, such as exposure and response prevention, should be applied fairly uniformly across patients.

Issues in Pharmacotherapy and Psychotherapy

A range of themes emerge from the discussion of pharmacotherapy and psychotherapy for each of the OCRDs.

A first important point is that pharmacotherapy treatment principles for OCD differ in subtle but important ways from those for the management of mood and anxiety disorders. Although a range of antidepressants are useful in many mood and anxiety disorders, in OCD and BDD there appears to be a more selective response to serotonergic antidepressants—that is, clomipramine and the selective serotonin reuptake inhibitors (SSRIs). Patients with OCD and BDD are typically able to tolerate standard starting dosing of medication (e.g., escitalopram 10 mg daily), unlike those with panic disorder (who often require very low initial doses of medication). However, patients with OCD, BDD, and illness anxiety disorder often require much higher doses, administered for longer durations, than those patients with major depression (Bloch et al. 2010; Phillips and Hollander 2008). These guidelines are well established in OCD; there are fewer rigorous data in BDD and illness anxiety disorder, but available data support this approach to pharmacotherapy. At the same time, many similar principles do apply across the mood disorders, anxiety disorders, and OCRDs; in particular, we would note the value of maintenance treatment in preventing relapse across these conditions.

It is worth emphasizing, however, that serotonergic antidepressants may not be effective for all of the OCRDs. Despite the seminal observation that clomipramine is more effective than desipramine in a range of OCRDs, data from trials of SSRIs in trichotillomania (hair-pulling disorder) have been surprisingly disappointing (although many were underpowered). Although few randomized controlled trials have focused on OCRDs with comorbid mood and anxiety disorders, it seems reasonable to use SSRIs in patients with trichotillomania (hair-pulling disorder) and a comorbid SSRI-responsive condition. There are some data indicating that SSRIs are useful in hoarding disorder, but again, there is a lack of randomized controlled trials in this area, and hoarding symptoms in patients with OCD appear less responsive to these agents (Bloch et al. 2014).

One hypothesis is that dopamine blockers are more effective in some of the OCRDs, perhaps particularly those characterized by body-focused repetitive behaviors, such as trichotillomania (hair-pulling disorder) and excoriation (skin-picking) disorder. In this regard, it is noteworthy that antipsychotic augmentation of SRIs may be particularly helpful in OCD patients with comorbid tics (compared with patients with OCD without comorbid tics). There is growing interest in the role of glutamatergic agents in the OCRDs, and although further work is needed, N-acetylcysteine can arguably be considered a first-line agent in the treatment of adult trichotillomania (hair-pulling disorder).

There are a number of similarities in the cognitive-behavioral approaches used for anxiety disorders and several of the OCRDs. Indeed, one of the rationales for placing the chapter on OCRDs immediately after the chapter on anxiety disorders was to emphasize overlaps in the phenomenology, psychobiology, and certain aspects of effective treatment approaches across these various conditions (Stein et al. 2011). Exposure, for example, is an important component of CBT treatment for anxiety disorders, OCD, BDD, and hoarding disorder and may also have a role in illness anxiety disorder. Some CBT approaches are also shared by several OCRDs; for example, response prevention is a crucial component of CBT for OCD and BDD and probably hoarding disorder and illness anxiety disorder, and habit reversal is recommended for OCRDs characterized by body-focused repetitive behaviors (trichotillomania [hair-pulling disorder] and excoriation [skin-picking] disorder) as well as for tic disorders.

At the same time, it must be emphasized that psychotherapy treatment principles should be specifically tailored to the OCRDs. There are important differences between CBT for OCRDs and CBT for the anxiety disorders, and CBT approaches within the OCRDs vary in important ways from disorder to disorder. For example, ritual prevention is important in the treatment of BDD, OCD, and probably also hoarding disorder and illness anxiety disorder, but it is not typically used to treat anxiety disorders. Regarding differences in CBT approaches to the individual OCRDs, exposure is an important component of treatment for both BDD and OCD, but in our experience exposure should be done more slowly and later in the treatment (after first learning cognitive restructuring and ritual prevention) when treating BDD.

We also use techniques such as mirror retraining for BDD, which is not relevant to OCD. Hoarding disorder and illness anxiety disorder require a somewhat different CBT approach than that used for other OCRDs. The CBT approach to trichotillomania (hair-pulling disorder) and excoriation (skin-picking) disorder differs from that for OCRDs with a prominent cognitive component and consists largely of habit reversal training (which is also an important component of treatment for tic disorders).

An additional set of considerations are those pertaining to the use of combined pharmacotherapy and psychotherapy. Although it makes intuitive sense that pharmacotherapy and psychotherapy are complementary, there is a surprising lack of data showing that combined treatment is more effective for OCD than either pharmacotherapy or psychotherapy alone at the start of treatment (data on combined treatment are virtually nonexistent for other OCRDs). From a clinical perspective, we usually recommend concomitant use of both treatments from the start for patients who have severe illness (e.g., are housebound because of their symptoms) or who are at risk for suicide. In our view, medication should always be used initially for patients with more severe symptoms or worrisome levels of suicidality; it may also be used for more mildly or moderately ill patients.

Pharmacotherapy alone may be chosen first for a variety of reasons, including the presence of comorbid mood and anxiety disorders, patient preference, and lack of availability of CBT therapists. CBT may be useful as a subsequent added intervention in many individuals with OCRDs who are hoping to improve their response even further (and those with treatment-refractory illness) and in patients who plan to reduce medication dosage. Alternatively, CBT alone can be considered as a first-line treatment for more mildly to moderately ill patients, although patients need to be prepared to do the work that is required for such treatments to be effective (e.g., homework assignments). Motivational interviewing techniques may be used to enhance motivation to participate in CBT. Such techniques are often needed for patients with hoarding disorder or with absent-insight or poor-insight BDD or OCD.

Special Populations and Gender Issues

In this section we briefly review three special populations: children and adolescents, the elderly, and patients with intellectual disability. Clinicians working with each of these populations may face a number of specific challenges, and a short review of such challenges therefore seems pertinent. We also briefly discuss gender issues in relation to the OCRDs.

Many psychiatric disorders can be conceptualized as neurodevelopmental, in that they have an early onset. Many of the OCRDs can begin prepubertally, and BDD, trichotillomania (hair-pulling disorder), excoriation (skin-picking) disorder, and OCD usually develop before adulthood, emphasizing the importance of this perspective. On the one hand, it is remarkable how similar the symptomatology of each of the OCRDs is across the different life stages. On the other hand, it is important for clinicians to be aware of key differences in presentations; in childhood, for example, patients are less likely to provide abstract religious or philosophical explanations (e.g., emphasizing moral purity) for their washing rituals. Children and adolescents with BDD appear to have poorer BDD-related insight than adults, perhaps reflecting less well developed metacognitive skills, which may mediate poor insight in some disorders.

It is also important for clinicians to be aware of the importance of subclinical hair pulling, rituals, and body image concerns in normal development and to not conflate these with trichotillomania (hair-pulling disorder), OCD, or BDD. The presence of normal concerns and rituals in childhood and the high prevalence of subclinical obsessions and compulsions in youth and adults reinforce the potential value of an evolutionary psychiatry perspective that speaks to the adaptive value of many behavioral responses (Stein and Nesse 2011).

However, it is equally if not more important to avoid making the opposite error, which is to assume that collecting, hair pulling, or body image concerns are likely normal when they occur in youth. BDD, for example, often goes undiagnosed in childhood and adolescence because clinicians or parents assume that appearance concerns are normative in this age group; misdiagnosis may result in suicide attempts and marked interference with normal adolescent development, including school dropout. It is important to assess diagnostic criteria for the relevant OCRD in any individual with OCRD-like symptoms, even if the symptoms initially appear to reflect normative concerns. Of relevance to this discussion, as noted earlier, it is common for individuals with these disorders to conceal or minimize OCRD symptoms because they are ashamed of them; thus, symptoms may actually be more severe than they appear to outside observers. The presence of clinically significant distress or impairment resulting from the obsessions/preoccupations or repetitive behaviors, in particular, signals the need for likely intervention.

Finally, we would emphasize that there are some differences in pharmacotherapy, as well as more notable and important differences in CBT, that clinicians need to be aware of when treating children. CBT for the OCRDs requires a developmentally appropriate approach. For example, CBT for youths often requires greater use of external reinforcement and rewards, and parents need to be more involved in treatment. Handouts or forms, which are important when doing CBT during sessions and for homework, must be age appropriate. Because youths have less well developed metacognitive skills, any cognitive restructuring that is done must be simpler than for adults; typically, more emphasis is placed on behavioral strategies. Treatment must also address adolescent developmental transitions and tasks; problems such as school refusal due to an OCRD need particular attention.

OCRDs do not commonly present for the first time in the elderly. When they do, it is particularly important to rule out the presence of an underlying medical disorder; hoarding behavior, for example, may be seen in elderly patients with early dementia. In other respects, however, the assessment and treatment of elderly patients with an OCRD may not differ very markedly from those of younger patients. From a pharmacotherapy perspective, clinicians may need to be more aware of potential drug-drug interactions and to be more cautious with higher doses of medication. From a psychotherapy perspective, in our experience patients who have had an OCRD for many years and then respond later in life to treatment may need support with the realization that they have lost so many years to the condition. This is particularly the case if the disorder has substantially interfered with the attainment of life goals, such as a career or relationships.

In patients with severe intellectual disability, stereotypic movement disorder may be an important problem, with a relatively early onset in life. In many ways, this disorder can arguably be considered the analogue of body-focused repetitive behavioral disorders that present later in life in individuals with normal intelligence. In our clinical experience, patients with mild intellectual disability may present with symptoms that are more reminiscent of OCD than of stereotypic movement disorder. Thus, for example, they may have very specific checking rituals that cause them distress (particularly if they cannot complete them) and that interfere with their daily activities. They may not be able to provide abstract explanations for why their rituals are important, as patients with OCD typically can, but in other respects their behaviors may be similar to typical compulsions. Although the literature on OCD in patients with intellectual disability is relatively sparse, in our experience standard pharmacotherapy (perhaps being more cautious about higher doses) and basic CBT techniques can be useful.

Across the OCRDs there are many pertinent gender issues to consider. In community studies, females predominate across the OCRDs. However, in clinical practice, gender ratios may be more balanced in OCD, BDD, and hoarding disorder clinics, with females predominating in body-focused repetitive behavior disorder clinics. This anecdotal observation raises the question of whether increased outreach is needed to women with OCRDs in order to facilitate treatment seeking.

In OCD, there is growing evidence that males have earlier onset of OCD and are more likely to have comorbid tics. In trichotillomania (hair-pulling disorder), onset may coincide with menarche. In several OCRDs, there is evidence of symptom exacerbation premenstrually or de novo onset in the peripartum period. It is important for clinicians to be particularly aware of gender issues in assessing and evaluating patients (e.g., in BDD, men are more likely to have a comorbid substance use disorder, including abuse of anabolic steroids). Although SRIs can be dosed similarly in males and females with OCRDs, it is important for clinicians to keep an eye on the growing literature indicating differences in dose requirements by sex for various psychotropics.

Future Directions

Much research on OCRDs has focused on efficacy rather than effectiveness trials; that is, the focus has been on earlier-stage (efficacy) trials conducted in academic settings using narrow inclusion criteria rather than on trials undertaken in clinical practice settings with broad inclusion criteria. This focus, in part, reflects the fact that far fewer treatment studies have been done on the OCRDs than on disorders such as the mood, anxiety, or psychotic disorders. The literature on pragmatic trials in mood and psychotic disorders has taught the field a great deal, and there is a need for similar work to take place in the OCRDs. There are surprisingly few longitudinal studies of the OCRDs; it is hoped that such work will emerge in future years. From a clinical perspective, it is perhaps relevant to be simultaneously proud of how much has been learned and humbled by how much remains to be understood; for many questions that our patients ask us, the evidence base does not exist to provide a very precise answer.

From a global public health perspective, the World Health Organization's revision of the *International Classification of Diseases* (ICD-11) is also important. ICD-11 is focused in particular on the use of the nomenclature in a broad range of settings, including use by nonspecialized clinicians working in primary care in low-resourced areas (a description that applies to the majority of the world's clinical population). DSM-5 and ICD-11 have broadly similar chapters and disorders in order to ensure that international practice, teaching, and research have a firm universal foundation. At the same time, the principles underlying DSM-5 and ICD-11 are somewhat different, reflecting their different mandates, and as a consequence there may be some differences between the two nomenclatures in the chapter on OCRDs. The ICD-11 principles remind clinicians of the importance of working with colleagues in primary care settings to improve diagnosis and treatment of these conditions.

While advances in global mental health characterize one important series of advances in psychiatry, another crucial set of advances is seen in work emphasizing the notion of psychiatry as a clinical neuroscience. The National Institute of Mental Health has emphasized the need for translational approaches to psychiatry research, with the possibility that such approaches will lead to improvements in clinical care, including personalized medicine (Insel et al. 2010). The Research Domain Criteria framework includes constructs such as cognitive inflexibility, which may ultimately lead to new ways of assessing and understanding symptoms across the OCRDs. Similarly, growing work on endophenotypes that cut across the different OCRDs may lead to advances in our knowledge of pathogenesis and to new treatment targets. Only time will tell whether such efforts will succeed, but in the interim, from a clinical perspective, these approaches are arguably important in giving both clinicians and patients hope for the future.

Consumer advocacy is already playing an important role in OCRDs. The International OCD Foundation and the Trichotillomania Learning Center, for example, provide up-to-date information on their Web sites, take calls from mental health consumers, and make referrals. In addition, these organizations have funded a range of significant research in the field. Importantly, the inclusion of excoriation (skin-picking) disorder in DSM-5 gathered momentum not only because of the increased research data available on this condition over recent decades but also because of clear feedback from consumer organizations and from individual patients indicating that such inclusion would improve diagnosis and treatment for many individuals around the world (Stein and Phillips 2013). In the future, we hope and expect that consumer participation in setting research agendas will grow, and we urge clinicians to be aware of the work of consumer organizations, to be involved with them, and to provide support.

References

American Psychiatric Association: Diagnostic and Statistical Manual of Mental Disorders, 3rd Edition, Revised. Washington, DC, American Psychiatric Association, 1987

American Psychiatric Association: Diagnostic and Statistical Manual of Mental Disorders, 4th Edition. Washington, DC, American Psychiatric Association, 1994

American Psychiatric Association: Diagnostic and Statistical Manual of Mental Disorders, 5th Edition. Arlington, VA, American Psychiatric Association, 2013

Bloch MH, McGuire J, Landeros-Weisenberger A, et al: Meta-analysis of the dose-response relationship of SSRI in obsessive-compulsive disorder. Mol Psychiatry 15(8):850–855, 2010 19468281

Bloch MH, Bartley CA, Zipperer L, et al: Meta-analysis: hoarding symptoms associated with poor treatment outcome in obsessive-compulsive disorder. Mol Psychiatry 19(9):1025–1030, 2014 24912494

Insel T, Cuthbert B, Garvey M, et al: Research domain criteria (RDoC): toward a new classification framework for research on mental disorders. Am J Psychiatry 167(7):748–751, 2010 20595427

LeBeau RT, Mischel ER, Simpson HB, et al: Preliminary assessment of obsessive-compulsive spectrum scales for DSM-5. J Obsessive Compuls Relat Disord 2:114–118, 2013

Leckman JF, Denys D, Simpson HB, et al: Obsessive-compulsive disorder: a review of the diagnostic criteria and possible subtypes and dimensional specifiers for DSM-V. Depress Anxiety 27(6):507–527, 2010 20217853

Lochner C, Stein DJ: Obsessive-compulsive spectrum disorders in obsessive-compulsive disorder and other anxiety disorders. Psychopathology 43(6):389–396, 2010 20847586

Phillips KA, Hollander E: Treating body dysmorphic disorder with medication: evidence, misconceptions, and a suggested approach. Body Image 5(1):13–27, 2008 18325859

Phillips KA, Hart AS, Simpson HB, et al: Delusional versus nondelusional body dysmorphic disorder: recommendations for DSM-5. CNS Spectr 19(1):10–20, 2014 23659348

Stein DJ, Nesse RM: Threat detection, precautionary responses, and anxiety disorders. Neurosci Biobehav Rev 35(4):1075–1079, 2011 21147162

Stein DJ, Phillips KA: Patient advocacy and DSM-5 (editorial). BMC Med 11:133, 2013 23683696

Stein DJ, Craske MG, Friedman MJ, et al: Meta-structure issues for the DSM-5: how do anxiety disorders, obsessive-compulsive and related disorders, post-traumatic disorders, and dissociative disorders fit together? Curr Psychiatry Rep 13(4):248–250, 2011 21603904

Storch EA, Kaufman DA, Bagner D, et al: Florida Obsessive-Compulsive Inventory: development, reliability, and validity. J Clin Psychol 63(9):851–859, 2007 17674398

Index

Page numbers printed in **boldface** *refer to tables, boxes, or figures.*